Promoting Health

This book is dedicated to the most important people in my life, my immediate family: Sara, Jon, Laura, and my four young grandchildren, Lyra, Milo, Raffy and Bella. You are my very own health promoters, bestowing on me high levels of wellbeing and inspiring me to live a healthy and long life.

Senior Content Strategist: Alison Taylor
Content Development Specialist: Veronika Watkins
Project Manager: Manchu Mohan
Designer: Paula Catalano
Illustration Manager: Emily Costantino

Ewles & Simnett's

Promoting Health

A Practical Guide

Seventh Edition

ANGELA SCRIVEN

FOREWORD BY SHIRLEY CRAMER CBE
Chief Executive, Royal Society for Public Health, London, UK

ELSEVIER
Edinburgh   London   New York   Oxford   Philadelphia   St Louis   Sydney   Toronto   2017

ELSEVIER

First edition 1985
Second edition 1992
Third edition 1995
Fourth edition 1999
Fifth edition 2003
Sixth edition 2010
Seventh edition 2017

ISBN: 978-0-7020-6692-4

British Library Cataloguing in Publication Data
A catalogue record for this book is available from the British Library

Library of Congress Cataloging in Publication Data
A catalog record for this book is available from the Library of Congress

Notice

Knowledge and best practice in this field are constantly changing. As new research and experience broaden our knowledge, changes in practice, treatment and drug therapy may become necessary or appropriate. Readers are advised to check the most current information provided (i) on procedures featured or (ii) by the manufacturer of each product to be administered to verify the recommended dose or formula, the method and duration of administration, and contraindications. It is the responsibility of the practitioner, relying on their own experience and knowledge of the patient, to make diagnoses, to determine dosages and the best treatment for each individual patient, and to take all appropriate safety precautions. To the fullest extent of the law, neither the Publisher nor the Editor assumes any liability for any injury and/or damage to persons or property arising out of or related to any use of the material contained in this book.

 your source for books,
journals and multimedia
in the health sciences

www.elsevierhealth.com

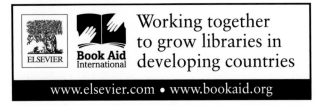
Working together
to grow libraries in
developing countries

www.elsevier.com • www.bookaid.org

The
Publisher's
policy is to use
**paper manufactured
from sustainable forests**

Printed in China
Last digit is the print number: 9 8 7 6 5 4 3 2 1

CONTENTS

v

FOREWORD

The challenges to the public's health are many and varied and have never been greater as our lives and environments are more complex and interdependent. Despite our best efforts and improved knowledge, the obesity problem is fast becoming an epidemic with high costs to the individual, families and society. Although smoking rates have fallen from their heights in the 1970s, we still have one in five people addicted to tobacco in the UK, and it remains our biggest single cause of death. Misuse of alcohol remains a major cause of long-term ill health, and mental health problems are on the increase in our stressed society. Effective health promotion is critical if we are to turn back the tide of ill health caused by noncommunicable disease, and this seventh edition of *Promoting Health: A Practical Guide* is an essential read for all those involved in health improvement and promotion.

The mantra is that 'Public health is everyone's business', and if we are to make a real difference to health and wellbeing then we need many more people to understand health improvement. This book, widely read in earlier editions by students, academics, policy makers and planners, is designed for a broad range of individuals involved in almost every sector. In the last year, the Royal Society for Public Health has highlighted the scale and scope of the wider workforce for the public's health which encompasses those who have the 'opportunity and ability to improve the public's health through their daily work'. Housing officers, firefighters, allied health professionals and community pharmacy are only a few of the professions who have enthusiastically embraced the health and wellbeing agenda. These groups, with teachers and the voluntary sector, could all benefit from this accessible and practical guide to health improvement.

There is a growing evidence base of what works in health promotion, and this is built upon each year across a range of disciplines. *Promoting Health: A Practical Guide* highlights current thinking which can be applied in different settings, ensuring that it is relevant for a variety of practitioners, and also captures the current policy context for all those who aim to improve the public's health.

This seventh edition also highlights the role of social media in promoting health and wellbeing. Many tools are now available to help individuals monitor and support their own wellbeing, as well as provide accurate and current information at any time. More is now being invested by internet-based companies in technology to support health and wellbeing than is being invested in pharmaceuticals which is a turn of the tide towards prevention.

Promoting Health: A Practical Guide provides a welcome and holistic text for health promotion at every level and for a wide group of readers. It is a wise investment at this time of exceptional challenge for the public's health.

SHIRLEY CRAMER, CBE
Chief Executive
Royal Society for Public Health

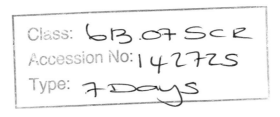

PREFACE

The aim of this book is to provide an accessible practical guide for public health practitioners and health promoters. It was first published in 1985, and in response to demand a new updated edition has been produced approximately every 5 years. This is the seventh edition. Earlier editions have also been published in German, Hungarian, Finnish, Greek, Indonesian, Italian and Swedish.

The book is addressed to all those who promote health including health promotion specialists and public health practitioners and other members of public health teams; hospital, community and occupational health nurses; health visitors and midwives; hospital doctors and general practitioners; dentists and dental hygienists; pharmacists; health service managers and the professions allied to medicine and health trainers and champions. It is also for the wide range of health promoters in statutory and nonstatutory agencies, for example, local authority staff such as environmental health officers and social workers, voluntary organisations, youth and community workers, teachers with a health education remit in schools, colleges and universities, probation officers, prison officers and police officers.

Health promotion and public health encompass a wide variety of disciplines and activities with the common purpose of improving the health of individuals and communities. This book is concerned with the what, why, who and how of health promotion and public heath practice. It aims to help you explore important questions such as the following:

- What is health and wellbeing?
- What are the determinants of health and wellbeing?
- What constitutes 21st century health promotion and public health practice? How does it fit with the wider public health movement?

- Who are the agents and agencies with remits for public health and health promotion?
- How are the needs identified when promoting health?
- How are priorities set for evidence-informed practice?
- How are health promoting public health campaigns and projects planned, managed and evaluated?
- How can health promoters and public health practitioners best carry out health promotion? What are the competencies they require?
- What are the key issues for public health and health promotion in the 21st century?

There is a focus on the theories, principles and competencies for practice, whatever your background and wherever you work. The range of health issues and the settings for health promotion (such as communities, schools, workplaces, GP surgeries and hospitals) is wide ranging, but it is beyond the scope of this book to cover all these in depth. Different professional groups will all have their own areas of expert knowledge and specialist skills to be employed alongside the specific competencies in promoting health addressed in this book.

The book is organised into three parts. *Part 1. Thinking About Health, Health Promotion and Public Health* deals with essential ideas of what health, health promotion, public health and health education are about, and the different approaches and ethical issues that need to be considered. The agencies and people who have a part to play in health promotion and public health are identified.

Part 2. Planning and Managing Health Promotion and Public Health Practice focuses on planning and evaluation at the level of a health promoter's daily work, beginning with a basic planning and evaluation framework. This is followed with a discussion of how to identify and assess needs and priorities, and develop skills to manage yourself and your work effectively.

Part 3. Competence in Health Promotion and Public Health Practice examines how you can develop your competence in carrying out a range of activities including enabling people to learn in one-to-one and group settings, enabling people towards healthier living, working with communities and changing policies and practices. The fundamentals of communication and of using communication tools are also addressed.

This seventh edition is fully revised and updated to take account of the new challenges and the changing context in which health is promoted in the 21st century. The text will examine the national strategies for health and new policies that have a bearing on the promotion of health. It is important to note, however, that policies and strategies for health frequently change, particularly when governments change, and there will be a general election during the life of this seventh edition with the UK also committed to leaving the EU, which will have an impact on public health strategies at the international level.

New issues that are highlighted are:

- changes to the structure and organisation of public health in the UK
- national standards for work in health promotion and public health
- new research on the comparative effectiveness of different approaches to health promotion and public health practice
- that the internet now plays a dominant role in public health. Websites, webinars, blogs and other relevant social media will be referenced at the end of each chapter. Social media such as Facebook, Twitter, Instagram and YouTube will

be considered in terms of their use as health-promoting assets
- changing approaches including social marketing, social media campaigns and pressure groups and nudging.

Several terms have been used to describe the people that health promotion targets. These terms include 'patients' (referring mainly to those who receive their health promotion in a healthcare environment), 'clients' (for patients and nonpatients) or simply users, individuals or groups. The term 'health promoters' is used to cover the multidisciplinary workforces that have remits for promoting health that were listed at the beginning of this Preface. It also covers those with a specialist remit to promote health. Since the sixth edition of the book, the term most commonly used in England to describe the specialist workforce is '**public health practitioners**'. Throughout this edition, the term 'health promoter' is used alongside the term 'public health practitioner' to reflect the multidisciplinary workforce that the book is targeting (see Chapters 2 and 3 for a detailed discussion on who promotes health and what the differences are between health promotion and public health).

The user-friendly style adopted in the previous editions has been retained. The overall aim of the book is the same, to keep you involved so that studying this book will be an active educational experience. Exercises are included to undertake as an individual or in a group, and examples and case studies are provided to help you to apply ideas to your own situation. Often, the exercises are designed to stimulate thought and discussion, and there may be no right answers. You will need to think it through, talk it over and reflect. In this way, the answers will have personal meaning and application.

ANGELA SCRIVEN

ACKNOWLEDGEMENTS

Linda Ewles and Ina Simnett, the authors of the first five editions of this book, produced a seminal text that has been used in the training and education of health promoters and public health practitioners over the last 30 years. Their book has shaped health promotion and public health practice in the UK over this time. In this, the seventh edition, some of the exercises and elements of the first six editions have been adjusted to reflect changes to public health policy and practice. I would like to thank Shirley Cramer for her Foreword, the health promoters who have provided case studies of their work and Veronika Watkins from Elsevier for her support and encouragement throughout the process of producing this new edition.

PART 1

Thinking About Health, Health Promotion and Public Health

PART SUMMARY

Part 1 has three purposes:

- It sets the context for the whole book by introducing key concepts, principles and ideas, and by providing you with a common language in which to communicate about health promotion and public health.
- It offers an introduction to the dimensions of health and the domains and scope of public health and health promotion, which enables you to focus on the wide range of activities and approaches being utilised by health promoters.
- It highlights important philosophical and ethical issues, which are explored in a practical context later in the book.

Health is an extremely difficult word to define, but it is clearly important that you know what it means. This is discussed in Chapter 1, along with a description of the major influences on health and inequalities in health. There is also an historical overview of some of the international and national movements that have worked towards better health.

In Chapter 2, health promotion and public health is defined and shown to encompass a wide range of activities. Frameworks are given for classifying the major areas of health promotion action. Public health competencies are outlined, and an exercise is provided to help you to explore the scope of your health promotion and public health practice work.

In Chapter 3, the agents and agencies of health promotion and public health practice are identified, and there is an opportunity to clarify your own health-promoting role.

In Chapter 4, the aims and values associated with different approaches to promoting health are analysed, a number of ethical dilemmas are examined and guidance is provided on how to make ethical decisions.

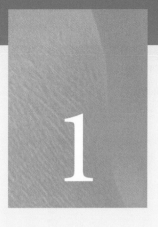

1 WHAT IS HEALTH?

CHAPTER CONTENTS

SUMMARY

This chapter starts with an exercise which enables you to examine what being healthy means to you and reviews the wide variation in perceptions and concepts of health. The interaction of the dimensions of health is considered (physical, mental, emotional, social, spiritual, cultural, environmental, societal), and health is explored as a holistic concept. Factors that influence health are identified, with a particular focus on medicine and inequalities in health. Case studies illustrate the factors that shape the health of people in differing circumstances. In the final section, there is an overview of the contribution of international and national movements towards better health.

WHAT DOES BEING HEALTHY MEAN TO YOU?

Being healthy means different things to different people, and much has been researched and written about people's varying perceptions and concepts of health (see, for example, Benyamini 2014; Mouratidi et al, 2015). It is important that public health practitioners and health promoters explore and define what being healthy means and what it might mean to the individuals and groups that you work with.

EXERCISE 1.1
What does being healthy mean to you?

In **Column 1**, tick any of the statements that describe important aspects of your health.

In **Column 2**, tick the six statements that you consider to be the most important aspects of being healthy.

In **Column 3,** rank these six in order of importance – put 1 by the most important, 2 by the next most important and so on down to 6.

If you are working in a group, compare your responses with others. Discuss the similarities and differences and the reasons for your choices. Analyse what your choices tell you about your perception of health.

Continued on following page

EXERCISE 1.1		
What does being healthy mean to you? *(Continued)*		
For me, being healthy involves:	Column 1	Column 2	Column 3
1. Being able to connect with family, friends, social networks and/or community	☐	☐	☐
2. Living to old age	☐	☐	☐
3. Feeling generally happy, in control and able to manage stress	☐	☐	☐
4. Having an adequate income	☐	☐	☐
5. Not being reliant on tablets or medicines	☐	☐	☐
6. Being the ideal weight for my height	☐	☐	☐
7. Taking regular exercise and feeling fit	☐	☐	☐
8. Living in my own sociocultural milieu	☐	☐	☐
9. Never smoking or using recreational drugs	☐	☐	☐
10. Not experiencing ill health or disease	☐	☐	☐
11. Having good levels of health literacy	☐	☐	☐
12. Being resilient and able to adapt to life's challenges	☐	☐	☐
13. Drinking only recommended safe levels of alcohol	☐	☐	☐
14. Having a home and a secure community to live in	☐	☐	☐
15. Having my body in good functional order	☐	☐	☐
16. Getting on well with other people most of the time	☐	☐	☐
17. Eating a nutritious diet and having access to clean water	☐	☐	☐
18. Enjoying some form of relaxation or recreation	☐	☐	☐
19. Having a job or meaningful occupation			
20. Having a good work-life balance			

Exercise 1.1 generally indicates that people can hold very different perceptions of health. What you choose is often a reflection of your particular circumstances, your experiences and/or your professional background. For example, if you are a migrant or a refugee you may consider living within your own sociocultural milieu as important to health, or if you work in a smoking cessation service you may prioritise not smoking as a crucial aspect of being healthy. As your circumstances change, your idea of what being healthy means to you might also change.

CONCEPTS OF HEALTH AND WELLBEING

Health is a difficult concept to define in absolute terms. The meaning can be culturally (Napier et al 2014; World Health Organization (WHO) 2015) and professionally determined and has changed over time. A variety of definitions and explanations of what it means to be healthy exists and can influence how health is promoted (Johannson et al 2009).

Lay Perceptions

It is important to understand the way lay people think about health and wellness, as this influences their health and wellness-related behaviours. Researchers have found a wealth of complex lay notions about health. Some lay perceptions are based on pragmatism, where health is regarded as a relative phenomenon, experienced and evaluated according to what an individual finds reasonable to expect, given their age, medical condition, and social situation. For them, being healthy may just mean not having a health problem which interferes with their everyday lives. The development and validation of a measure of lay definitions of health, the wellness beliefs scale, confirmed three distinct wellness beliefs: belief in the importance of biomedical (absence of illness), functional (ability to carry out daily tasks), and wellbeing (vitality) indicators of wellness. Whatever the lay understandings of health and wellbeing are based on, however, they illustrate that lay accounts are unique, and strategies for public health must be individualised (Bishop & Yardley 2010). To take just two examples:

1. The health and illness beliefs of the oldest demonstrate that a moral, hierarchical approach to health problems exists which may represent resistance to adopt the 'sick role', while seeking to maintain control over health as functional dependence and frailty increases (Elias & Lawton 2014).
2. Although generally willing to discuss health inequalities, many of the lay study participants tended to explain health inequalities in terms of individual behaviours and attitudes rather than social/structural conditions (Putland et al 2011).

Concepts and understanding of health, illness and disease have generally been linked with people's social and cultural situations. Knowledge of illness, prevention and treatment can also be powerful in shaping people's concept of health. Standards of what may be considered healthy also vary. An elderly woman may say she is in good health on a day when her chronic arthritis has eased up enough to enable her to get to the shops. A man who smokes may not regard his early morning cough as a symptom of ill health because to him it is normal. People assess their own health subjectively, according to their own norms and expectations, and may also trade-off different aspects of health. A common example is that individuals may accept the physical health damage from smoking as the price they pay for the emotional and/or social benefits.

Because of this variety and complexity of the ways in which health and wellbeing are perceived, it is difficult to objectively measure health when based on lay accounts.

For more about measuring health, see Chapter 7, finding and using evidence.

Concepts of Health

Concepts of health have changed over time. In the late 19th and 20th century, as medical discoveries were made and medical practice developed, there was a preoccupation with a mechanistic view of the body and consequently with physical health. Earlier still, there have been centuries of many philosophies of health in different civilisations, such as Greek, where a more holistic view of

health has been held. See Rosen (2015) for a history of public health and the legacy of Greek views on health, science and medicine. Since the 1970s, the concept of health has been thoroughly discussed within the philosophy of medicine, with several categories of definitions developed ranging from merely physiological interpretations to more holistic, including a number of dimensions such as mental and/or social, with the inclusion of the term wellbeing. Three levels of health have been mooted by Lerner and Berg (2015): Individual, Population and Ecosystem. But they argue that only health at the individual level might be seen as a true concept of health and that health at the other levels are more a tool for the surveillance and measurement of processes or states. One way of examining the various meanings and understandings that have been given to the term health is to use broad categories or models. Five models are identified in the following text and include the *medical model*, the *holistic model*, the *biopsychosocial model*, the *ecological model* and the *wellness model*.

The Medical Model

- The medical model (sometimes called a biomedical model) dominated thinking about health for most of the 20th century.
- Health is defined and measured as the absence of disease and the presence of high levels of function.
- This approach uses the sciences such as physiology, anatomy, pathophysiology, pharmacology, biology, histopathology and biochemistry.
- In its most extreme form, the medical model views the body as a machine to be fixed when broken.
- It emphasises treating specific physical diseases, does not accommodate mental or social problems well, and de-emphasises prevention, or prevention is seen as disease prevention rather than tackling the wider determinants of health or promoting optimal wellbeing. It is often referred to as reductionist.

The Holistic Model

- The holistic model was exemplified by the WHO constitution, which referred to health as a state of complete physical, mental and social wellbeing and not merely the absence of disease or infirmity (WHO 1948).
- This broadened the medical model perspective and highlighted the idea of positive health,

although the WHO did not originally use that term and linked health to wellbeing and a range of dimensions, not just physical.

■ Holistic health is difficult to measure. This is less because of the complexity of measuring wellbeing (see the wellness model in the following text) but more because doing so requires some subjective assessments that contrast sharply with the objective indicators favoured by the medical model.

The Biopsychosocial Model

■ The biopsychosocial model (see Fig. 1.1) advances the medical model by incorporating some aspects of the holistic model, specifically the social, psychological and emotional dimensions.

■ It recognises that health and wellbeing cannot be understood in isolation from the social and cultural environment.

■ It acknowledges and takes into account individual and group circumstances that might affect health. (See Engels 1978 for the origins of this model and Henriques 2015 for a useful critique.)

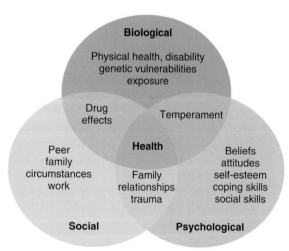

FIG. 1.1 ■ The biopsychosocial model. *(Source: http://www.pierluigimasini.it/2016/02/01/lapproccio-biopsicosociale-in-medicina/)*

The Ecological Model

Social ecology provides a framework for understanding how individuals and their social environments

mutually affect each other. The ecological health model (sometimes referred to as the socioecological health model) informs public health and health promotion as it emphasises the linkages between multiple factors (or determinants) affecting health across the lifespan. Typically, they are grouped into categories:

■ **Individual**, sometimes called intrapersonal factors, such as genetics and individual behaviours.

■ **Interpersonal,** which include social support, family, friends and peer characteristics.

■ **Institutional and community environments**, for example work sites, schools, service systems and transportation. Risk factors to health here may include the level of unemployment, population density, or the existence of a local drug trade.

■ **Broader social, economic, and political influences**, which could encompass a range of factors from social policies that maintain socioeconomic inequalities, laws and regulations and social and cultural norms, to racism and discrimination (Wendal et al 2012; Rodermann 2013).

The Wellness Model

In 1984 a WHO discussion document proposed moving away from viewing health as a state toward a dynamic model that presented it as a process or a force (WHO 1984). This was amplified in the *Ottawa Charter for Health Promotion*, which proposed that health is the extent to which an individual or group is able to realise aspirations and satisfy needs and to change or cope with the environment, with health seen as a positive concept, emphasising social and personal resources (WHO 1986).

Related to this is the notion of resiliency, such as the success with which individuals and communities adapt to changing circumstances (see Antonovsky's (1979 and 1987) Sense of Coherence theory and Becker et al 2010 for an update). Overall, therefore, there has been a change from measuring health as the absence of disease or illness, to wellbeing, which is influenced by a diverse range of conditions, such as quality of life, material circumstances and various types of capital. There is a growing interest in population wellbeing as an objective of governments. The Organisation for Economic Cooperation and Development (OECD) has been instrumental in

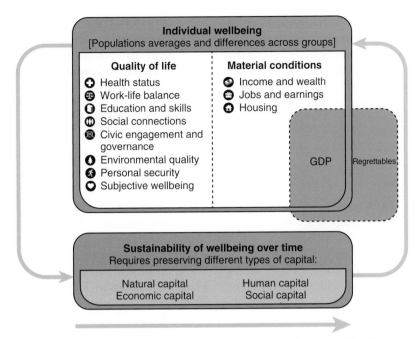

Individual wellbeing
[Populations averages and differences across groups]

Quality of life
- ✚ Health status
- ⚖ Work-life balance
- ✎ Education and skills
- ⚭ Social connections
- ⊗ Civic engagement and governance
- ♨ Environmental quality
- ⚐ Personal security
- ◓ Subjective wellbeing

Material conditions
- ◉ Income and wealth
- ⊜ Jobs and earnings
- ⌂ Housing

GDP   Regrettables

Sustainability of wellbeing over time
Requires preserving different types of capital:

Natural capital   Human capital
Economic capital   Social capital

FIG.1.2 ■ OECD Framework for measuring wellbeing. *(Source: OECD 2016)*

producing a framework for measuring wellbeing in populations (see Fig. 1.2) and a range of wellbeing indicators (OECD 2016). The UK has measurements against national indicators of wellbeing (Office for National Statistics (ONS) 2016).

There are advantages and disadvantages to each of the five models and explanations of the meaning of health. The medical model has credence because diseases represent a major global public health problem, and disease states need to be treated and can be readily diagnosed and counted. But this approach is narrow, negative and reductionist, and in an extreme form implies that people with disabilities are unhealthy and that health is only about the absence of morbidity. A further potential limitation to the medical model is its omission of a time dimension. Should we consider as equally healthy two people in equal functional status, one of whom is carrying a fatal gene that may lead to early death?

The holistic, psychosocial, ecological and wellness models recognise a wider set of determinants of health. They also allow for more subtle discrimination of people who succeed in living productive lives despite a physical impairment. The visually impaired or diabetic, for example, may still be able to satisfy aspirations, be productive, have a good quality of life and wellbeing, and so be considered healthy. One disadvantage has been that the more holistic the conceptions of health, the more they run the risk of excessive breadth, but the measurements of wellbeing are now more established (see, for example, OECD (2015) for the latest measurements on wellbeing across 11 different dimensions of life and Godwin (2014) for the global youth wellbeing index).

It is important to note that the WHO (1948) constitution definition of health mentioned under the Holistic Model has been heavily criticised, mainly on two grounds: It is unrealistic and idealistic, and it implies a static position. Some criticisms of the WHO definition focus on its lack of operational value and the problem created by use of the word *complete*. An editorial in the Lancet (2009) is just one example of the range of criticisms levied against the WHO definition. Nonetheless, the WHO's focus on wellbeing encourages nations to expand the conceptual framework of their health systems beyond the traditional boundaries set by the physical condition of individuals and their diseases, and it challenges political, community and professional organisations devoted to improving or preserving health to pay more attention to wellbeing and the social determinants of health (see WHO 2012 for evidence of this).

In exploring the concept of health further, it is useful to consider the identification of the different dimensions of health which began with the WHO definition but have been subsequently expanded. The dimensions now include:

Physical health. This is perhaps the most obvious dimension of health and is concerned with the mechanistic functioning of the body.

Mental health. Mental health refers to the ability to think clearly and coherently. It can be distinguished from emotional and social health, although there is a close association between the three.

Emotional health. This means the ability to recognise emotions such as fear, joy, grief and anger, and to express such emotions appropriately. Emotional (or affective) health also means coping with stress, tension, depression and anxiety.

Social health. Social health means the ability to make and maintain relationships with other people.

Spiritual health. For some people, spiritual health might be connected with religious beliefs and practices; for other people, it might be associated with personal creeds, principles of behaviour and ways of achieving peace of mind and being at peace with oneself.

Societal health. So far, health has been considered at the level of the individual, but a person's health is inextricably related to everything surrounding that person. It is impossible to be healthy in a sick society that does not provide the resources for basic physical and emotional needs. For example, people obviously cannot be healthy if they cannot afford necessities like food, clothing and shelter, but neither can they be healthy in countries of extreme political oppression where basic human rights are denied. Women cannot be healthy when their contribution to society

is undervalued, and neither black nor white can be healthy in a racist society where racism undermines human worth, self-esteem and social relationships. Unemployed people cannot be healthy in a society that values only people in paid employment, and it is very unlikely that health can be fully achieved in areas that lack basic resources such as clean water or services and facilities such as health care, transport and recreation.

The identification of these different aspects of health is a useful exercise in raising awareness of the complexity and the holistic nature of health. But in practice it is obvious that dividing people's health into categories such as physical and mental can impose artificial divisions and unhelpful distortions. Sexual health, for example, can cross all these boundaries proving that the dimensions of health are interrelated.

When the WHO broadened their definition, as noted in the wellness model outlined earlier in the chapter, they also identified key aspects of health, encompassing ideas of:

- personal growth and development (realise aspirations)
- meeting personal basic needs (satisfy needs)
- the ability to adapt to environmental changes (resilience to change and ability to cope with the environment)
- a means to an end, not an end in itself (a resource for everyday life, not the objective of living)
- not just absence of disease (a positive concept)
- a holistic concept (social and personal resources…physical capacities).

These aspects of health have much to offer the public health practitioner and health promoter. They recognise that health is a dynamic state, that each person's potential is different and that each person's health needs vary. Working for health is both an individual and a societal responsibility, and involves empowering people to improve their quality of life. Table 1.1 sums up this section by offering a broad comparison of the medical and social models of health.

TABLE 1.1	
Comparison of the Medical and Social Models of Health	
Medical Model	**Social Model**
Negative (health is the absence of disease, illness, infirmity, disability)	Positive (health is more than the absence of disease, illness, infirmity, disability and is associated with wellbeing)
Narrow or simplistic understanding of health (reductionist)	Broad or complex understanding of health (holistic)
Medically biased definitions focusing on the absence of disease, illness, infirmity or disability	More holistic definitions of health taking a wider range of factors into account such as mental, social, spiritual dimensions of health
Doesn't take into account the broader determinants of health	Takes into account wider influences on health such as the environment and the impact of inequalities
Strongly influenced by scientific knowledge and is expert led, top-down in approach	Takes into account lay knowledge and understanding and can be bottom up in approach.
Emphasizes personal, individual responsibility for health	Emphasizes collective, social responsibility for health

Source: Adjusted from Warwick-Booth et al 2012

Exploring the concepts and competing explanations of health is a preliminary stage in understanding the determinants of health. Before moving on to a consideration of what affects health, it might be useful to undertake Exercises 1.2 and 1.3 and answer the associated questions.

EXERCISE 1.2
Dimensions of health and wellbeing

1. Go back to your answers in Exercise 1.1 'What does being healthy mean to you?' Tick if any of the following dimensions of health are reflected in the statements you ticked in Column 1:

Physical	☐	Emotional	☐
Mental	☐	Spiritual	☐
Social	☐	Societal	☐
Cultural	☐	Environmental	☐

2. Are any of these dimensions more important to you than the others? How do they relate to each other?
3. Consider Table 1.1. Do you think you have more of an affinity with a social or a medical model of health?
4. Which of the five models of health outlined earlier in the chapter would fit under the social model of health and why?
5. If you have had professional training in health or a related area of work, what difference has this made to your conceptions of health?
6. What do you think being healthy may mean to someone who:
   - has a permanent physical disability such as deafness or paralysis?
   - has an illness or infection for which there is currently no known cure such as diabetes, arthritis, HIV or schizophrenia?
   - lives in poverty?
7. Identify three or four key ideas about being healthy that you have learned from this exercise.

EXERCISE 1.3
What shapes people's health and wellbeing?

Read the case studies and answer the following questions:
- What factors might be affecting the health and wellbeing of each of the people in these case studies?
- Which one statement in Exercise 1.1 do you think each would choose as important to them?
- What might be done to promote and improve their health and wellbeing?
- Construct a list of the health and wellbeing determinants emerging from the case studies.

Continued on following page

What shapes people's health and wellbeing? *(Continued)*

Rose is 75, single and has always lived in the same small town. She has no immediate family, but she is active in the local community. Having worked all her adult life, she had thought that her state pension and her small occupational pension would be sufficient in her retirement, but she is finding paying the bills difficult. She is worried about her fuel bills, which increase each year, and has recently sold her car, as she can't afford the running costs.

Linda, 48, and **Andy**, 51, live together in a small bungalow and have a medium-sized mortgage. Due to their disabilities, they have both been unable to work and rely heavily on care and support services. They have mounted up considerable debts. Now, the couple is anxious about facing a review of their benefits under new welfare reforms that could cut their income.

Mary is 40 and exhausted from working long hours for minimum wage to try to provide for her four children, aged 3 to 14, and her 80-year-old mother, who is in the early stages of Alzheimer's. The three generations of the family share a damp and overcrowded three-bedroom council flat in the centre of a large city. Mary finds it difficult to pay for school uniforms and school trips. Her 14-year-old son has been bullied at school and has become withdrawn and violent.

John is 19 and lives in a town where there are 12 times as many people claiming job seeker's allowance as there are job vacancies. Despite having passed a number of GCSEs and A-levels and having applied for hundreds of jobs over the last 2 years, John is still unemployed. He has to live with his parents and finds this increasing a difficult situation. He wants his independence. He smokes cigarettes and has started to front load and binge drink when he goes out with his mates on the weekend.

Fiona is a successful criminal lawyer and a partner in a large law firm. She is 39 and works very long hours, often sleeping in the office overnight. To cope with stress, she exercises every day for a least an hour. She is often too busy to eat and just grabs coffee and snacks when she can. Her weight has dropped to the point where her body mass index (BMI, or height to weight ratio) is dangerously low. She has no time to socialise, and although she would like to have a boyfriend and start a family, her work-life balance doesn't allow for this.

Jayne is 39 and is a refugee. She is a single mother and unemployed. She lives with her two sons, both of whom have learning disabilities. The family has lived in temporary accommodation since arriving in the UK a year ago. Jayne has no family or friends in the area and feels isolated and anxious. She is increasingly concerned about not being able to provide a nutritious diet for her children.

Some of the case studies are adjusted from the Poverty and Social Exclusion Website referenced under the websites at the end of the chapter.

DETERMINANTS OF HEALTH AND WELLBEING

A state of health or wellbeing or ill health, however defined, is the result of a combination of factors having a particular effect on individuals or population groups at any one time. To work towards better health, we need to identify these influential factors.

Exercise 1.4 will have identified a range of factors which affect health and wellbeing. These might include genetics, gender, family, religion, culture, friends, income, advertising, public health campaigns, social media, health literacy, social cohesion and inclusion, socioeconomic grouping, race, age, employment, working and living conditions, health and social services, self-esteem, access to leisure facilities and other resources, education, national public health and social policies, geographical location, environmental pollution, war, migration and many more. (See Kickbush 2012 for a radical assessment of 21st century determinants of health and wellbeing and their implications for the promotion of health.)

Health and Medicine

There is much debate about the relative importance of the many and varied social determinants of health and wellbeing (see, for example, Marmot et al 2012). There have also been concerns that medicine might have less

A framework for the determinants of health?

Many models and frameworks have been developed over time which categorise and explain the interaction between the various factors that influence health and wellbeing. See, for example, Fig. 1.3, has been taken from the Australian Institute of Health and Welfare and forms part of their report on Understanding Health and Illness (2014):

- Critically assess the framework in Fig. 1.3. Do you feel all of the determinants have been included? Are there determinants which are missing or are there some that you would remove or modify?
- Undertake an internet search to consider other frameworks and models of determinants. Construct a model/framework that categorises the determinants in your particular geographical region or community.

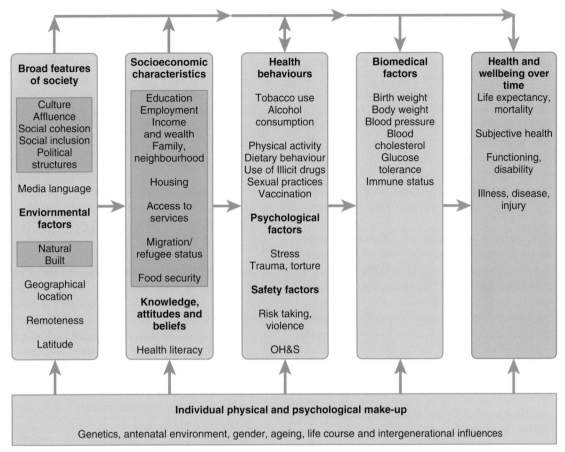

FIG. 1.3 ■ An example of a framework for the determinants of health. *Note:* Shading highlights selected social determinants of health. *(Source: Australian Institute of Health and Welfare 2014)*

effect on the population's overall health improvement than promoting lifestyle changes or socioeconomic reforms, although the arguments are complex. Faust and Menzel (2011) offer a range of multidisciplinary empirical and moral debates about what is the right prevention/treatment balance, which is a multifaceted debate. The National Health Service (NHS) in the UK is often seen as a treatment and care service for people who are ill, not as the major means of improving public health (Baggott 2015 and Boyce et al 2010 offer further discussion of the NHS and prevention policies).

Some people have claimed that the practice of scientific medicine has, in fact, done considerable harm. Examples are the side-effects of treatment, complications that set in after surgery and patient dependence on prescribed drugs. But more important, perhaps, is that control over health and illness has been taken away from people themselves, who become dependent on doctors and medical drugs. Aspects of life that are natural, such as pregnancy and childbirth, menopause, and ageing, have become medicalised, and the responsibility for health has shifted from the lay public to the medical profession. These arguments that medicine is, at best, a treatment and care service for the ill and, at worst, a means of undermining people's competence and confidence to improve their health reached a peak around 1980, led in part by the work of Illich (1977), but they are still relevant today (Collyer 2014).

The Wider Determinants of Health

In the UK, the Black Report (Townsend & Davidson 1982) showed that, for almost every kind of illness and disability in the UK, people in the upper socioeconomic groups had a greater chance of avoiding illness and staying healthy than those in the lower socioeconomic groups. It also established the differences in the risks to men and women, and variations in the apparent health consequences of living in different parts of the country.

All this pointed to the fact that the major determinants of health were socioeconomic conditions, geographical location and gender. Evidence from the late 1990s (Acheson 1998) demonstrated that the health gap was widening, so that while overall population health may be improving, the rate of improvement is not equal across all sections of society. The gap in the health status between the lower socioeconomic groups and the higher socioeconomic groups continues to increase.

Work comparing data across different countries has shown another slant on the issue of inequalities. It is not the richest societies that have the best health, but those that have the smallest income differences between rich and poor. It is the *relative* difference in income levels which is crucial. The reason seems to be that small income differences across society mean an egalitarian society that has a strong community life and better quality of life in terms of strong social networks, less social stress, higher self-esteem, less depression and anxiety and more sense of control (Hosseinpoor et al 2015 for global health inequality monitoring; Marmot 2015).

The Marmot Review (2010) on UK inequalities has resulted in a range of evidence papers for action (Public Health England (PHE) 2014). There are also practice resources aimed at local action by directors of public health and public health teams, people working in local authority services that may influence health and wellbeing, and health and wellbeing boards (PHE 2015).

One way of addressing health inequalities and inequities is by building *social capital*. Social capital is the term used to describe investment in the social fabric of society, so that communities develop high levels of trust and many networks for the exchange of information, ideas and practical help. Social capital is produced when, for example, there are neighbourhood schemes of child care and crime prevention, community groups and social activities that engage a wide range of interests and people. Low levels of social capital have been linked to socioeconomic inequalities in health (Uphoff et al 2013).

Differences in health experience may not be due entirely to socioeconomic determinants. There are important differences in rates of illness and death between ethnic groups, which may be related to differences in income, education and living conditions, cultural factors or genetic make-up. There are also differences associated with age, sex, occupation and where people live (ONS 2015). Addressing the distribution of wealth in society, reducing the gap between rich and poor and tackling socioeconomic disadvantage are clearly political issues, and the 2010 strategic review of health inequalities (Marmot et al 2010) demonstrates the UK government's continued commitment to reducing health inequalities.

IMPROVING HEALTH – HISTORICAL OVERVIEW

A number of conclusions can be drawn from the previous discussion. First, health is a complex concept, meaning different things to different people. Second, health status is linked with people's ability to reach their full potential. Finally, health is affected by a wide range of factors, which may be broadly classified as:

- lifestyle factors to do with individual health and risk-taking behaviour (which may be strongly influenced by socioeconomic and cultural experiences)
- broader social, economic, cultural, political and environmental factors such as whether people live in an egalitarian society, what social support networks are available, and how they live in terms of employment, income and housing.

Early public health work in the first half of the 20th century in the UK concentrated on structural reforms such as slum clearance, improved sanitation and clean air. Then in the 1950s and 1960s the focus shifted towards the need for changes in individual health behaviour, for example, family planning, venereal disease (the original term to describe sexually transmitted infections), accident prevention, immunisation, cervical smear checks, weight control, alcohol consumption and smoking. This emphasis on the lifestyle approach meant a concentration of effort on health education, which was reflected in government statements at the time (see, for example, Department of Health and Social Security 1976). Over time, this emphasis has been heavily criticised because it distracts attention from the social and economic determinants of health and tended to blame individuals for their own ill health. For example, people with heart disease could be blamed for it because they were overweight and smoked, but the complex social reasons for being overweight and smoking, what Marmot (2005) refers to as the causes of the causes, were ignored. Reasons may have included lack of education, no help available to stop smoking, eating and smoking used as a way of coping with stresses such as poor housing or unemployment, lack of availability of cheap nutritious foods, and so on. This blaming people for their health behaviour became known as ***victim-blaming*** (see Dougherty (1993) and Caraher (1995) for early discussions of victim-blaming and Tengland (2016) for more recent use of the term). In the 1980s a broader approach was used in conjunction with what was called the new public health movement (WHO 1986). It encompassed health education but also political and social action to address issues such as poverty, employment, discrimination and the environment in which people live. It also, importantly, focused on the grass-roots involvement of people in shaping their own health destiny.

See Chapter 3 for nformation on people and organisations working to improve public health.

INTERNATIONAL INITIATIVES FOR IMPROVING HEALTH

More is said about the role of the WHO and other international organisations in Chapter 3.

The WHO took a leading role in the evolution of health promotion in the 1980s and 1990s. It stated in 1978 that the main target of governments in the coming decades should be the attainment for all citizens of the world by the year 2000 of a level of health that will permit them to lead a socially and economically productive life (WHO 1978). This was the beginning of what came to be known as the *Health for All* (HFA) movement. It led to the development of a strategy for the WHO European Region in 1980 (WHO 1985).

This regional strategy called for fundamental changes in the health policy of member countries, including a much higher priority for health promotion and disease prevention. It called for not only health services but all public sectors with a potential impact on health to take positive steps to maintain and improve

health. Specific regional targets were published; these have been subsequently updated and the movement is now called *Health 21* (see WHO 2012 for an assessment of Health for All and Health 21 in a contemporary context). The targets emphasise the following HFA principles:

- Reducing inequalities in health
- Positive health through health promotion and disease prevention
- Community participation
- Cooperation between health authorities, local authorities and others with an impact on health
- A focus on primary health care as the main basis of the healthcare system

A major milestone for health promotion was the publication in 1986 of the *Ottawa Charter,* launched at the first WHO international conference on health promotion held in Ottawa, Canada (WHO 1986). This identified five key themes for health promotion:

1. Building healthy public policies
2. Creating supportive environments
3. Developing personal skills through information and education in health and life skills
4. Strengthening community action
5. Reorienting health services toward prevention and health promotion.

(See McQueen & Salazar (2011) and Potvin & Jones (2011) for an overview of the influence of Ottawa.)

The Jakarta declaration in 1997 (WHO 1997) reiterated the importance of the *Ottawa Charter* principles and added priorities for health promotion in the 21st century:

- Promote social responsibility for health
- Increase investment for health development
- Expand partnerships for health promotion
- Increase community capacity and empower the individual
- Secure an infrastructure for health promotion.

The Bangkok Charter for Health in a Globalized World is the most recent WHO declaration (WHO 2005). The Charter builds on Ottawa by asserting that progress towards a healthier world requires strong political action, broad participation and sustained advocacy.

The call is to ensure that health promotion's established repertoire of proven effective strategies will need to be fully utilised, with all sectors and settings acting to:

- **advocate** for health based on human rights and solidarity
- **invest** in sustainable policies, actions and infrastructure to address the determinants of health
- **build capacity** for policy development, leadership, health promotion practice, knowledge transfer and research, and health literacy
- **regulate and legislate** to ensure a high level of protection from harm and enable equal opportunity for health and wellbeing for all people
- **partner and build alliances** with public, private, nongovernmental and international organisations and civil society to create sustainable actions.

It is clear that the Charters briefly outlined previously are targeting the wider determinants of health, and are not focused on a narrow understanding of health and how it can be achieved.

NATIONAL INITIATIVES

See Chapter 3, section on national health strategies, for more about national strategies for health and how they are implemented.

Influenced by the WHO Charters, an important development for the UK in the early 1990s was the advent of national strategies for health improvement. The first was *The Health of the Nation* in England (Department of Health 1992) and comparable strategies for Wales, Scotland and Northern Ireland. These were the first national strategies to focus on health and health gain rather than illness and health services, and to take a broader view of health.

The most recent of these strategies are:

- 2010: In England the Department of Health published Healthy Lives Healthy People: Our strategy for public health in England (Department of Health 2010).
- 2014: The National Assembly for Wales (NAW) Public Health White Paper: Listening to you – your health matters (NAW 2014).
- 2014: Northern Ireland Public Health Agency Making Life Better 2012–2023 is the 10-year

public health strategic framework providing direction for policies and actions to improve the health and wellbeing of people in Northern Ireland (PHA 2014).
- 2016: The Scottish Office (SO) has just published 2015 Review of Public Health in Scotland, Strengthening the Function and Re-Focussing Action for a Healthier Scotland (SO 2015).

WHERE ARE WE NOW?

It is clear from the previous discussion that there is a broad understanding of the wider determinants of people's health, and there are international and national health strategies which recognise the wider determinants and are revised on an ongoing basis. There is a stronger international, national and local emphasis on prevention, health improvement and reducing inequalities, with health promotion and public health playing a bigger part in the remits of many health and social welfare professions. In the UK, health and wellbeing issues feature more in public policy debate at both central and local government and in the health service. But as yet these positive developments have failed to narrow the health gap between socioeconomic groups both between and within nations. Health promoters and public health practitioners in the UK are still faced with entrenched inequality in health status and huge problems of poverty, unemployment and homelessness (Marmot et al 2010; Buck & McGuire 2015). This raises questions about the distribution of wealth both within and between countries and confirms that public health is a political issue (for further detailed critical debates on inequalities in health, see Marmot 2015 and Smith et al 2016).

PRACTICE POINTS

- Health and being healthy mean different things to different people, and you need to explore and understand what they mean to you and to the individuals and population groups you work with.
- A wide range of factors at many levels influence and determine people's health.
- There are wide inequalities in the health status of people from different socioeconomic and ethnic groups, age groups, sexes and people who live in different geographical locations.

- Improving people's health means addressing the social, environmental, political and economic factors that affect their health, as well as individual health behaviour and lifestyle.

- International and national strategies and movements have emerged to tackle the complex lifestyle, socioeconomic and environmental interrelating determinants of health, and to target the reduction of inequalities in health.

REFERENCES

Acheson D 1998 Independent inquiry into inequalities in health. London, The Stationery Office.

Antonovsky A 1979 Health, stress and coping. San Francisco, Jossey-Bass.

Antonovsky A 1987 Unravelling the mystery of health – how people manage stress and stay well. San Francisco, Jossey-Bass.

Australian Institute of Health and Wellbeing 2014 Understanding health and illness. http://www.aihw.gov.au/australias-health/2014/understanding-health-illness/.

Baggott R 2015 Understanding health policy. 2nd ed. Cambridge, Polity Press.

Becker CM, Glascoff MA, Felts WM 2010 Salutogenesis 30 years later: where do we go from here? International Electronic Journal of Health Education 25–32.

Benyamini Y 2014 Health and illness perception. In: The Oxford Handbook of Health Psychology. Oxford, OUP USA.

Bishop FL, Yardley L 2010 The development and initial validation of a new measure of lay definitions of health: the wellness beliefs scale. Psychology & Health 25(3):271–287.

Boyce T, Peckham S, Hann A, Trenholm S 2010 A pro-active approach. Health promotion and ill-health prevention. London, Kings Fund.

Buck D, McGuire D 2015 Inequalities in life expectancy: changes over time and implications for policy. London, Kings Fund.

Caraher M 1995 Nursing and health education: victim blaming. British Journal of Nursing 4(20):1190–1192, 1209–1213.

Collyer F 2014 The Palgrave handbook of social theory in health illness and medicine. London, Palgrave.

Department of Health 1992 The health of the nation: a strategy for health in England. London, The Stationery Office.

Department of Health 2010 Healthy Lives, Healthy People: our strategy for public health in England. Stationary Office.

Dougherty CJ 1993 Bad faith and victim-blaming: the limits of health promotion. Health Care Analysis 1(2):111–119.

Editorial 2009 The Lancet 373(9666):781.

Elias T, Lawton K 2014 Do those over 80 years of age seek more or less medical help? A Qualitative Study of Health and Illness Beliefs and Behaviour of the Oldest Old. Sociology of Health and Illness 36(7):970–985.

Engels GL 1978 The biopsychosocial model and the education of health professionals. Annals of the New York Academy of Sciences 310:169–181.

Faust HS, Menzel PT eds. 2011 Prevention vs. treatment: what's the right balance? Oxford, OUP.

Godwin N 2014 The Global Youth Wellbeing Index. Center for Strategic and International Studies and International Youth Foundation.

Henriques G 2015 The biopsychosocial model and its limitations. Psychology Today. https://www.psychologytoday.com/blog/theory-knowledge/201510/the-biopsychosocial-model-and-its-limitations.

Hosseinpoor AR, Bergen N, Schlotheuber A 2015 Global Health Action 2015, 8:29034. http://dx.doi.org/10.3402/gha.v8.29034.

Illich I 1977 Limits to medicine – medical nemisis: the expropriation of health. Harmondsworth, Pelican.

Institute of Health Equity 2016 Publications. http://www.instituteofhealthequity.org/articles.

Johansson H, Weinehall L, Emmelin M 2009 "It depends on what you mean": a qualitative study of Swedish health professionals' views on health and health promotion. BMC Health Service Research. 9:91.

Kickbush I 2012 21st century health determinants: a new challenge for health promotion. Global Health Promotion 19(3):5–7.

Lerner H, Berg C 2015 The concept of health in one health and some practical implications for research and education: what is one health? Infection, Ecology and Epidemiology 5:10.

Marmot M, Atkinson T, Bell J, et al 2010 Fair society, healthy lives: strategic review of health inequalities in England – the Marmot review. London, Institute of Health Equity, University College London. http://www.dh.gov.uk/en/Publichealth/Healthinequalities/DH_094770.

Marmot M, Allen J, Bell R, Bloomer E, Goldblatt P 2012 On behalf of the Consortium for the European Review of Social Determinants of Health and the Health Divide. WHO European Review of Social Determinants of Health and the Health Divide. The Lancet 380:1011–1029.

Marmot M 2015 The health gap: the challenge of an unequal world. London, Bloomsbury Publishing.

Marmot M 2005. Social Determinants of Health Inequalities. Lancet 365:1099–104.

McQueen D, Salazar L 2011 Health Promotion, The Ottawa Charter and "Developing Personal Skills": A Compact History of 25 Years. Health Promotion International 26(suppl 2):194–201.

Mouratidi P, Bonoti F, Leondari A 2015 Children's perceptions of illness and health: an analysis of drawings. Health Education Journal 75(4):434–447.

Napier AD, Ancarno C, Butler B, et al 2014 Culture and health. The Lancet 384(9954):1607–1639.

National Assembly for Wales 2014 Public health white paper–listening to you, your health matters. Cardiff, NAW.

Nettleton S 2013 The sociology of health and illness. Cambridge, Polity Press.

Office for National Statistics 2015 Trend in life expectancy at birth and at age 65 by socio-economic position based on the National Statistics Socio-economic Classification, England and Wales: 1982–1986 to 2007–2011. http://www.ons.gov.uk/peoplepopulationandcommunity/birthsdeathsandmarriages/lifeexpectancies/bulletins/trendinlifeexpectancyatbirthandatage65bysocioeconomicpositionbasedonthenationalstatisticssocioeconomicclassificationenglandandwales/2015-10-21.

Office for National Statistics 2016 Personal well-being in the UK: 2015 to 2016. http://www.ons.gov.uk/peoplepopulationandcommunity/wellbeing/bulletins/measuringnationalwellbeing/2015to2016.

Organisation for Economic Co-operation and Development 2015 How's Life? Measuring well-being Paris, OECD Publishing.

Organisation for Economic Co-operation and Development 2016 Measuring well-being and progress: well-being research. http://www.oecd.org/statistics/measuring-well-being-and-progress.htm.

Potvin L, Jones CM 2011 Twenty-five years after the Ottawa Charter: the critical role of health promotion for public health. Canadian Journal of Public Health 102(4):244–248.

Public Health Agency (HSC) 2014 Making Life Better 2012–2023. http://www.publichealth.hscni.net/making-life-better.

Public Health England 2014 Local action on health inequalities: evidence papers. https://www.gov.uk/government/publications/local-action-on-health-inequalities-evidence-papers.

Public Health England 2015 Local action on health inequalities: practice resources. https://www.gov.uk/government/collections/local-action-on-health-inequalities-practice-resources.

Putland C, Baum FE, Ziersch AM 2011 From causes to solutions - insights from lay knowledge about health inequalities. Public Health 11:67.

Rodermann M 2013 John Hopkins School of Public Health: The Ecological Model in Public Health. http://www.jhsph.edu/research/centers-and-institutes/womens-and-childrens-health-policy-center/eco-model/eco-model.html.

Rosen G 2015 A history of public health. Baltimore, John Hopkins University Press.

Scottish Office 2015 Review of public health in Scotland: Strengthening the function and re-focussing action for a healthier Norwich, The Stationery Office.

Smith KE, Hill S, Bambra C 2016 Health inequalities: critical perspectives. Oxford, Oxford University Press.

Tengland PA 2016 Behavior change or empowerment: on the ethics of health-promotion goals. Health Care Analysis 24(1):24–46.

Townsend P, Davidson N 1982 Inequalities in health: Black Report. Harmondsworth, Penguin.

Uphoff EP, Pickett KE, Cabieses B, Small N, Wright JA 2013 Systematic Review of the Relationships Between Social Capital and Socioeconomic Inequalities in Health: A Contribution to Understanding the Psychosocial Pathway of Health Inequalities. The Official Journal of the International Society for Equity in Health:54.

Warwick-Booth L, Cross R, Lowcock D 2012 Contemporary health studies: An introduction. Cambridge, Polity Press.

Wendal ML, Whitney RG, McLeroy KR 2012 Ecological approaches. http://oxfordindex.oup.com/view/10.1093/obo/9780199756797-0037.

World Health Organization 1948 Constitution of the World Health Organization. www.who.int/governance/eb/who_constitution_en.pdf.

World Health Organization 1978 Alma Ata Declaration. Geneva, WHO.

World Health Organization 1984 Health promotion: a discussion document on the concepts and principles. Copenhagen, WHO.

World Health Organization 1985 Regional targets for health for all. Geneva, WHO.

World Health Organization 1986 The Ottawa charter for health promotion. Geneva, WHO. http://www.who.int/hpr/hpr/documents/ottawa.html.

World Health Organization 1997 The Jakarta declaration on leading health promotion into the 21st century. Geneva, WHO. http://www.who.int/hpr/hpr/documents/jakarta/english.html.

World Health Organization 1999 Health 21: health for all in the 21st century. Copenhagen, WHO.

World Health Organization 2005 The Bangkok charter for health promotion in a globalized world. Geneva, WHO. http://www.who.int/healthpromotion/conferences/6gchp/bangkok_charter/en/index.html.

World Health Organization 2012 The European Health Report 2012: Charting the way to wellbeing. Copenhagen, WHO.

World Health Organization 2015 Beyond bias: exploring the cultural contexts of health and well-being measurement, WHO European Region. Copenhagen, WHO.

WEBSITES

OECD Data on wellbeing measures http://www.oecd.org/statistics/howslife.htm

Poverty and Social Exclusion http://www.poverty.ac.uk/tags/case-study

BLOGS

This blog is written by Sir Michael Marmot, UCL Institute of Health Equity, with up-to-date discussion on inequalities in health. http://marmot-review.blogspot.co.uk/

This is a public health forum for discussing public health in the European Region of WHO. http://discussion.euro.who.int/profiles/blog/list

A Public Health England "Public Health Matter" Blog, Health and Wellbeing category. https://publichealthmatters.blog.gov.uk/category/hwb//

FACEBOOK

OECD Facebook pages, for a series of videos on health and wellbeing, in particular "When it comes to quality of life, what matters most to you" discussing the better life index. https://www.facebook.com/theOECD/videos

2

WHAT IS HEALTH PROMOTION?

CHAPTER CONTENTS

SUMMARY

This chapter starts with a discussion of the definitions of health promotion, public health and the related terms of health improvement, health development, health education and social marketing. This is followed by an examination of the position of health promotion within the multidisciplinary public health movement. An outline of the scope of health promotion work is offered, with frameworks for activities for promoting health. Broad areas of practice covered by professional health promoters and the core competencies needed are set out with an outline of the framework for national occupational standards. Exercises are included to help you explore the range of public health and health promotion activities and the extent of your own health promotion work.

DEFINING HEALTH PROMOTION

Health promotion as a term was used for the first time in the mid-1970s (Lalonde 1974) and quickly became an umbrella term for a wide range of strategies designed to tackle the wider determinants of health. There is no clear, universally adopted consensus of what is meant by health promotion. Some definitions focus on activities, others on values and principles and are often imprecisely defined, with Tannahill (2009) arguing that there are so many definitions that the term 'health promotion' has become meaningless. This is not the case. Health promotion involves promoting the health and wellbeing of individuals, communities and whole population groups. Promotion in this context means improving, advancing, supporting, advocating for, empowering and placing health higher on personal, public and political agendas.

Given that major socioeconomic determinants of health are often outside individual or even collective control, a fundamental aspect of health promotion is that it aims to empower people to have more control over aspects of their lives that affect their health. These twin elements of improving health and having more control over it are fundamental to the aims and activities of health promotion. The World Health Organization (WHO) definition of health promotion

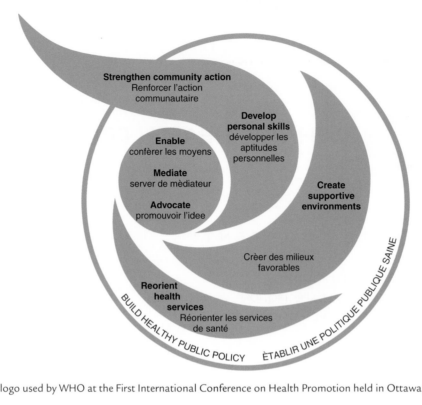

FIG. 2.1 ■ The logo used by WHO at the First International Conference on Health Promotion held in Ottawa, Canada, in 1986. *(WHO, 1986)*

as it appears in the Ottawa Charter has been widely adopted and encompasses this: Health promotion is the process of enabling people to increase control over, and to improve, their health (WHO 1986). It could be argued that the WHO definition is too elusive and as such is unfit for purpose. It was, however, accompanied with a logo and an explanation which indicated more clearly what the process of enabling people to increase control over and improve their health would entail (Fig. 2.1).

The logo and the Ottawa Charter present five key action areas and three strategies for health promotion, which further explain the nature and purpose of health promotion (see Box 2.1 for further details):

Action Areas

- Build healthy public policy
- Create supportive environments for health
- Strengthen community action for health
- Develop personal skills
- Reorient health services.

Strategies

- Enable
- Mediate
- Advocate.

EXERCISE 2.1

Consider the definition, logo, action areas and strategies previously outlined and expanded on in Box 2.1, and answer the following questions:

1. How relevant do you feel the Ottawa Charter is to public health action in the 21st century?

2. Consider the local, national and international public health policies that you are familiar with and assess whether the ideas and values contained within the Ottawa Charter have influenced public health policy development.

3. Are there any of the action areas and strategies outlined in the Ottawa Charter which are embedded in your professional remit and/or practice, and if so, what are they?

4. Do you consider yourself to be a health promoter? Please explain your answer.

BOX 2.1
THE OTTAWA CHARTER (WHO 1986)

Build Healthy Public Policy – Health promotion goes beyond health care. It puts health on the agenda of policy makers in all sectors and at all levels, directing them to be aware of the health consequences of their decisions and to accept their responsibilities for health. Health promotion policy combines diverse but complementary approaches including legislation, fiscal measures, taxation and organizational change. It is coordinated action that leads to health, income, and social policies that foster greater equity. Joint action contributes to ensuring safer and healthier goods and services, healthier public services, and cleaner, more enjoyable environments. Health promotion policy requires the identification of obstacles to the adoption of healthy public policies in non-health sectors and ways of removing them. The aim must be to make the healthier choice the easier choice for policy makers as well.

Create Supportive Environments – Our societies are complex and interrelated. Health cannot be separated from other goals. The inextricable links between people and their environment constitutes the basis for a socioecological approach to health. The overall guiding principle for the world, nations, regions and communities alike is the need to encourage reciprocal maintenance – to take care of each other, our communities and our natural environment. The conservation of natural resources throughout the world should be emphasized as a global responsibility. Changing patterns of life, work and leisure have a significant impact on health. Work and leisure should be a source of health for people. The way society organizes work should help create a healthy society. Health promotion generates living and working conditions that are safe, stimulating, satisfying and enjoyable. Systematic assessment of the health impact of a rapidly changing environment – particularly in areas of technology, work, energy production and urbanization – is essential and must be followed by action to ensure positive benefit to the health of the public. The protection of the natural and built environments and the conservation of natural resources must be addressed in any health promotion strategy.

Strengthen Community Actions – Health promotion works through concrete and effective community action in setting priorities, making decisions, planning strategies and implementing them to achieve better health. At the heart of this process is the empowerment of communities – their ownership and control of their own endeavours and destinies. Community development draws on existing human and material resources in the community to enhance self-help and social support and to develop flexible systems for strengthening

public participation in and direction of health matters. This requires full and continuous access to information, learning opportunities for health, as well as funding support.

Develop Personal Skills – Health promotion supports personal and social development through providing information and education for health, and enhancing life skills. By so doing, it increases the options available to people to exercise more control over their own health and over their environments, and to make choices conducive to health. Enabling people to learn throughout life to prepare themselves for all of its stages and to cope with chronic illness and injuries is essential. This has to be facilitated in school, home, work and community settings. Action is required through educational, professional, commercial and voluntary bodies, and within the institutions themselves.

Reorient Health Services – The responsibility for health promotion in health services is shared among individuals, community groups, health professionals, health service institutions and governments. They must work together towards a healthcare system which contributes to the pursuit of health. The role of the health sector must move increasingly in a health promotion direction, beyond its responsibility for providing clinical and curative services. Health services need to embrace an expanded mandate which is sensitive and respects cultural needs. This mandate should support the needs of individuals and communities for a healthier life and open channels between the health sector and broader social, political, economic and physical environmental components. Reorienting health services also requires stronger attention to health research as well as changes in professional education and training. This must lead to a change of attitude and organization of health services which refocuses on the total needs of the individual as a whole person.

Moving into the Future – Health is created and lived by people within the settings of their everyday life; where they learn, work, play and love. Health is created by caring for oneself and others, by being able to take decisions and have control over one's life circumstances, and by ensuring that the society one lives in creates conditions that allow the attainment of health by all its members. Caring, holism and ecology are essential issues in developing strategies for health promotion. Therefore, those involved should take as a guiding principle that, in each phase of planning, implementation and evaluation of health promotion activities, women and men should become equal partners.

It has been argued that the Ottawa Charter has established a radical international agenda for public health, strongly influencing the values public health pursues and that public health has integrated health promotion (Potvin & Jones 2011). However, the social model of

health (see Chapter 1) that health promotion embraces can be in sharp contrast to a more medically dominated public health approach. While some are less optimistic about the influence of health promotion, particularly in the UK (see, for example, Dixey 2012), others see an important future for health promotion in advancing the wellbeing, wellness and quality of life agenda within public health (Edington et al 2015).

The Connection Between Health Promotion and Public Health

There has been considerable debate about the relationship between health promotion as a set of professional activities – internationally guided by WHO charters and declarations such as the Ottawa Charter previously discussed – and public health, which in England is regulated by the Faculty of Public Health.

What is Public Health?

In the UK, the Faculty of Public Health (FPH) defines public health as the science and art of promoting and protecting health and wellbeing, preventing ill health and prolonging life through the organised efforts of society (FPH 2016).

The Faculty's approach is that public health:

- is population-based
- emphasises collective responsibility for health, its protection and disease prevention
- recognises the key role of the state, linked to a concern for the underlying socioeconomic and wider determinants of health, as well as disease
- emphasises partnerships with all those who contribute to the health of the population.

The Faculty proposes three domains of public health outlined in Table 2.1 and nine areas of public health practice.

The nine key areas are:

- surveillance and assessment of the population's health and wellbeing
- assessing the evidence of effectiveness of health and healthcare interventions, programmes and services
- policy and strategy development and implementation
- strategic leadership and collaborative working for health
- health improvement
- health protection
- health and social service quality
- public health intelligence
- academic public health.

Functions of the Local Public Health System can be found on the FPH website (see the reference at the end of the chapter) in addition to current manifestos and details on public health standards.

Internationally, public health is seen as multifaceted and targeting numerous social, environmental and behavioural determinants, including the impacts of globalisation, economic constraints, living conditions, demographic changes and unhealthy lifestyles (Lomazzi 2016). The World Federation of Public Health Associations (WFPHA) in collaboration with the WHO have developed a global charter for the public's health, and in doing so they point to the major influence of Ottawa Charter for Health Promotion (WHO 1986) in improving health throughout the world. The purpose of the public health Charter is to provide a succinct and practical implementation guideline to public

---

TABLE 2.1

Faculty of Public Health Domains of Public Health

THREE DOMAINS OF PUBLIC HEALTH PRACTICE

Health Improvement	Improving Services	Health Protection
■ Inequalities	■ Clinical effectiveness	■ Infectious diseases
■ Education	■ Efficiency	■ Chemicals and poisons
■ Housing	■ Service planning	■ Radiation
■ Employment	■ Audit and evaluation	■ Emergency response
■ Family/community	■ Clinical governance	■ Environmental health hazards
■ Lifestyles	■ Equity	
■ Surveillance and monitoring of specific diseases and risk factors		

Source: Adjusted from FPH (2016)

health associations to work with other Non-Government Organizations (NGOs), universities, civil society and governments to plan and implement strategies for better health outcomes. The WFPHA conceptualises global public health for a new health era, more dedicated to preventive solutions rather than a disease-specific focus. The Global Charter for the Public's Health provides new insights into the direction of public health and provides guidance for a group of core services: Protection, Prevention and Promotion, and a group of enabler functions: Governance, Advocacy, Capacity and Information (Moore et al 2016; WFPHA 2016; see Fig. 2.2).

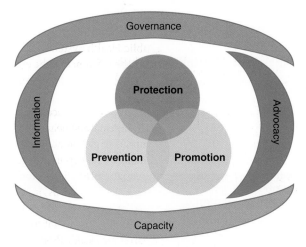

FIG. 2.2 ■ WFPHA charter core services and functions of public health. *(Source: WFPHA 2016)*

EXERCISE 2.2

Examine the UK FPH public health domains plus their nine key areas of public health, the WFPHA Global Charter for the Public's Health pronouncements and associated Fig. 2.2 and answer the following:

- Which FPH domains and key areas of practice do you not consider to be health promotion, and why?
- Where does health promotion fit in the WFPHA global public health charter?
- What conclusions can you draw from Exercises 2.1 and 2.2 in terms of the difference between public health and health promotion?
- Do you consider yourself to be working in health promotion or public health or both? Explain your answers.

See Chapter 3 for an overview of the health promotion and public health workforce.

It's important to note that, in addition to health promotion and public health, a range of other terms have been used to describe the process of enabling individuals and communities to improve their health. These include health development, health improvement, health education and social marketing. Health development is used in a number of ways. There are public health teams and units that refer to themselves as health development departments (see, for example, the Health and Social Care Northern Ireland (HSCNI) South Eastern Health and Social Care Trust Health Development Department Guide 2016), and there is a Health Development Consultancy (HDC), which supports health promoters and public health practitioners by producing a range of resources for use in practice (HDC 2016). Health improvement is frequently used by national health agencies (see Welsh Government 2016). The term covers a wide range of activity, principally focused on improving the health and wellbeing of individuals and communities (much like health promotion). Health education comprises the consciously constructed opportunities for learning involving some form of communication designed to improve health literacy, including improving knowledge and developing life skills which are conducive to individual and community health. It has been described as a core public health discipline (Auld et al 2011). In the 1970s, the range of activities undertaken in the pursuit of better health began to diverge from health education. There was also criticism that the health education approach was too narrow, focused too much on behavioural change and could become victim-blaming (see Chapter 1, Historical Overview) and increasingly work was being undertaken on wider issues such as political action to change public policies. Such activities went beyond the scope of traditional health education, and the term 'Health Promotion' came into use to describe the wider range of health interventions used to tackle the broader determinants of health.

Like health education, social marketing is a health promoting strategy to achieve and sustain behaviour goals on a range of social issues. There are a number of definitions of social marketing, but the National Social Marketing Centre (NSMC) in the UK uses the following: Social marketing is an approach used to develop activities aimed at changing or maintaining people's behaviour for the benefit of individuals and society as a whole (NSMC 2016). See the following text for further discussion of social marketing.

THE SCOPE OF HEALTH PROMOTION

The questions in Exercise 2.3 give examples of the wide range of activities that may be classified as health promotion. Answering 'yes' to each one indicates a broad view of what may be included: mass media advertising, campaigning on health issues, patient education, self-help, environmental safety measures, public policy issues, health education, preventive and curative medical procedures, codes of practice on health issues, health-enhancing facilities in local communities, workplace health policies and personal and social education for young people. Answering 'no' indicates that you identify criteria that you believe exclude these activities from the realms of health promotion. For example, you may have said 'no' to Item 2 because a sugar tax might impact negatively on families living in poor financial circumstances, thus putting their health more at risk.

Frameworks and models for classifying health-promoting activities have helped to determine the scope of health promotion (see, for example, Tannahill 2009). Drawing on these, Fig. 2.3 identifies the activities that contribute to health gain and maps out all those activities which aim to improve people's health and wellbeing. There are two sets of activities: those about providing services for people who are ill or who have disabilities, and positive health activities, which are about personal, social and environmental changes aiming to prevent ill health, to improve wellbeing and develop healthier living conditions and lifestyles. These two sets of activities overlap, because they both contribute to health gain, and they are often closely related in practice. Ten categories of activities are identified, comprising two illness and disability services and eight types of positive health activities.

Illness and Disability Services

Personal social services. This includes all those social services aimed at addressing the needs of sick people and people with disabilities or disadvantages

---

EXERCISE 2.3

Exploring the scope of health promotion

Consider each of the following activities and decide whether you think each is, or is not, health promotion:

	Yes	No
1. Using TV, radio, cinema and social media for advertisements to encourage people to drink safely.	☐	☐
2. Campaigning for a tax on sugar.	☐	☐
3. Explaining to patients how to carry out their doctor's advice.	☐	☐
4. Setting up a self-help group for people who have been sexually abused as children.	☐	☐
5. Providing advice on environmental threats including pollution and noise.	☐	☐
6. Leading on the development, implementation and evaluation of health improvement programmes across organisations, partnerships and communities to improve population health and wellbeing and reduce health inequalities.	☐	☐
7. Identifying the causes and distribution of ill health, interpreting the results and reporting on their implications.	☐	☐
8. Immunising children against infectious diseases such as measles.	☐	☐
9. Protesting to local and national politicians about a breach in the voluntary code of practice for alcohol advertising.	☐	☐
10. Running low-cost gentle exercise classes for older people at local leisure centres.	☐	☐
11. A celebrity chef advocating for healthier menu choices at school canteens.	☐	☐
12. Teaching a school-based programme of personal, social, economic and health education.	☐	☐
13. Providing support to people with learning disabilities living in the community.	☐	☐
14. Tackling community issues based on local needs assessment such as childhood obesity and smoking.	☐	☐

What were your reasons for deciding whether an activity is or is not 'health promotion'?

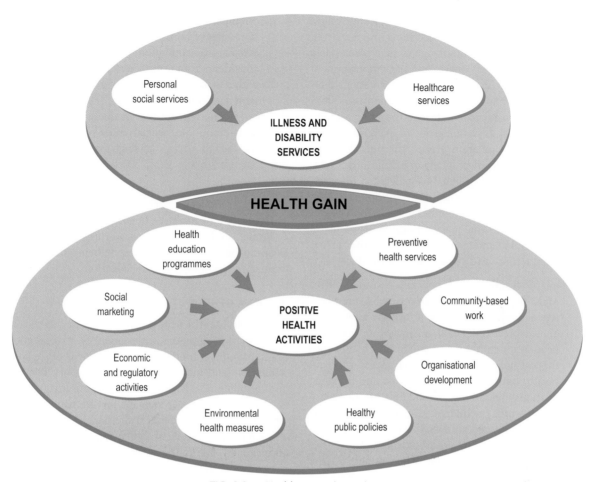

FIG. 2.3 ■ Health promoting actions.

whose health, wellbeing and quality of life is improved by those services. This includes, for example, community care of mentally ill people.

Healthcare services. This includes the major work of the health services: treatment, cure and care in primary care and hospital settings.

An important question when considering the boundaries of service provision by health promoters is, 'If all illness and disability services improve health and produce varying amounts of health gain, are they all called health promotion?' For example, is giving someone with osteoarthritis a full hip replacement considered health promotion?

It is helpful to go back to the WHO (1986) definition of health promotion, which is about enabling people to increase control over and improve their health. Are things that need to be done to people (like a full hip replacement) excluded from this definition, so it is not health promotion? They are health gain activities. What about those aspects of care and treatment that are about enabling people to take control over their health and improve it (such as educating patients in the skills of diabetes self-care)? Creating a health-promoting environment by, for example, modifying a home to make it suitable for a person with disabilities or providing affordable housing for homeless people might also be seen as health promotion.

Positive Health Activities

Health Education Programmes

These are planned opportunities for people to learn about health and wellbeing, and to undertake voluntary changes in their behaviour. Such programmes may include providing information, exploring values and attitudes, making health decisions and acquiring skills to enable behaviour change to take place. They involve developing self-esteem and self-empowerment so that people are enabled to take action about their health. This can happen on a personal one-to-one level such as health visitor/client, teacher/pupil; in a group such as a smoking cessation group or exercise class; or reaching large population groups through the mass media, social media, health fairs or exhibitions.

See Chapters 10 through 14 for detailed information on carrying out these health-promotion activities.

Health education programmes may also be a part of health care and personal social services, and because of this, it is useful to understand the concepts of primary, secondary, tertiary and quantenary health education.

- Primary health education. This would reflect McKinley's (1979) vision of upstream, preventative activity. It is directed at healthy people and aims to prevent ill health arising. Most health education for children and young people falls into this category, dealing with such topics as sexual health, nutrition and social skills and personal relationships, aiming to build up a positive sense of self-worth in children. Primary health education is concerned not merely with helping to prevent illness but with positive wellbeing.
- Secondary health education. There is also often a major role for health education when people are ill. It may be possible to prevent ill health moving to a chronic or irreversible stage and to restore people to their former state of health. This is known as secondary health education, educating patients about their condition and what to do about it. Restoring good health may involve the patient changing behaviour (such as stopping smoking) or complying with a therapeutic regime and, possibly, learning about self-care and self-help. Clearly, health education of the patient is of great importance if treatment and therapy are to be effective and illness is not to recur.
- Tertiary health education. There are, of course, many patients whose ill health has not been, or could not be, prevented and who cannot be completely cured. There are also people with permanent disabilities. Tertiary health education is concerned with educating patients and their carers about how to make the most of the remaining potential for healthy living, and how to avoid unnecessary hardships, restrictions and complications. Rehabilitation programmes contain a considerable amount of tertiary health education with a focus on improving quality of life.
- Quantenary health education. This concentrates on facilitating optimal states of empowerment and emotional, social and physical wellbeing during a terminal stage (see Hancock 2001; Scriven 2005).

It is not always easy to see where people fit into this primary, secondary or tertiary framework because a person's state of health is open to interpretation. For example, is educating an overweight person who appears to be perfectly well, despite being overweight, primary or secondary health education?

Social Marketing

The NSMC identifies the primary aim of health-related social marketing as the achievement of a social good (rather than commercial benefit) in terms of specific, achievable and manageable behaviour goals, relevant to improving health and reducing health inequalities. Social marketing is a systematic process using a range of marketing techniques and approaches (a marketing mix) phased to address short-, medium- and long-term issues. The following six features and concepts are pertinent to understanding social marketing:

- Customer or consumer orientation. A strong customer orientation with importance attached to understanding where the customer is starting from, their knowledge and attitudes and beliefs, along with the social context in which they live and work.
- Behaviour and behavioural goals. Clear focus on understanding existing behaviour and key influences upon it, alongside developing clear behavioural goals. These can be divided into actionable and measurable steps or stages, phased over time.
- Intervention mix and marketing mix. Using a mix of different interventions or methods to achieve a particular behavioural goal. When used at the strategic level, this is commonly referred to as the intervention mix, and when used operationally, it is described as the marketing mix.
- Audience segmentation. Clarity of audience focus using audience segmentation to target effectively.

Exchange. Use of the exchange concept, understanding what is being expected of people, and the real cost to them.

Competition. This means understanding factors that impact on people and that compete for their attention and time (adjusted from NSMC 2016).

Social marketing uses the total process planning model summarised in Fig. 2.3. The front-end scoping stage drives the whole process. The primary concern is establishing clear actionable and measurable behaviour goals to ensure focused development across the rest of the process. The ultimate effectiveness and success of social marketing rests on whether it is possible to demonstrate direct impact on behaviour. It is this feature that sets it apart from other communication or awareness-raising approaches, such as health education, where the main focus is on imparting information and enabling people to understand and use it. For more details on how to engage in health-related social marketing, refer to the NSMC website referenced at the end of this chapter and Lee and Kotler (2015).

Preventive Health Services

These include medical services that aim to prevent ill health, such as immunisation, family planning and personal health checks, as well as wider preventive health services such as child protection services for children at risk of abuse.

Community-Based Work

This is a bottom-up approach to health promotion, working with and for people, involving communities in health work such as local campaigns for better facilities. It includes community development, which is essentially about communities identifying their own health needs and taking action to address them. The sort of activities that may result could include forming self-help and pressure groups and developing local health-enhancing facilities and services.

See Chapter 15, Working with communities.

Organisational Development

This is about developing and implementing policies within organisations to promote the health of staff and customers. Examples include implementing policies on equal opportunities, providing healthy food choices at places of work and working with commercial organisations to develop and promote healthier products.

See Chapter 16, Influencing and implementing policy.

Healthy Public Policies

Developing and implementing healthy public policies involves statutory and voluntary agencies, professionals and the public working together to develop changes in the conditions of living. It is about seeing the implications for health in policies about, for example, equal opportunities, housing, employment, transport and leisure. Good public transport, for example, would improve health by reducing the number of cars on the road, decreasing pollution, using less fuel and reducing the stress of the daily grind of travelling for commuters. It could also reduce isolation for those who do not own cars and enable people to have access to shopping and leisure facilities, all measures that improve wellbeing (see Scriven 2007 for a detailed overview of healthy public policies).

See Chapter 16, Influencing and implementing policy.

Environmental Health Measures

Environmental health is about making the physical environment conducive to health, whether at home, at work or in public places. It includes public health measures such as ensuring clean food and water and controlling traffic and other pollution.

Economic and Regulatory Activities

These are political and educational activities directed at politicians, policy makers and planners involving lobbying for and implementing legislative changes such as food labelling regulations, pressing for voluntary codes of practice such as those relating to alcohol advertising or advocating financial measures such as increases in tobacco taxation.

A FRAMEWORK FOR HEALTH PROMOTION ACTIVITIES

Building on Fig. 2.3, there are two points to make about the use of the framework of health-promotion activities in Fig. 2.4. The first is that it illustrates that health promotion has an established relationship to both public health and health and social care practice, but it also includes a specialist field of activities that are vital to the public

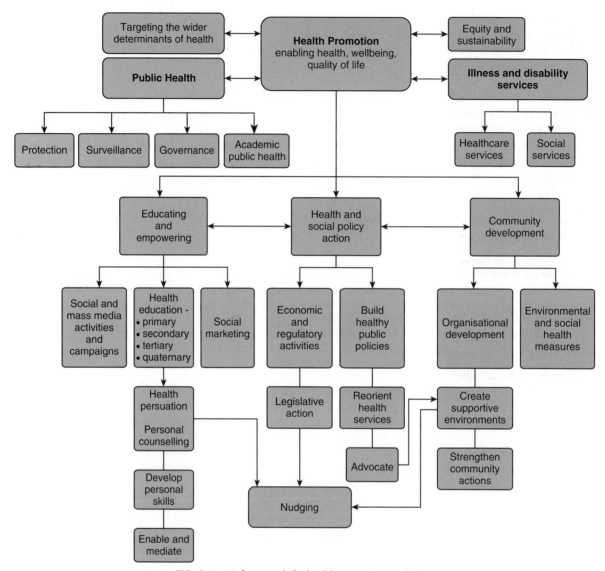

FIG. 2.4 ■ A framework for health promotion activities.

health agenda and to population health and wellbeing. The second point to consider when using the framework is that health promotion does not always fall neatly into categories. For example, would a public health practitioner who was supporting a local women's health group be engaged in a health education programme because they provided health information to the group and set up stress management sessions, or in community-based work because some members of the group had got together to lobby their local health services for better sexual health advice clinics for young people?

Obviously areas of activity overlap, but this is not important. What is important is to appreciate the range of activities encompassed by health promotion, the link between health promotion, public health, health care and social services and the many ways in which you can contribute to health improvements.

This framework reflects planned, deliberate activities, but it is important to recognise that a great deal of health promotion happens informally and incidentally. For example, health-related depictions in TV soaps and dramas are becoming more authentic and prompt people to seek support (see, for example, MIND 2014), and product advertising campaigns can have positive health messages such as promoting moderate drinking (the Heineken 2016 'Moderate Drinkers Wanted' commercial). There are, therefore, health-promotion activities which are not likely to be planned with specific health promotion aims in mind. They may, however, be significant influences for behavioural and lifestyle changes.

See Chapter 11, section on mass media.

EXERCISE 2.4

Identifying your health promotion work

Look at Fig. 2.4 and position your professional activities across the framework. Are there aspects of your work which you consider to be health promotion or public health practice that are not covered by this framework? If so, what are they and how would you incorporate them into the framework?

AREAS OF COMPETENCIES IMPORTANT TO PROMOTING HEALTH

To engage in the activities outlined in the framework in Fig. 2.4, health promoters and public health practitioners require a range of competencies. Competencies can be defined as a combination of the essential knowledge, abilities, skills and values necessary for the practice of health promotion. Core competencies are the minimum set of competencies that constitute a common baseline for all health promotion roles (Barry et al 2011). There are two aspects of health promotion work to consider. One is the specialist aspect such as immunising a child, taking a cervical smear test, recording blood pressure or undertaking microbiological tests for food hygiene purposes. All of these are the subject of specialist training and outside the scope of this book.

The other aspect of promoting health is about working with people to promote health and wellbeing in many different situations with a variety of different aims. To do this, health promoters need to have knowledge of particular methods and acquire specialist competencies. The CompHP was developed in Europe in 2012 with the aim of establishing competencies and a certification system for health promotion (Barry et al 2012). The competencies framework covers a range of areas as indicated in Fig. 2.5, with all of these competencies covered in this book, including the following:

Managing, Planning and Evaluating

All these are addressed in Part 2: Planning and managing for effective practice, Chapters 5 through 9.

Managing resources for health promotion and public health practice, including budgets, materials, time and people/teams, is crucial. Systematic planning is needed for effective and efficient health promotion. All health promotion work also requires evaluation, and different evaluative methods are appropriate for different approaches.

Communicating and Educating

Communication and educating are addressed in Chapters 10 through 14.

Health promotion is about people, so competence in communication is essential and fundamental. A high level of competence is needed in one-to-one communication and in working with groups in various ways, both formal and informal.

Effective communication is an educational competence, but health promoters also need to understand how people receive information and learn. For example, patient education requires communication and educational competencies.

Marketing and Publicising

Marketing and publicising are covered in Chapter 11.

This requires competence in, for example, marketing and advertising, using the social media, local radio and getting local press coverage of health issues. It may be used when undertaking any health promotion or public health practice activities that would benefit from wider publicity.

Facilitating, Networking, Partnership Working

This means enabling others to promote their own and other people's health, using various means such as sharing skills and information and building up confidence and trust. These competencies are particularly important when working with communities. They are also vital for working with other agencies and forming partnerships for health that cross barriers of organisations and disciplines.

Facilitating, networking and partnership working are addressed in Chapters 9, 13 and 15.

Influencing Policy and Practice

Influencing policies and practices that affect health can be at any level, from national (such as policies set by government or political parties about, for example, housing, transport and future directions for the NHS) to the level of day-to-day work (such as what sort of health promotion programmes will be run in a GP practice, or what resources will be devoted to specific health promotion activities in an environmental health department).

Influencing policy and practice is addressed in Chapter 16.

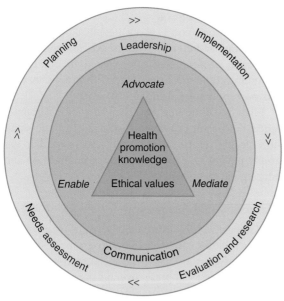

FIG. 2.5 ■ CompHP Core Competencies Framework for Health Promotion. *(Source: Barry et al 2012)*

COMPETENCIES IN PUBLIC HEALTH AND HEALTH PROMOTION

A number of initiatives in the UK and in Europe have resulted in a clear set of competencies for public health and health promotion. At an international level, the Galway Consensus Statement based on building global capacity in health promotion (Morales et al 2009) sets out eight domains of core competency in health promotion, and these have been consolidated in the CompHP discussed earlier.

The UK Public Health Skills and Knowledge Framework (PHSKF; PHE 2016) with an overview in Table 2.2 is applicable to all those in the multidisciplinary public health workforce. PHSKF is reflective of the prevailing public health landscape and is an important tool in developing public health capabilities needed in future. The Framework consists of three areas (A Technical, B Context, C Delivery) each with a set of four or five functions, with each function having approximately six subfunctions. Function A2 is about the enterprise behind health promotion, including community development, advocacy, behaviour change and sustainable efforts to address the wider determinants of health. Within these functions are reference to elements of WHO's Ottawa Charter for Health Promotion (1986) and Marmot's proportionate universalism (Marmot et al 2010; Carey et al 2015). All public health workers will be contributing to some of these functions. It is noted, however, that there is a specialist workforce who are particularly knowledgeable and skilled in this area, health promotion or improvement specialists.

Exercise 2.5 is designed to encourage you to think about your health promotion and public health practice work and how it contributes to the wider public health function. It will also help you to think about the differences between health promotion and public health.

EXERCISE 2.5

Mapping your health promotion and public health work against the UK Public Health Skills and Knowledge Framework (PHSKF)

Study Table 2.2 and note with the appropriate numbers from the PHSKF your level of activity in the public health Areas and Functions using the following Likert scale. If you currently do not have a health promotion or public health role, identify those areas where you would like further training.

Very high level	High level	Fair level	Some level	No activity

What were the results of this mapping in terms of your understanding of the differences between health promotion and public health?

Explain the difference between public health and health promotion.

TABLE 2.2

UK Public Health Skills and Knowledge Framework (PHSKF)

Function	Area A TECHNICAL					
A1 Measure, monitor and report population health and wellbeing; health needs; risks; inequalities; and use of services	A1.1 identify data needs and obtain, verify and organise that data and information	A1.2 Interpret and present data and information	A1.3 manage data and information in compliance with policy and protocol	A1.4 Assess and manage risks associated with using and sharing data and information, data security and intellectual property	A1.5 Collate and analyse data to produce intelligence that informs decision making, planning, implementation, performance monitoring and evaluation	A1.6 Predict future data needs and develop data capture methods to obtain it
A2 Promote population and community health and wellbeing, addressing the wider determinants of health and health inequalities	A2.1 Influence and strengthen community action by empowering communities through evidence-based approaches	A2.2 Advocate public health principles and action to protect and improve health and wellbeing	A2.3 Initiate and/or support action to create environments that facilitate and enable health and wellbeing for individuals, groups and communities	A2.4 Design and/or implement universal programmes and interventions while responding proportionately to levels of need within the community	A2.5 Design and/or implement sustainable and multi-faceted programmes, interventions or services to address complex problems	A2.6 Facilitate change (behavioural and/or cultural) in organisations, communities and/or individuals
A3 Protect the public from environmental hazards, communicable disease, and other health risks, while addressing inequalities in risk exposure and outcomes	A3.1 Analyse and manage immediate and longer-term hazards and risks to health at an international, national and/or local level	A3.2 Assess and manage outbreaks, incidents and single cases of contamination and communicable disease, locally and across boundaries	A3.3 Target and implement nationwide interventions designed to offset ill health (e.g. screening, immunisation)	A3.4 Plan for emergencies and develop national or local resilience to a range of potential threats	A3.5 Mitigate risks to the public's health using different approaches such as legislation, licensing, policy, education, fiscal measures	

Continued on following page

TABLE 2.2
UK Public Health Skills and Knowledge Framework (PHSKF) (Continued)

Area A TECHNICAL

Function						
A4 Work to, and for, the evidence base, conduct research, and provide informed advice	A4.1 Access and appraise evidence gained through systematic methods and through engagement with the wider research community	A4.2 Critique published and unpublished research, synthesise the evidence and draw appropriate conclusions	A4.3 Design and conduct public health research based on current best practice and involving practitioners and the public	A4.4 Report and advise on the implications of the evidence base for the most effective practice and the delivery of value for money	A4.5 Identify gaps in the current evidence base that may be addressed through research	A4.6 Apply research techniques and principles to the evaluation of local services and interventions to establish local evidence of effectiveness
A5 Audit, evaluate and re-design services and interventions to improve health outcomes and reduce health inequalities	A5.1 Conduct economic analysis of services and interventions against health impacts, inequalities in health and return on investment	A5.2 Appraise new technologies, therapies, procedures and interventions and the implications for developing cost-effective equitable services	A5.3 Engage stakeholders (including service users) in service design and development, to deliver accessible and equitable person-centred services	A5.4 Develop and implement standards, protocols and procedures, incorporating national 'best practice' guidance into local delivery systems	A5.5 Quality assure and audit services and interventions to control risks and improve their quality and effectiveness	

Area B CONTEXT

Function					
B1 Work with, and through, policies and strategies to improve health outcomes and reduce health inequalities	B1.1 Appraise and advise on global, national or local strategies in relation to the public's health and health inequalities	B1.2 Assess the impact and benefits of health and other policies and strategies on the public's health and health inequalities	B1.3 Develop and implement action plans with and for specific groups and communities, to deliver outcomes identified in strategies and policies	B1.4 Influence or lead on policy development and strategic planning, creating opportunities to address health needs and risks, promote health and build approaches to prevention	B1.5 Monitor and report on the progress and outcomes of strategy and policy implementation making recommendations for improvement

B2 Work collaboratively across agencies and boundaries to improve health outcomes and reduce health inequalities	B2.1 Influence and co-ordinate other organisations and agencies to increase their engagement with health and wellbeing, ill-health prevention and health inequalities	B2.2 Build alliances and partnerships to plan and implement programmes and services that share goals and priorities	B2.3 Evaluate partnerships and address barriers to successful collaboration	B2.4 Collaborate to create new solutions to complex problems by promoting innovation and the sharing of ideas, practices, resources, leadership and learning	B2.5 Connect communities, groups and individuals to local resources and services that support their health and wellbeing	
B3 Work in a competitive contract culture to improve health outcomes and reduce health inequalities	B3.1 Set commissioning priorities balancing particular needs with the evidence base and the economic case for investment	B3.2 Specify and agree service requirements and measurable performance indicators to ensure quality provision and delivery of desired outcomes	B3.3 Commission and/or provide services and interventions in ways that involve end users and support community interests to achieve equitable person-centred delivery	B3.4 Facilitate positive contractual relationships managing disagreements and changes within legislative and operational frameworks	B3.5 Manage and monitor progress and deliverables against outcomes and processes agreed through a contract	B3.6 Identify and de-commission provision that is no longer effective or value for money
B4 Work within political and democratic systems and with a range of organisational cultures to improve health outcomes and reduce health inequalities	B4.1 Work to understand, and help others to understand, political and democratic processes that can be used to support health and wellbeing and reduce inequalities	4.2 Operate within the decision making, administrative and reporting processes that support political and democratic systems	4.3 Respond constructively to political and other tensions while encouraging a focus on the interests of the public's health	4.4 Help individuals and communities to have more control over decisions that affect them and promote health equity, equality and justice	4.5 Work within the legislative framework that underpins public service provision to maximise opportunities to protect and promote health and wellbeing	

Continued on following page

TABLE 2.2

UK Public Health Skills and Knowledge Framework (PHSKF) *(Continued)*

Area C DELIVERY

Function					
C1 Provide leadership to drive improvement in health outcomes and the reduction of health inequalities	C1.1 Act with integrity, consistency and purpose, and continue my own personal development	C1.2 Engage others, build relationships, manage conflict, encourage contribution and sustain commitment to deliver shared objectives	C1.3 Adapt to change, manage uncertainty, solve problems and align clear goals with lines of accountability in complex and unpredictable environments	C1.4 Establish and coordinate a system of leaders and followers engaged in improving health outcomes, the wider health determinants and reducing inequalities	C1.5 Provide vision, shape thinking, inspire shared purpose and influence the contributions of others throughout the system to improve health and address health inequalities
C2 Communicate with others to improve health outcomes and reduce health inequalities	C2.1 Manage public perception and convey key messages using a range of media processes	C2.2 Communicate sometimes complex information and concepts (including health outcomes, inequalities and life expectancy) to a diversity of audiences using different methods	C2.3 Facilitate dialogue with groups and communities to improve health literacy and reduce inequalities using a range of tools and technologies	C2.4 Apply the principles of social marketing and/or behavioural science to reach specific groups and communities with enabling information and ideas	C2.5 Consult and listen to individuals, groups and communities likely to be affected by planned intervention or change
C3 Design and manage programmes and projects to improve health and reduce health inequalities	C3.1 Scope programmes/projects stating the case for investment, the aims, objectives and milestones	C3.2 Identify stakeholders, agree requirements and programme/project schedule(s) and identify how outputs and outcomes will be measured and communicated	C3.3 Manage programme/project schedule(s), resources, budget and scope, accommodating changes within a robust change control process	C3.4 Track and evaluate programme/project progress against schedule(s) and regularly review quality assurance, risks and opportunities to realise benefits and outcomes	C3.5 Seek independent assurance throughout programme/project planning and processes within organisational governance frameworks
C4 Prioritise and manage resources at a population/systems level to achieve equitable health outcomes and return on investment	C4.1 Identify, negotiate and secure sources of funding and/or other resources	C4.2 Prioritise, align and deploy resources towards clear strategic goals and objectives	C4.3 Develop workforce capacity and mobilise the system-wide paid and volunteer workforce, to deliver public health priorities at scale	C4.4 Design, implement, deliver and/or quality assure education and training programmes, to build a skilled and competent workforce	C4.5 Adapt capability by maintaining flexible in-service learning and development systems for the workforce

Source: Adjusted from Public Health England (2016)

PRACTICE POINTS

- Health promotion and public health practice encompasses a wide range of approaches that are united by the same goal, to enable people to increase control over and improve their health.
- It is important for you to identify the full scope of your health promotion and public health practice work and to see how this fits with the work of your organisation or employer and the wider remit of public health.
- PHSKF provides a competencies (skills and knowledge) map which can be used by organisations, managers, education and training providers, and individuals to improve the quality of public health and health promotion work.

REFERENCES

Auld ME, Radius SM, Galer-Unti RJ, Hinman JM, Gotsch AR, Mail PD 2011 Distinguishing between health education and health information dissemination. American Journal of Public Health 101(3):390–391.

Barry M, Battel-Kirk B, Davison H et al 2011 CompHP developing competencies and professional standards for health promotion capacity building in Europe. St Denis Cedex, IUHPE, Paris.

Barry M, Battel-Kirk B, Davison H, et al 2012 The CompHP Project Handbooks. http://www.iuhpe.org/images/PROJECTS/ACCREDITATION/CompHP_Project_Handbooks.pdf.

Carey G, Crammond B, De Leeuw E 2015 Towards health equity: a framework for the application of proportionate universalism. International Journal for Equity in Health 14:81.

Dixey R 2012 Health promotion: Global principles and practice. Oxfordshire, CABI Publishing.

Edington DW, Schultz AB, Pitts JS, Camilleri A 2015 The future of health promotion in the 21st century: a focus on the working population. American Journal of Lifestyle Medicine. Vol xx no x. http://edingtonassociates.com/wp-content/uploads/2016/02/AJLM605789.pdf.

Faculty of Public Heath 2016 What is public health. http://www.fph.org.uk/what_is_public_health.

Hancock T 2001 Healthy people in healthy communities in a healthy world: The science, art and politics of public health in the 21st century. Paper presented at the launch of the OU School of Health and Social Welfare Health Promotion and Public Health Research Group, 12 September 2001. Milton Keynes, The Open University.

Health Development Consultancy (HDC) Healthy Lifestyle Resources. http://www.healthdc.co.uk/resources/.

Heineken 2016 Moderate Drinkers Wanted TV, cinema, and internet commercial. http://tvadsongs.uk/heineken-advert-song-i-need-a-hero-commercial/.

HSCNI 2016 South Eastern Health and Social Care Trust Health Development Department Guide. http://www.setrust.hscni.net/pdf/HD_Directory(1).pdf. Accessed June 2016.

Lalonde M 1974 A new perspective on the health of Canadians. Ottawa, Information Canada http://www.phac-aspc.gc.ca/ph-sp/pdf/perspect-eng.pdf.

Lee NR, Kotler P 2015 Social marketing: changing behaviors for good, 5th edn. London, Sage.

Lomazzi, M 2016 A Global Charter for the Public's Health-the public health system: role, functions, competencies and education requirements. European Journal of Public Health 26(2):210–2.

Marmot M, Atkinson T, Bell J et al 2010 Fair society, healthy lives: strategic review of health inequalities in England – the Marmot review. London, Institute of Health Equity, University College London. http://www.dh.gov.uk/en/Publichealth/Healthinequalities/DH_094770.

McKinlay JB 1979 A case for refocusing upstream: the political economy of health. In: Javco EG, (eds) Patients, physicians and illness. Basingstoke, Macmillan.

MIND 2014 Time for change: lets end mental health discrimination. Making a drama out of a Crisis. https://www.time-to-change.org.uk/sites/default/files/Making_a_drama_out_of_a_crisis.pdf.

Morales AS-M, Battel-Kirk B, Barry MM et al 2009 Perspectives on health promotion competencies and accreditation in Europe. Global Health Promotion 16(2):21–30.

NSMC 2016 What is social marketing. http://www.nsmcentre.org.uk/content/what-social-marketing-1.

Potvin L, Jones CM 2011 Twenty-five years after The Ottawa Charter: the critical role of health promotion for public health. Canadian Journal of Public Health 102(4):244–248.

Public Health England 2016 Public health skills and knowledge framework. https://www.gov.uk/government/uploads/system/uploads/attachment_data/file/545012/Public_Health_Skills_and_Knowledge_Framework_2016.pdf.

Scriven A 2005 Promoting health: policies, principles and perspectives. In: Scriven A (ed) Health promoting practice: the contribution of nurses and allied health professions. Basingstoke, Palgrave.

Scriven A 2007 Healthy public policies: rhetoric or reality. In: Scriven A, Garman G (eds) 2007 public health: social context and action. Maidenhead, Open University Press.

Tannahill A 2009 Health promotion: the Tannahill model revisited. Public Health Volume 122(12):1387–1391.

Welsh Government 2016 Health improvement. http://gov.wales/topics/health/improvement/?lang=en.

World Federation of Public Health Associations 2016 A global charter for the public's health. http://www.wfpha.org/wfpha-projects/14-projects/171-a-global-charter-for-the-public-s-health-3.

World Health Organization 1986 The Ottawa Charter for Health Promotion. Geneva, WHO. http://www.who.int/healthpromotion/conferences/previous/ottawa/en/index4.html.

WEBSITES

Functions of the Local Public Health System 2016. http://www.fph.org.uk/uploads/Functions%20of%20the%20local%20PH%20system%20FINAL%20200514.pdf.

BLOGS

Faculty of Public Health Blog, Better Health For All 2016. https://betterhealthforall.org/. Accessed June 2016.

The National Social Marketing Centre Blog. The National Social Marketing Centre Blog. http://www.thensmc.com/blog. Accessed June 2016.

FACEBOOK

Royal Society for Public Health. https://www.facebook.com/royalsocietyforpublichealth/. Accessed June 2016.

International Social Marketing Association (iSMA). https://www.facebook.com/socialmarketingassociation/. Accessed June 2016.

TWITTER

Faculty of Public Health FPH@FPH.
Association of Directors of Public Health ADPH@ADPHUK.

YOUTUBE

Heineken 2016 Moderate Drinkers Wanted TV, cinema, and internet commercial. https://www.youtube.com/watch?v=cpwd4A5myx0.

WHO PROMOTES HEALTH?

CHAPTER CONTENTS

SUMMARY

In this chapter, some of the key agents and agencies of public health and health promotion are identified and their roles discussed. Included are international and national organisations, the government, local authorities, the National Health Service (NHS) and voluntary and Non-Government Organisations (NGO). The chapter ends with an exercise on identifying and mapping key local health promoters and public health professionals in your geographical area.

This chapter provides an overview of the people and organisations that support and enable better individual and population health. The aim here is to identify the agents and agencies through which planned, deliberate public health and health promotion programmes and policies are delivered. It must be recognised that these agents and agencies change over time and that there are government reorganisations of health and public health systems on a fairly regular basis. Those working to promote health need to be very familiar with local and national systems. At the time of writing, the four countries that make up the UK – England, Wales, Scotland and Northern Ireland – have slightly different health and public health systems. Box 3.1 sums up the current organisational structures in the four countries. Many of the health promoters and public health practitioners discussed later in the chapter either work in these health and public health systems or establish collaborative partnerships with the people who do.

EXERCISE 3.1

1. Critically compare the different health structures outlined in Box 3.1 and identify the key differences in the organisation of public health between England, Wales, Scotland and Northern Ireland.

2. If you were a government Minister for Health, how would you structure the statutory health promotion and public health services? For example, would you have a lead agency for public health and, if so, what would you call it? Would you locate responsibility for public health within the NHS or the local authority? What areas of public health would you prioritise? Offer a rational for each of your decisions.

BOX 3.1
AN OVERVIEW OF THE UK HEALTH AND PUBLIC HEALTH SYSTEMS

ENGLAND

Health services in England are centrally funded from the Department of Health. The NHS provides healthcare services through NHS trusts and foundation trusts (including mental health and ambulance trusts), as well as some charities and social enterprises. All GPs in England are part of a clinical commissioning group which is responsible for planning and commissioning the services their patients need.

NHS England oversees the NHS commissioning budget of approximately £80 billion, and its area teams are responsible for commissioning the following services:

- GP
- Dental
- Pharmacy
- Some optical services
- Screening and immunisation programmes
- Public health services in England are primarily delivered through:
  - Public Health England (PHE)
  - local authorities (LAs) that have public health responsibilities

PHE was formed in 2013. Its mission is to protect and improve the nation's health and wellbeing and reduce health inequalities. The Health and Social Care Act (2012) gave some local authorities mandatory requirements for commissioning public health services such as sexual health, NHS health checks and the National Child Measurement Programme, and for providing public health advice through clinical commissioning groups. Each of these LAs has a health and wellbeing board which sets the local strategic direction for public health and a strategy based on the needs of the local population. Local authorities also have statutory responsibilities to ensure systems are in place to protect the health of the population and to provide information and advice in the event of a health protection incident or outbreak (see Fig. 3.1).

WALES

As a devolved administration, Wales receives a block grant from the UK central government which is then distributed between the different departments including NHS Wales. The main difference for patients in Wales is that prescriptions for medicines are free for everyone.

NHS Wales delivers services through seven health boards and three NHS trusts, each one responsible for providing all healthcare services within a particular geographical area. The three NHS trusts in Wales with an all-Wales focus are The Welsh Ambulance Services Trust for emergency services; Velindre NHS Trust which offers specialist services in cancer care; and Public Health Wales.

The seven health boards work together with community health councils, which represent patients and user groups. Public Health Wales makes a commitment to:

- improving health and reducing health inequalities
- improving the quality, equity and effectiveness of services
- protecting people from infectious and environmental hazards.

Each of the seven health boards in Wales has a director of public health who works closely with Public Health Wales. The directors of public health are responsible for providing professional advice and leadership within their health boards and for working in partnership with their related local authorities.

SCOTLAND

As a devolved administration, Scotland receives a block grant from the UK central government, which is then distributed between the different departments including NHS Scotland.

NHS Scotland is made up of 14 health boards which are responsible for delivering the acute and primary healthcare services their populations need. There are also eight special health boards that cover services such as ambulance services, Scotland's health improvement agency (called NHS Health Scotland) and NHS Education for Scotland.

Public Health in Scotland

Each health board has a public health department where responsibility lies for monitoring and improving the health of their populations.

NHS Health Scotland is one of the special health boards, and its overall aim is to improve Scotland's health by focusing on the inequalities. NHS Health Scotland is the main health improvement agency in Scotland and covers every aspect of health improvement across all health topics, settings and life stages.

More than 50 organisations are involved in health protection in Scotland over two 'tiers':

- Local authorities and NHS boards
- Government, NHS special boards, Scottish Environment Protection Agency, Scottish Water, the Food Standards Agency and the Health and Safety Executive.

Health Protection Scotland provides the following advice and services to the rest of NHS Scotland:

- The national blood transfusion service
- Advice on healthcare environments and equipment
- Monitoring hazards and exposures affecting people's health
- Providing guidance on tackling healthcare-associated infections
- Coordinating screening programmes.

BOX 3.1
AN OVERVIEW OF THE UK HEALTH AND PUBLIC HEALTH SYSTEMS *(Continued)*

NORTHERN IRELAND

The health system differs in Northern Ireland in that both health and social care are provided through an integrated service, and prescriptions for medical care are free for everyone. Northern Ireland receives a block grant from the UK Treasury which funds the Department of Health, Social Services, and Public Safety for Northern Ireland (DHSSPS). The DHSSPS has overall responsibility for providing health and social care services in Northern Ireland including public health and public safety.

Health and Social Care Board

Working under the DHSSPS, a Health and Social Care Board is responsible for commissioning services, resource management, performance management and service improvement. The Health and Social Care Board works to identify and meet the needs of the Northern Ireland popula-tion through its five local commissioning groups who cover the same geographical areas as five health and social care trusts that deliver health and social care services. A separate trust – Northern Ireland Ambulance Trust – provides ambulance services across Northern Ireland.

Public Health in Northern Ireland

The Public Health Agency (PHA) is responsible for:
- health protection
- screening
- health and social care research and development
- safety and quality
- improving health and social wellbeing.

It also provides public health, nursing and allied health professional advice to support the Health and Social Care Board and its local commissioning groups.

Source Adjusted from Health Careers 2016a
Please refer to each country's health and public health websites referenced at the end of this chapter for further details and updates.

NATIONAL PUBLIC HEALTH AGENCIES

The Government

The national public health strategies for health in England, Wales, Scotland and Northern Ireland demonstrate a commitment towards the pursuit of improved health and a reduction in health inequalities for the populations they serve. To this end, in England, key public health agencies have been established such as the National Institute for Health and Care Excellence (NICE) and Public Health England (PHE; see the following text). Government tackles health issues such as drug and substance misuse (Department of Health (DoH) 2013a) and obesity and healthy eating (DoH 2015). In relation to obesity, the government action in England involves giving people advice on a healthy diet and physical activity through the Change 4 Life programme; improving labelling on food and drink to help people make healthy choices with a consistent front of pack labelling system that makes it clear what is in food and drink; and encouraging restaurant businesses to include calorie information on their menus so that people can make healthy choices. For full details on the obesity strategy, see DoH (2015) and for the Childhood Obesity, see Plan for Action DoH (2016).

The National Institute for Health and Care Excellence (NICE)

The National Institute for Health and Care Excellence (NICE) is a non-departmental public body providing national guidance and advice to improve health and social care for England. The way NICE was established in legislation means that the guidance is officially England-only. However, there are agreements to provide certain NICE products and services to Wales, Scotland and Northern Ireland. Decisions on how the guidance applies in these countries are made by the devolved administrations who are often involved and consulted with in the development of NICE guidance. NICE also provides resources to help maximise use of evidence and guidance for key groups including general practitioners (GPs), local government and public health professionals (NICE 2016). Their evidence sections Lifestyle and Wellbeing and Population Groups are of particular importance to those promoting health with guides on topics and approaches such as behaviour change.

Public Health England

Public Health England (PHE) provides national leadership and expert services to support public health through:

- coordinating a national public health service and delivering some of these elements
- building an evidence base to support local public health services
- supporting the public to make healthier choices
- providing leadership to the public health delivery system
- supporting the development of the public health workforce (see Table 3.1 for the main public health functions of PHE).

Fig. 3.1 identifies how PHE relates to other parts of the NHS.

Health Services

Statutory health services are very important agents for public health and the promotion of health globally, nationally and locally. The NHS in the UK has a significant role in improving and protecting public health. Fig. 3.1 shows the structure of the health services in England.

Fig. 3.1 shows the relationship between the DoH, PHE, NICE, local authorities (with their Health and Wellbeing Boards responsible for the local health and wellbeing strategy) and the delivery of public health. Community services include health centres, clinics and services in people's homes. Mental health services provide health and social care for people with mental health problems. These services are provided through primary care, such as GP services, or through more specialist care. This might include counselling and other psychological therapies, community and family support, or general health screening. For example, people experiencing bereavement, depression, stress or anxiety can get help from their GP and be referred to a specialist mental health service (NHS Choices 2016).

Hospital services employ medical teams and a range of other health-promoting professions such as physiotherapists, radiographers, podiatrists, speech and language therapists, counsellors, occupational therapists and psychologists.

Primary care is the first point of health services contact for most people and includes GPs, dentists, pharmacists and optometrists, as well as NHS walk-in centres and the NHS 111 telephone service. Secondary care is a range of specialist services, usually based in a hospital as opposed to being in the community, and patients are usually referred to secondary care by a primary care provider such as a GP. Both primary and secondary care services have health promotion functions. In the Five Year Forward View (NHS England 2014b), the government has identified what it calls the health and wellbeing gap. The emphasis is on prevention based on concerns that health inequalities are widening, and there is an increase in what is regarded as avoidable illness. In the future, NHS primary and secondary care services may be called upon to prioritise health promotion and other preventative strategies.

The structures in Scotland, Wales and Northern Ireland differ (see Box 3.1 for the overview). In addition to Box 3.1, Understanding the New NHS (NHS England 2014a) offers a succinct outline of the provision in these three countries. In the interests of keeping the text in this book short, the examples used are drawn from England but readers in all countries will

TABLE 3.1			
The Public Health and Health Promotion Functions of PHE			
The main public health functions of PHE are:			
Health protection	Health improvement	Knowledge and information	Operations
For example, notifiable disease outbreak prevention, recording and management and major incident response	Responsible for developing a 21st-century health and wellbeing service addressing health inequalities, for example, health promotion and screening services	For example, disease registration, research and development	Ensuring delivery of consistently high-quality services, for example, the national microbiology unit

Source: Adjusted from NHS England 2014a

The structure of the NHS in England
(showing emerging devolution)

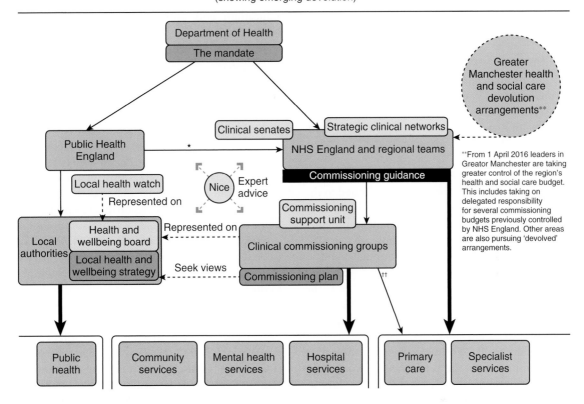

FIG. 3.1 ■ Public health and the structure of the NHS in England. *(Source: Kings Fund 2016)*

*Screening/immunisation programmes run by NHS England.

†† In 2016/17 a total of 114 CCGs will have assumed full responsibility for the commissioning of primary medical care services under delegated commissioning arrangements. Nearly all CCGs are expected to have taken on delegated arrangements by 2017/18.

**From 1 April 2016 leaders in Greater Manchester are taking greater control of the region's health and social care budget. This includes taking on delegated responsibility for several commissioning budgets previously controlled by NHS England. Other areas are also pursuing 'devolved' arrangements.

need to familiarise themselves with the structure in the country where they work by undertaking Exercise 3.2.

Online Public Health Resources: NHS Direct Wales, NHS Choices

NHS Direct Wales is a telephone helpline open 24 hours a day with an associated webpage. The webpage offers multiple categories of public health advice and guidance including information on a range of health issues, a directory of local services, a travel health category and a Live Well section which offers a wide range of health promotion information and advice to help users improve their lifestyle. There is information on alcohol, smoking, physical activity, healthy eating, sexual health and much more. The Live Well section also offers advice

on vaccinations and pregnancy, and offers tools to support lifestyle changes such as alcohol unit and body mass index (BMI) calculators. NHS Choices for England is very similar in terms of the health promoting resources it provides. There are podcasts from ITunes relating to their Couch to 5 K challenge, strength and flex workouts and a very useful Health News section.

NHS Walk-In Centres (WICS)

NHS walk-in centres (WICs) offer convenient access to a range of treatments for minor illnesses and injury. WICs are managed by Clinical Commissioning Groups (CCGs). Nurse-led centres often provide health promotion and advice, which could include stop-smoking support, blood pressure checks and emergency contraception. For an evaluation of WICS, see Monitor (2014).

Other National and Local Public Health Agencies

Non-Government Organisations

There are a number of NGOs concerned specifically with public health and health promotion in the UK such as The Royal Society for Public Health, the UK Public Health Association and The Institute of Health Education and Health Promotion.

The Royal Society for Public Health (RSPH). The RSPH is an independent organisation dedicated to the promotion and protection of population health and wellbeing. It advises on policy development; provides education and training services; encourages scientific research; disseminates information through publications, reports, blogs, Facebook, Twitter and webpages; and runs public health campaigns. The RSPH is the largest multidisciplinary public health organisation in the UK and advocates for the importance of specialised health promotion and public health practitioners within public health. Their campaigns demonstrate their commitment to the principles of health promotion. For example, their 'Dream it. Try it. Live it.' (RSPH 2016) campaign aims to empower young people to adopt healthy behaviours and raise awareness of the benefits of living healthier, more active lives. The campaign covers a range of topics including mental wellbeing, physical activity, healthy eating, body image and the importance of sleep, and it is led by a team of young volunteers linked to the youth health champion qualification with support from RSPH staff. These volunteers direct the campaign as well as conduct interviews, research, make and edit promotional videos, write blogs and work with a wide range of public health and corporate organisations. It is a multimedia campaign using Twitter, Instagram, YouTube and Snapchat. Updates are also posted on the youth health movement website. See website references at the end of this chapter.

The Institute of Health Promotion and Education (IHPE). The IHPE is a professional association which brings together people with a professional interest in health education and health promotion. The Institute

offers comprehensive information resources (such as the International Journal of Health Promotion and Education) and professional development support (IHPE 2016).

Voluntary and Charitable Organisations and Pressure Groups

There are very many international and national voluntary and charitable organisations concerned with public health and health promotion. National examples of these are The Advisory Council on Alcohol and Drug Education (TACADE) and the National Association for Mental Health (MIND). Most of these organisations produce educational material, and some run training courses for professionals and/or the public. Some organisations act mainly as pressure groups such as Friends of the Earth. See Bull et al (2014) for a critical and detailed examination of the role of the charity sector in supporting individual and population health in the UK.

Professional Associations

Professional associations such as the British Medical Association (BMA), the Royal College of Nursing (RCN), the Chartered Institute for Environmental Health (CIEH) and the Faculty of Public Health (FPH) have been highly influential in policy and legislative changes and in practice support and training of their members in public health and health promotion.

Trade Unions

Trade unions are active in promoting health, wellbeing and safety at work, both through negotiating workplace conditions and through their health and safety representatives (Trade Union Council 2015). In the UK, the Health and Safety Executive (HSE) also oversees the implementation of health and safety at work legislation and provides a range of resources and information on workplace health.

Commercial and Industrial Organisations

These have a role in safeguarding public health. Examples include companies providing water and refuse removal. In recent years in the UK, some facilities with a public health protection function have been privatised. This has raised public health dilemmas, for example, 'Should water companies have the right to cut off supplies to consumers who do not pay their bills when a possible consequence of this is the occurrence and spread of infectious diseases such as dysentery?'

Manufacturers and Retailers

Manufacturers and retailers are a powerful influence on public health. For example, in the UK, millions of families use a major supermarket every week. Food manufacturers have both the technical expertise to make healthier products and the marketing expertise to influence purchasing habits. If the full strength of these skills is directed towards activities to encourage and enable people to make healthier food choices, the public health benefits could be great. The Public Health Responsibility Deal (DoH 2011) was established to maximise these benefits. By working in partnership, public health, commercial and voluntary organisations agreed on practical actions to secure more progress, more quickly, with less cost than legislation across a range of public health issues including food, alcohol, physical activity and health at work (see Panjwani and Carraher 2014, Evaluation of the Public Health Responsibility Deal).

The Mass Media

The mass media refers to all major outlets distributing public health information across a variety of formats including television, print, radio and online. Mass media can facilitate targeted health campaigning or can contribute indirectly. The trend towards developing an online presence as well as the traditional newspapers or TV channels demonstrates a move towards the immediacy of web-based communications. The mass media are intensively employed in public health including the production and distribution of booklets, pamphlets, exhibits, newspaper and magazine articles, and radio and television programmes, plus the various online and social media outlets (such as YouTube, Facebook, Twitter, websites and Instagram). These media are employed to promote the uptake of health information and knowledge, to change health attitudes and values and to encourage the establishment of new health behaviour (Catalán-Matamoros 2011). Dosemagen and Aase (2016) use a range of arguments to demonstrate the value of the social media to public health.

See Chapter 11 for more about the mass media and social media in public health and health promotion

including a consideration of some of the negative influences.

Churches and Religious Organisations

Churches and religious organisations can play an important part in developing values, attitudes and beliefs that affect health. The findings of one American study show how a church-based health promotion initiative can achieve success and outline factors to consider when designing church-based health-promotion interventions (Banerjee et al 2015).

INTERNATIONAL PUBLIC HEALTH AGENCIES

The European Community

Ranging from influence over world trade laws affecting health to population health issues such as obesity to the use of comparative data to affect health policy, the European Union's (EU) EU's public health policies are an important influence on national and local policies (Greer & Kurzer 2013). The Europe 2020 strategy (European Commission 2016) aims to turn the EU into a smart, sustainable and inclusive economy promoting growth for all, one prerequisite of which is a population in good health. Specific EU public health action includes EU-wide laws and standards for health products, services and patients; giving EU countries tools to help them cooperate and identify best practices (such as in health promotion activities, tackling risk factors, disease management); and funding health projects through the EU health programme.

The EU backs preventive action against diseases including:

- responsible food labelling so consumers know what they are eating
- action against breast, cervical and colorectal cancer; EU-wide screening programmes provide quality assurance guidelines for treatment, pooling knowledge and resources
- measures to promote a healthy diet and exercise, encouraging governments, NGOs and industry to work together, making it easier for consumers to change their lifestyles
- combating smoking through legislation on tobacco products, raising awareness, advertising and sponsorship.

The policy paper Investing in Health (EU Commission 2013) endorses investing in people's health, particularly through health-promotion programmes, as a way of reducing inequalities and tackling social exclusion. In addition, the EU helps national governments to prepare more effectively for serious health threats affecting more than one country and to coordinate their response, for example, by enabling vaccines and other medical inputs to be purchased jointly. The European Centre for Disease Prevention and Control in Stockholm assesses emerging threats so the EU can respond rapidly. It pools knowledge on current and emerging threats and works with national counterparts to develop disease monitoring across Europe (for more details, see European Centre for Disease Prevention and Control 2016).

The World Health Organization (WHO)

The WHO has a significant role in guiding both European and global health policy. It has issued many statements in the form of declarations and charters addressing important and broad areas of health promotion and public health-related policy. It is responsible for Health 2020, the new European policy for health and wellbeing (WHO 2016), and coordinates European networks such as School and Youth Health/Health Promoting Schools and Healthy Cities.

The WHO's role in guiding the promotion of health is discussed in Chapter 1, and Health 2020 is outlined in Chapter 16.

Other International Agencies

The International Union for Health Promotion and Education (IUHPE)

The IUHPE is a unique worldwide, independent and professional association of individuals and organisations committed to improving the health and wellbeing of the people through education, community action and the development of healthy public policy. It is a leading global network working to promote health and contribute to the achievement of equity in health between and within countries. It advances the knowledge base and improves the quality and effectiveness of health promotion and health education practice. The IUHPE works across all continents and decentralises its activity through regional offices. It works in close cooperation with the major intergovernmental

and NGOs such as WHO, to influence and facilitate the development of health promotion strategies and projects.

As an international health promotion agency, it works towards:

- greater equity in the health of populations between and within countries of the world
- effective alliances and partnerships to produce optimal health promotion outcomes
- accessible evidence-based knowledge to inform practice
- excellence in policy and practice for effective quality health promotion
- high levels of capacity in individuals, organisations and countries to undertake health-promotion activities.

To achieve these goals, the IUHPE pursues the following objectives:

- Increased investment in health promotion by governments, intergovernmental and NGOs, academic institutions and the private sector
- An increase in organisational, governmental and inter-governmental policies and practices that result in greater equity in health between and within countries
- Improvements in policy and practice of governments at all levels, organisations and sectors that influence the determinants of the health of populations
- Strong alliances and partnerships among all sectors based on agreed ethical principles, mutual understanding and respect
- Activities that contribute to the development, translation and exchange of knowledge and practice that advance the field of health promotion (including world conferences)
- The wide dissemination of knowledge to health promotion practitioners, as well as to policy makers, government officials and other key individuals and organisations
- A strong and universally accessible knowledge base for effective, quality health promotion
- Improved mechanisms for the exchange of ideas, experience and knowledge that promote health and wellbeing

- A global forum for mutual support and professional advancement of members
- Capacity-building opportunities for individuals and institutions to better carry out health-promotion initiatives and advocacy efforts (IUHPE 2016).

In the dissemination of knowledge, the IUHPE is very active. It has an international journal, Global Health Promotion, and has associated journals which rank amongst the most important peer-reviewed journals in the field of health promotion.

European Public Health Alliance (EPHA)

EPHA is Europe's leading NGO advocating for better population health. It is a member-led organisation made up of public health NGOs, patient groups, health professionals and disease groups working together to improve health and strengthen the voice of public health in Europe. EPHA is a member of, among others, the Social Platform, the Health and Environment Alliance (HEAL) and the EU Civil Society Contact Group. Their mission is to bring together the public health community to provide thought leadership and facilitate change, to build public health capacity, to deliver equitable solutions to European public health challenges and to improve health and reduce health inequalities.

Their vision is of a Europe with universal good health and wellbeing where all have access to a sustainable and high quality health system: A Europe whose policies and practices contribute to health, both within and beyond its borders.

What they do:

- Monitor the policy-making process within the EU institutions and support the flow of information on health promotion and public health policy developments amongst all interested players including politicians, civil servants, NGOs, stakeholders and the public
- Promote greater awareness amongst European citizens and NGOs about policy developments and programme initiatives that effect the health of those living in the EU, allowing them to contribute to the policy-making process
- Train, mentor and support NGOs, local health organisations, those working with disadvantaged

communities, and enable engagement with the EU.
- Participate in policy debates and stakeholder dialogues to raise the profile of health in all policy areas, supporting collaboration and partnerships between NGOS and other organisations active at European, national and local levels on health promotion and public health (EPHA 2016)

World Federation of Public Health Associations (WFPHA)

The WFPHA is an international NGO composed of multidisciplinary national public health associations. It is the only worldwide professional society representing and serving the broad field of public health. WFPHA's mission is to promote and protect global public health. It does this throughout the world by supporting the establishment and organisational development of public health associations and societies of public health through facilitating and supporting the exchange of information, knowledge and the transfer of skills and resources, and through promoting and undertaking advocacy for public policies, programs and practices that will result in a healthy and productive world. WFPHA brings together public health professionals interested and active in safeguarding and promoting the public's health through professional exchange, collaboration and action. WFPHA is accredited as an NGO in official relation with the WHO. It collaborates with the WHO to advance the field of public health through the promotion of pro-health policies, strategies and best practices around the world. The Federation also holds consultation status with the United Nations Economic and Social Council (ECOSOC). It is the only worldwide professional society representing and serving the broad area of public health as distinct from single disciplines or occupations (WFPHA 2016). They have developed the Global Charter for Public Health, which is discussed in Chapter 2.

Agents of Health Promotion

National and local policy in the UK has focused on the development of a multidisciplinary public health workforce (see, for example, PHE 2014 for an overview of organising the public health multidisciplinary teams). The extent and nature of the public health workforce will vary within countries. In England, the Centre for Workforce Intelligence (CFWI) was commissioned by PHE, Health Education England (HEE) and the DoH to gather information on the core public health workforce. In the report, they point to the public health system in England going through a transitional period following changes brought about by the Health and Social Care Act (2012) including the shift of responsibility for most public health commissioning from the NHS to local authorities and the establishment of a central agency in PHE. These changes are now embedded. Table 3.2 demonstrates what are considered to be public health core roles and gives an estimation of the workforce numbers in England. The largest four groups of the core public health workforce listed in Table 3.2 will have key health promotion functions, although health promotion is not mentioned in their titles.

TABLE 3.2
Mapping the Core Public Health Roles in England

Core Public Health Roles	Numbers
Health Visitors	11,000
Public Health Practitioners	Up to 10,000
Environmental Health Professionals	5,500-8,500
School Nurses	4,000
Public Health Scientists	1,500-2,500
Public Health Consultants, Specialists and Registrars Including Directors of Public Health	1,450-1,650
Intelligence and Knowledge Professionals	1,000-1,300
Public Health Managers	600-1,200
Other Public Health Nurses	350-750
Public Health Academics	200-300

Source: Adjusted from Centre for Workforce Intelligence 2014

In addition to the core public health workforce, many groups will contribute to health promotion and public health but will not necessarily have either public health or health promotion, or even health, in their professional titles. Fig. 3.2 identifies a broader range of agents and agencies with a remit for promoting statutory, non-statutory, national and international public health. Most will have a variety of health-promoting functions or engage in a range of health-promoting activities.

The agents and agencies identified in Fig. 3.2 may work together in collaborative partnerships in an effort to make their work more effective. Partnership working has been a dominant theme in national and international health promotion and public health policies with government strategies and guidelines continuing to focus on the importance of partnerships for health between agencies and across government departments (see Chapter 9 for more on public health partnership).

Directors of Public Health

The director of public health is the lead officer for public heath functions within local authorities. They have specialist public health expertise and access to specialist resources spanning the three domains of public health: health improvement, health protection and health care (such as the population health aspects of NHS-funded clinical services). The director has a critical role in public health needs assessment which drives commissioning and clinical commissioning. They will also lead on health protection and champion health across the whole of the authority's business (Health and Social Care Act 2012).

Health Promotion Specialists

Health promotion specialists (sometimes known by other professional titles such as public health practitioners; see the following text) are usually located within the public health teams. Health promotion specialists would normally hold postgraduate qualifications in health promotion and would be responsible for the provision of expert advice, leadership, partnership development, training, programme development (including strategy and policy) and resources to support local health promotion initiatives. They liaise with other health promotion agents and agencies to ensure that public health activities, wherever initiated, are coordinated and supported. For an overview of the work of health promotion specialists, see Prospects (2016).

Public Health Practitioners

In England, the term 'public health practitioner' is used to describe members of the core public health

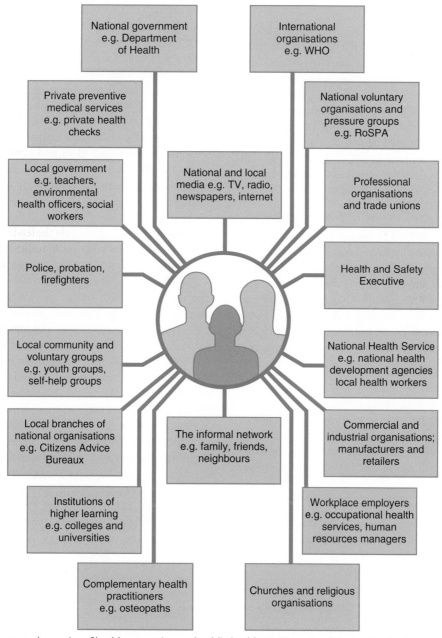

FIG. 3.2 ▪ Agents and agencies of health promotion and public health. RoSPA = Royal Society for the Prevention of Accidents.

workforce with public health skill and knowledge working in various areas of public health including health improvement and health protection. They may support healthy lifestyle programmes or work in local communities or public health teams specialising in health protection. They may also play an important role in national and local health campaigns or work in the public health knowledge and intelligence teams in local or national government organisations (Centre for Workforce Intelligence 2016).

Public Health Specialists

Public health specialists work as system leaders at strategic or senior management level in public health teams or at a senior level of expertise such as epidemiology. They come from a variety of professional backgrounds before entering a five-year training programme, which covers all aspects of public health, and are registered with the Faculty Public Health and required to maintain registration through appraisal and revalidation. They have both leadership skills and technical skills and work across all of the three public health domains outlined in Chapter 2 (FPH 2016).

Health Trainers and Community Health Champions

The health trainer's (HT) role is well established in England. HTs assist clients to assess their lifestyles and wellbeing, set goals for improving their health, agree on action-plans, and provide practical support and information that will help people change their behaviour. This could include promoting the benefits of taking regular exercise and eating healthily, reducing alcohol intake, breastfeeding, practicing safe sex and stopping smoking and substances. Their role generally includes:

- helping people identify how their behaviours may be affecting their health
- supporting individuals to create a health plan to help make changes to improve their health
- helping individuals to become more knowledgeable about things that can affect their health and wellbeing
- signposting to other agencies and professionals.

Health trainers are trained and knowledgeable about the health issues that affect the community they are working in. Their clients may be identified from existing community and support groups, through referral (such as from a health professional at a children's centre) or via self-referral. Clients often come from hard-to-reach disadvantaged groups such as the homeless, travellers and those with drug, alcohol and addiction problems. While much of a health trainer's work will be on a one-to-one basis, they sometimes work with groups of people, for example, delivering group sessions on behaviour change and health improvement. Health trainers may also be assisted in their work by members of the community who have been trained to be health trainer champions (HTCs). HTCs are usually volunteers who have undertaken health improvement training at level 2 with the Royal Society of Public Health and who can help health trainer services extend their reach within communities.

Health trainers often work for private companies that provide a health trainer service for the NHS or for a local authority. They may also work directly for the NHS, a local authority or a charity, in the prison service or the armed services (Health Careers 2016b). See also Health Trainers England (2016a) for case studies on health trainers and Case Study 3.1 for an example of the work that they undertake. The Royal Society of Public Health, in their critical assessment of Health Trainer activity, report that the services are an important strategic and tactical asset in reducing health inequalities and that this workforce has an almost unique ability to leave a legacy with their clients in terms of improved health awareness and understanding (Shircore 2013). Other countries in the UK have considered using health trainers (see Price and Lester 2012).

CASE STUDY 3.1

Building Community Health Champions, NHS Sheffield, UK.

Sheffield has a population of more than 550,000, and about one-fifth of the population lives in the most deprived quintile of neighbourhoods. It faces problems such as low life expectancy, high smoking rates, child obesity and lower breastfeeding levels.

Community health champions (CHCs) are volunteers engaged with a variety of services to improve their own health and the health of others in their community through a diverse range of activities. The champions, many of whom are recruited from disadvantaged communities or with personal experience of ill health, draw on their own local knowledge and life experience to motivate people to take part in healthy social activities, establish groups to meet local needs or signpost people to relevant services. The community health champions are an example of

Building Community Health Champions, NHS Sheffield (Continued)

a sustainable programme that is having an impact in some of the city's most disadvantaged communities. Since 2008, 600 voluntary champions have been recruited who are working in 22 voluntary and community organisations and reaching more than 10,000 people. The champions are achieving positive results for their own health and wellbeing and for others in their neighbourhoods and networks. The model has seen great success in Sheffield with evaluation reports showing improved outcomes overall such as:

- increased confidence
- improved self-esteem and self-belief
- improvements in health and lifestyle such as people eating healthily, losing weight and becoming more active
- better awareness and knowledge of health issues
- improved mental health and wellbeing.

Evaluation of the CHC programme has shown that many individuals move along pathways to education, paid employment and enterprise. A Social Return on Investment assessment has indicated savings of £2.07 for every £1 spent on the programme (without measuring the impact on the people who the champions support). The evidence from the Sheffield champions programme is summarised in the NICE Shared Learning database, and there are YouTube videos which show how the programme has made a difference in Sheffield.

MUST DO'S AND TOP TIPS FROM SHEFFIELD

- Work in partnership with organisations rooted in the communities
- Recruit from the communities where you hope to see an impact

- Provide first-class training at the outset and supplement this to meet identified needs throughout the time that CHCs spend with the programme
- Integrate with other staff and volunteers to provide joined-up services
- Monitor and evaluate throughout using recognised and credible agencies such as universities
- Value the volunteers and recognise their potential to be agents of change within their communities.

HOW DID SHEFFIELD DO THIS?

The Sheffield Community Health Champions Programme started in 2008 with funding from the Big Lottery (Altogether Better). It aimed to promote physical activity, healthy eating and general health and wellbeing, especially in communities with the greatest health inequalities. At the end of the lottery grant period, Sheffield City Council (SCC) and NHS Sheffield took over the funding of this programme. Since April 2014, funding has come through the SCC as part of the public health grant. With the help of the initial funding, a voluntary sector consortium was commissioned to run the programme. They contracted with voluntary, community and faith sector organisations who recruited and hosted the volunteers to become CHCs. Training, supervision and support was provided, and each champion undertook to provide 70 to 100 hours of their time over 6 months. The skills and experience that the champions acquired have given many of them the confidence and ability to move into paid employment. This has been particularly notable in the recruitment of health trainers in Sheffield.

Source Health Trainers England 2016b

General Practitioners

General practitioners (GPs) provide a comprehensive range of diagnosis and treatment medical services for patients registered with their practice and for those outside the practice in an emergency. They refer patients to other healthcare workers as necessary, for example, to counsellors, practice nurses, health visitors, physiotherapists or consultants specialising in a particular disease area. GPs and their practice teams have a crucial role to play in promoting health and preventing disease. Every consultation is an opportunity to detect early warning signs that could prevent illness and disease. The Royal College of General Practitioners (RCGP) agrees that GPs should be proactive in carrying out public health activities and interventions. However, a study undertaken by the Kings Fund (2016) found that GPs in England were focusing mainly on secondary prevention despite the enormous potential for general practice to take a more proactive role in ill-health prevention. Public health guidance from NICE advises primary care professionals such as GPs to opportunistically and proactively carry out activities such as brief interventions (see Chapter 14 for a GP Case Study of a brief intervention). But, for example, in the case of smoking, GPs frequently respond to requests for help giving up smoking rather than proactively engaging existing smokers. The Kings Fund study found that, while the RCGP expects GPs to possess a wide range of skills related to health promotion, many GPs say that they lack these skills. It was also found that the method GPs use to address public health and ill-health prevention is to provide information and advice, whereas other interventions can be more effective (Boyce et al 2010). See also Scriven and Wylie (2010) for an examination of the health promotion competencies recommended for the medical curriculum.

Nurses and Midwives

Specialist public health nurses have specific health-promoting roles, and every nurse and midwife can make every contact count and become a health-promoting practitioner. Maximising the impact of nursing and midwifery on improving and protecting the public's health is one of the six key action areas of the national nursing midwifery and care strategy Compassion in Practice, launched in December 2012 (DoH 2012) with an update Compassion in Practice 2 years on (NHS England 2014c). Fig. 3.3 demonstrates the range of roles of nurses in promoting health and wellbeing.

Kemppainen et al (2012) in their research on hospital nurses' contribution to health promotion concludes that nursing is an appropriate profession in which to promote health, but that nurses have not yet demonstrated a clear and obvious role in implementing health promotion activities beyond giving information to patients.

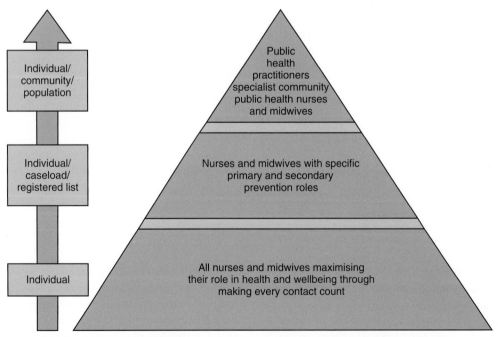

FIG. 3.3 ■ Nurses' involvement in health promotion. *(Source: Public Health England 2013)*

Other Health Professions

There are many other health professionals with health-promoting health functions such as dentists (see, for example, Watts et al (2014) for an interesting discussion of the role of the dental team in promoting health equity) and hospital and retail pharmacists. Each year, pharmacies are required participate in up to six campaigns at the request of NHS England. This involves the display and distribution of leaflets and undertaking prescription-linked interventions on major areas of public health concern such as encouraging smoking cessation (PSNC 2016), and the full range of professions allied to medicine (Needle et al 2011) have a significant part to play in health promotion.

HEALTH PROMOTION AGENTS AND AGENCIES OUTSIDE THE NHS

Local Authorities

The Health and Social Care Act (2012) gives responsibility for health improvement to upper tier and unitary local authorities. Local leadership and responsibility for public health in England therefore lies with local authorities. They have a ring-fenced government grant and a specialist public health team led by a director of public health. Upper tier authorities are supported by the existing expertise within district councils such as environmental health. Local authorities have considerable freedom in terms of how they choose to improve their population's health, although they have to have regard to the Public Health Outcomes Framework and the extant evidence regarding public health measures.

A small number of steps and public health services are mandatory. Steps to be taken to protect the health of the local population:

- Ensuring NHS commissioners receive the public health advice they need
- Appropriate access to sexual health services
- The National Child Measurement Programme
- NHS Health Check assessment.

Many local authority staff outside of the public health team have health-promotion functions such as recreation and leisure officers, housing officers, regeneration, youth and community workers, trading standards and community safety officers.

Environmental Health Officers/Practitioners

Environmental health officers/practitioners are at the forefront of public health as every aspect of environmental health is designed to improve the public's health, wellbeing and safety. Their work can make a real difference to people's health and wellbeing. The areas that environmental health professionals work to meet statutory regulations include:

- noise and environmental pollution
- food safety and hygiene
- workplace (occupational) health
- housing standards.

For further details, see Chartered Institute of Environmental Health (2016).

Personal, Social and Health and Economic (PSHE) Teachers and Schools

Schools are an important setting to develop the knowledge, skills and attributes young people need to keep themselves healthy and to thrive as individuals, family members and members of society. Personal, social, health and economic education is the curriculum area which develops these skills (Department for Education 2013). The PSHA is a national body with grant funding from the government and is at the forefront of the development of PSHE (PSHA 2014; 2016) and provides a wide range of research and resources for teachers and schools. The Health Promoting Schools initiative (WHO 2016) also strives to improve the health of school personnel, families and community members as well as pupils.

Social Services

The social services cover both social work and social care, providing an important range of health-promoting interventions to people who may fall outside the remit of health services. The client categories are the most vulnerable in society including the mentally ill; the elderly; children who are abused, neglected or without support; the physically sick and disabled; and people with learning disabilities. The services are provided within diverse settings, including people's homes, with social workers problem solving (as advisor, broker or advocate), offering psychosocial therapy, enabling behaviour change and engaging in crisis intervention (Spicker 2014; 2016).

Complementary and Alternative Medicine Practitioners

Whilst there is no universally agreed definition of complementary and alternative medicine (CAM), NHS Choices (2017) suggests that, when a non-mainstream practice is used together with conventional medicine, it's considered complementary, and when a non-mainstream practice is used instead of conventional medicine, it is considered complementary. Those practising CAM include homoeopaths, chiropractors, osteopaths, acupuncturists, reflexologists and practitioners of herbal medicine, yoga, massage and shiatsu, among others. These practitioners can play a part in promoting health, often using a more holistic approach. Therapies may be available from the NHS, either by a member of the primary care team or through referral to a complementary practitioner. There is potential for collaboration and closer integration between health promotion and complementary therapies with Hawk et al (2015) highlighting that behaviours related to diet, physical activity and stress reduction are important factors in determining the health of the public and are also areas of importance and emphasis for many CAM practitioners.

OTHER LOCAL ORGANISATIONS AND GROUPS

There are numerous individuals, groups and organisations at the local level that promote particular aspects of health. Some notable ones are described here.

Universities and Colleges

Universities and colleges are not only responsible for the training of health promotion and public health professionals, they are key organisations for undertaking public health research. Moreover, The Healthy Universities Network under its international charter establish that health-promoting universities and colleges are well placed to transform the health, wellbeing and sustainability of our current and future societies (International Conference on Health Promoting Universities and Colleges 2015).

Community Groups

A huge range of community groups exists that undertake health-promotion activities on public health matters. In the UK, the government has clear aspirations for the voluntary and community sector as partners in public health, particularly in tackling health inequalities. The sector already operates extensively within health and social care with the statutory sector spending significant sums of money per year on services provided by voluntary and community organisations (Curry et al 2011).

Employers

Employers can be active in developing and implementing health-promoting policies in the workplace. Human resource officers and occupational health staff, in particular, are vital to implementing public health interventions (Young & Bhaurnik 2011).

Police, Probation and Prison Officers

The police protect the public from crime and violence, take action to prevent misuse of drugs and alcohol and help to ensure road safety. Prison officers and probation officers are involved in the health and wellbeing of prisoners and their families, and may be involved in initiatives such as health-promoting prisons (Woodall et al 2014).

Fire and Rescue Authorities

The varied role of the Fire and Rescue Authorities (FRAs) in improving public health is outlined through a series of case studies in the publication Beyond Fighting Fires (Local Government Association 2015). It is clear from these case studies that FRAs have a key role to play in ensuring that their communities are safe through responding to emergencies and also through their extensive preventative work as diverse as falls prevention in the home to obesity.

It is clear from the wide range of health promotion and public health agencies and agents outlined in this chapter, that some strategies, such as partnership working, will improve capacity. The continued building of multiprofessional understanding, partnerships and capabilities and pulling together of the different professional groups under the banner of health promotion is vital to future success. To do this effectively, it is important to know who are the health promotion and public health professionals working within your area. Exercise 3.2 requires you to make a public health professional map of your locality.

EXERCISE 3.2

Finding Out About Your Local NHS, Local Authority and the Wider Range of Public Health Agents and Agencies

Exercise 3.2 is designed to help you to find out how your local public health system is organised and to identify the health promotion agents and agencies which are important for your work. There is much to gain by having good local knowledge of health promoters you can refer clients to or work with in partnerships.

1. Find out about the structure of the public health teams in the area where you work:
   - What is the name and function of the local statutory organisation with responsibility for public health?
   - What regional and/or national organisations are responsible for public health where you work?
2. Find out about the agencies and agents on your patch:
   - Think of the geographical patch where you work, and identify its boundaries as clearly as you can. It might be the area served by a GP practice, the catchment area of a hospital or the population of a Local Authority or Health Trust.
   - Identify as many health promotion agents and agencies on your patch as you can using Fig. 3.2 and the information about agents and agencies in health promotion in this chapter as checklists.

It is likely that you will know some very well and others not at all. Identify those you would find it helpful to know more about and plan to find out about them. If there are some you know nothing about, such as the voluntary and community groups on your patch, identify people who are likely to know about them (such as health promotion or public health practitioners/specialists) and contact them to find out more.

PRACTICE POINTS

- It is important to understand the work of a whole range of agents and agencies with a health promotion and public health function, informal and formal, local, national and international.
- Think about how you can best work collaboratively with other people and agencies.
- Ensure that you are clear about your role and responsibilities in health promotion within the wider public health workforce.
- Consider how you could improve your health promotion and public health practice roles through education and training or through identifying what helps and hinders your health promotion and public health work and how your work could be improved.

REFERENCES

Banerjee A, Kin R, Strachan PH et al 2015 Factors facilitating the implementation of church-based heart health promotion programs for older adults: A qualitative study guided by the precede-proceed model. American Journal of Health Promotion 29(6):365–373.

Boyce T, Peckham S, Hann A, Trenholm S 2010 A pro-active approach. Health promotion and ill-health prevention: An inquiry into the quality of general practice in England. London, Kings Fund.

Bull D, Bagwell S, Nicholls A, Shiel F 2014 Supporting good health: The role of the charity sector. London, NPC.

Catalán-Matamoros D 2011 The role of mass media communication in public health. In: Smigorski K (ed) Health management—Different approaches and solutions in tech. http://cdn.intechopen.com/pdfs/24998/InTechThe_role_of_mass_media_communication_in_public_health.pdf.

Centre for Workforce Development 2014 Mapping the core public health workforce. http://www.cfwi.org.uk/publications/mapping-the-core-public-health-workforce.

Centre for Workforce Intelligence 2016 Understanding the public health practitioner workforce: A CFWI study. London, CfWI.

Chartered Institute of Environmental Health 2016 Public health and the environmental health professional. https://www.healthcareers.nhs.uk/explore-roles/public-health/environmental-health-professional and the http://www.cieh.org/.

Curry N, Mundle C, Sheil F, Weaks L 2011 The voluntary and community sector in health: Implications of the proposed NHS reforms. London, Kings Fund NCVO.

Department for Education 2013 Guidance for personal, social, health and economic education. https://www.gov.uk/government/publications/personal-social-health-and-economic-education-pshe/personal-social-health-and-economic-pshe-education.

Department of Health 2011 The Public Health Responsibility Deal. London, The Stationery Office.

Department of Health 2012 Compassion in Practice: Nursing, Midwifery and care staff, our vision and strategy. London, Stationary Office.

Department of Health 2013a 2010 to 2015 government policy: Drug misuse and dependency. London, The Stationery Office.

Department of Health 2015 2010 to 2015 government policy: obesity and healthy eating. https://www.gov.uk/government/publications/2010-to-2015-government-policy-obesity-and-healthy-eating/2010-to-2015-government-policy-obesity-and-healthy.

Department of Health 2016 Childhood Obesity A Plan for Action. https://www.gov.uk/government/uploads/system/uploads/attachment_data/file/546588/Childhood_obesity_2016__2__acc.pdf

Dosemagen S, Aase L 2016 How social media is shaking up public health and healthcare. The Blog, The Huffington Post. http://www.huffingtonpost.com/shannon-dosemagen-/how-social-media-is-shaki_b_9090102.html.

European Centre for Disease Prevention and Control 2016 What we do. http://ecdc.europa.eu/en/aboutus/what-we-do/Pages/Mission.aspx.

European Public Health Association 2016 About us. http://epha.org/about-us/.

EU Commission 2013 Investing in health. http://ec.europa.eu/health/strategy/docs/swd_investing_in_health.pdf.

EU Commission 2016 Europe 2020—For a healthier EU. http://ec.europa.eu/health/europe_2020_en.htm.

Faculty of Public Health 2016 The unique contribution of public health specialists. http://www.fph.org.uk/uploads/The%20unique%20contribution%20of%20Public%20Health%20Specialists%20FINALSept16%20RA.pdf.

Greer SL, Kurser P 2013 European Union Public Health Policy: Regional and global trends. Oxon, Routledge.

Hawk C, Adams J, Hartvigsen J 2015 The role of CAM in public health, disease prevention, and health promotion evidence-based complementary and alternative medicine. Volume 2015, Article ID 528487. http://dx.doi.org/10.1155/2015/528487.

Health Careers 2016a UK Health Systems. https://www.healthcareers.nhs.uk/about/working-health/uk-health-systems.

Health Careers 2016b Health Trainers. https://www.healthcareers.nhs.uk/explore-roles/public-health/health-trainer.

Health and Social Care Act 2012, c.7. http://www.legislation.gov.uk/ukpga/2012/7/contents/enacted.

Health Trainers England 2016a Case Studies. http://healthtrainersengland.com/evidence/case-studies/.

Health Trainers England 2016b Sheffield Community Health Champions. http://healthtrainersengland.com/wp-content/uploads/2014/06/Sheffield-Community-Health-Champions.pdf.

IHPE 2016 Home Page. http://ihpe.org.uk/.

International Conference on Health Promoting Universities and Colleges 2015 Okanagan Charter: An international charter for health promoting universities & colleges. https://open.library.ubc.ca/cIRcle/collections/53926/items/1.0132754.

International Union of Heath Promotion and Education 2016 Objectives. http://www.iuhpe.org/index.php/en/iuhpe-at-a-glance/objectives.

Kemppainen V, Tossavainen K, Turunen H 2012 Nurses' roles in health promotion practice: An integrative review. Health Promotion International. http://dx.doi.org/10.1093/heapro/das034.

Kings Fund 2016 How is the new NHS structured? http://www.kingsfund.org.uk/audio-video/how-new-nhs-structured.

Local Government Association (LGA) 2015 Beyond fighting fires: The role of the fire and rescue service in improving the public's health. London, LGA.

Monitor 2014 Walk in centre review: Final report and recommendations. http://www.monitor.gov.uk.

Needle J, Petchey R, Benson J, Scriven A, Lawrenson J, Hilari K 2011 The allied health professions and health promotion: A systematic literature review and narrative synthesis. London, HMSO.

NHS Choices 2016. http://www.nhs.uk/NHSEngland/thenhs/about/Pages/authoritiesandtrusts.aspx.

NHS Choices 2017 Complementary and alternative medicine: defining CAMS http://www.nhs.uk/Livewell/complementary-alternative-medicine/Pages/complementary-alternative-medicines.aspx

NHS England 2014a Understanding the New NHS. London, BMJ. https://www.england.nhs.uk/wp-content/uploads/2014/06/simple-nhs-guide.pdf.

NHS England 2014b Five-year forward view. https://www.england.nhs.uk/wp-content/uploads/2014/10/5yfv-web.pdf.

NHS England 2014c Compassion in Practice—2 years on. https://www.england.nhs.uk/wp-content/uploads/2014/12/nhs-cip-2yo.pdf.

NICE 2016 NICE Pathways—Mapping our guidance. https://pathways.nice.org.uk/.

Panjwani C, Caraher M 2014 The public health responsibility deal: Brokering a deal for public health, but on whose terms? Health Policy 114(2):163–173.

Personal, Social and Health Education Association 2014 PSHE Association Annual Survey Responses Summary 2014. London, PSHA. https://www.pshe-association.org.uk/sites/default/files/u6/impactnonstatutory_0.pdf.

Personal, Social and Health Education Association 2016 Curriculum for life: The case for statutory PSHE education. London, PSHA.

Pharmaceutical Services Negotiating Committee 2016 Public Health (Promotion of Healthy Lifestyles). http://psnc.org.uk/services-commissioning/essential-services/public-health/.

Price S, Lester C 2012 Health trainers: A rapid review of evidence. Cardiff, NHS Wales and Public Health Wales.

Prospects 2016 https://www.prospects.ac.uk/job-profiles/health-promotion-specialist.

Public Health England 2013 Nursing and midwifery contribution to public health improving health and wellbeing. London, PHE.

Public Health England 2014 Public health in the 21st century: organising and managing multidisciplinary teams in a local government context. London, Stationary Office.

Royal Society for Public Health 2016 Dream It, Try It, Live It. http://www.youthhealthmovement.org.uk/dream-try-live.html.

Scriven, A & Wylie A 2010 Health Promotion in the Medical Profession: what are the essential competencies and who decides in Wylie A Holt T 2010 Health Promotion in Medical Education: From Rhetoric to Action. Milton Keynes, Radcliffe.

Shircore R 2013 Health trainers half-year review 1st April–30th September 2013. London, Royal Society of Public Health.

Spicker P 2014 Social Policy: Theory and Practice, 3rd edn. Bristol, Policy Press.

Spicker P 2016 The personal social services: Social work and social care. http://www.spicker.uk/social-policy/pss.htm.

Trade Union Council 2015 Work and well-being: A trade union resource. London, TUC.

Watts RG, Williams DM, Sheiham A 2014 The role of the dental team in promoting health equity. British Dental Journal 216, 11–14.

Woodall J, Dixey R, South J 2014 Control and choice in English prisons: Developing health-promoting prisons. Health Promotion International 29(3):474–482.

World Federation of Public Health Associations 2016 About WPHA. http://www.wfpha.org/about-wfpha.

World Health Organization 2016 What is a Health Promoting School? http://www.who.int/school_youth_health/gshi/hps/en/.

Young V, Bhaurnik C 2011 Health and well-being at work: A survey of employers. London, Department of Work and Pensions.

WEBSITES

British Medical Association http://www.bma.org.uk.
CIEH http://www.cieh.org.
Friends of the Earth http://www.foe.co.uk.
http://www.fphm.org.uk.
http://www.hse.gov.uk.
International Union of Health. Promotion and health education, for full details of the organisation's work. http://www.iuhpe.org.
MIND http://www.mind.org.uk.
NHS Choices England http://www.nhs.uk/pages/home.aspx.
NHS Direct Wales http://www.nhsdirect.wales.nhs.uk/.
NHS England https://www.england.nhs.uk/.
NHS Scotland http://www.scot.nhs.uk/.
NHS Wales http://www.wales.nhs.uk/.
NICE purpose and structure https://www.nice.org.uk/about.
Northern Ireland Health and Social Care http://online.hscni.net/.
Northern Ireland HSC Public Health Agency http://www.publichealth.hscni.net/.
Public Health England https://www.gov.uk/government/organisations/public-health-england.

Public Health Wales http://www.publichealthwales.wales.nhs.uk/.
Royal College of Nursing http://www.rcn.org.uk.
TACADE http://www.tacade.com.
UK Public Health Association http://www.ukpha.org.uk/.
Youth Health Movement website, with access to their Blog, Facebook, and Twitter pages. http://www.youthhealthmovement.org.uk/dream-try-live.html.

BLOGS

Gateway Family Services, for further information on health trainers http://gatewayfs.org/blog/.
Public Health Register blog http://www.ukphr.org/blog/.
IUHPE Blog http://ihpe.org.uk/blog/.

FACEBOOK

Example of Facebook page for Health Trainers (showing some of the work of Health Trainers in Southampton, UK) https://www.facebook.com/SouthamptonHealthTrainers/?fref=ts.

VALUES AND ETHICAL CONSIDERATIONS IN HEALTH PROMOTION AND PUBLIC HEALTH

SUMMARY

In this chapter, some key philosophical issues about aims and values in health promotion and public health practice will be identified and explored. Two fundamental dilemmas about the aims of health promotion will be addressed. First, whether health promoters and public health practitioners should aim to change the individual's lifestyle choices or to change society, and second, whether they should set out to ensure compliance with health promotion and public health programmes or enable clients to make an informed choice. A framework of five approaches to health promotion is provided as a tool for analysing key aims and values along with exercises and case studies. Ethical issues are discussed, four ethical principles are described and there is a series of questions designed to help health promoters and public health practitioners to make ethical choices. Exercises on making ethical decisions are included.

This chapter establishes some of the philosophical issues linked to the promotion of individual and population health. You are encouraged to think deeply about why you are engaging in specific activities, what

values are reflected in your work and what ethical dilemmas are presented. Guidelines on how to approach ethical decision making are considered, and some key principles of practice are explored.

Health promotion and public health interventions, if successful, will influence the lives of individuals and communities, and it would be irresponsible to develop and engage in health promotion and public health without understanding the values and ethics that should underpin interventions.

EXPLORING THE AIMS OF HEALTH PROMOTION AND PUBLIC HEALTH PRACTICE

Should health promoters and public health practitioners aim to change individual behaviour and lifestyles or instead aim to influence the socioeconomic determinants that directly influence people's lifestyles, behaviour and health, or both? Public health action often focuses on changing the attitudes and behaviour of individuals and communities towards healthier lifestyles, whilst neglecting the influence of the socioeconomic, political and physical environments on people's lives, what Marmot (2016) calls the causes of the causes. This focus on lifestyle influences on health and the need to change behaviour can result in victim-blaming, which is a significant ethical dilemma that health promoters and public health practitioners need to address (see, for example, Holland 2014).

It is important to note that individuals often can change behaviour and may want to take responsibility to improve their health. Health promotion is an essential tool in enabling that process, by promoting people's self-esteem, confidence and empowering them to take more control over their own health. Proponents of the lifestyle behavioural change approach also maintain that medical and health experts have knowledge that enables them to know what is in the best interests of their patients and the public at large, and that it is their responsibility to persuade people to make healthier choices. Furthermore, society has vested that responsibility in health professionals, and the general public often seeks advice and help in health matters; it is not necessarily a matter of persuading them against their will. Sometimes, too, individuals may not be in a position to take responsibility because they may, for example, be too young, too ill or have severe learning difficulties. See McDaid et al (2014) for a fuller debate on the advantages and disadvantages of a behavioural change approach.

There are several points to be taken into account if the aim to change lifestyle is pursued:

- You cannot assume that lay people believe that health professionals know best. Sometimes health experts are proven wrong, and new evidence can contradict existing health messages. For example, over the years there has been much contradictory advice on what constitutes good nutrition with some people finding the barrage of information confusing, resulting in a backlash that results in people ignoring advice (Nagler 2014).
- There is a danger of imposing alien or opposing values. For example, a doctor may perceive that the most important thing for a patient's physical health is to lose weight and cut down on alcohol consumption, but drinking beer in the pub with friends may be far more important in terms of overall wellbeing to the overweight, middle-aged, unemployed patient. Who is right?

- Linked to this, a health promoter advocating lifestyle changes can be seen as making a moral judgment on clients' failure to change, that it is their own fault if, for example, they develop an obesity-related or smoking-related illness.
- Promoting a lifestyle change approach may produce negative and counterproductive feelings in the targeted individual or community such as guilt for failing to comply or of rebelliousness and anger at being told what to do resulting in resistance to comply (Kumar 2011).
- It cannot be assumed that individual behaviour is the primary cause of ill health. This is a limited view, and there is a danger that focusing on the individual's behaviour distracts attention from the significant and politically sensitive determinants of health such as the social and economic factors of racism, relative deprivation, poverty, housing and unemployment as outlined in Chapter 1 in the section What Affects Health?
- Finally, it also cannot be assumed that individuals have genuine freedom to choose healthy lifestyles. Freedom of choice is often limited by socioeconomic influences (Marmot 2016). Economic factors may affect the choice of food; for example, fresh fruit and wholemeal bread are relatively more expensive than biscuits and white bread (see Lambie-Mumford et al 2014 and the Food Ethics Council website referenced at the end of the chapter).

Social factors are also important. Freedom of choice about smoking for adolescents where both parents smoke, for example, is a complex issue (Mays et al 2014). Also, how much freedom do people really have to change other health-demoting factors such as stressful living or working conditions and unemployment? It is easy to blame an individual for their own ill health or poor lifestyle choices – becoming victim-blaming – when in reality they might be the victims of their socioeconomic circumstances. In some disadvantaged situations and where resources of time, energy and income are limited, health choices may become health compromises. What a health promoter or public health practitioner may see as irresponsibility may actually be what the client sees as the most responsible action in the circumstances. For example, mothers confronted with the day-to-day pressures of parenting may smoke as a way of relieving their stress. Research by Sperlich and Maina (2014) indicates that the single mothers in their study were utilising smoking as a way of coming to terms with negative and self-blaming ruminative thoughts.

Part 3 of this book is about how to promote health in a way that is sensitive to these issues. Chapter 16 looks at what you can do to challenge and change health-related policies.

It is crucially important that everyone engaged in health promotion and public health practice should be aware of these ethical concerns and have an opportunity to consider them in relation to their own work, particularly if they are engaged in interventions that aim to change individual lifestyles. Exercise 4.1 is designed to help you to think through your views on the aims of health promotion and public health practice.

EXERCISE 4.1

Analysing Your Philosophical Position on Health Promotion and Public Health Practice

Consider the following statements A and B:

A: The key aim of health promotion and public health practice is behaviour change: To inform people about the ways in which their behaviour and lifestyle can affect their health, to ensure that they understand the information, to help them explore their values and attitudes and (where appropriate) to help them to change their behaviour.

B: The key aim of health promotion and public health practice is to influence the wider determinants of health: To raise awareness of the many socioeconomic policies at a national and local level (such as welfare, employment, housing, food, transport) that are not conducive to good health and to work actively towards a change in those policies.

1. Taking statement A:
   - List arguments in support of this view.
   - List any points about the limitations of this view and any arguments against it.
2. Do the same with statement B.
3. Do you think that the views in A and B are complementary or incompatible? Why?
4. Imagine these two views at either end of a spectrum:

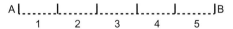

$$A |\ldots\ldots|\ldots\ldots|\ldots\ldots|\ldots\ldots|\ldots\ldots| B$$
$$\quad 1 \quad\quad 2 \quad\quad 3 \quad\quad 4 \quad\quad 5$$

Indicate the two positions on the scale of 1 to 5 which most closely reflect (a) what you actually do in practice and (b) what you would like to do if you were free to prioritise work exactly as you would choose.

Aiming for Compliance or Informed Choice?

Another key question about the aims of health promotion centres on what you aim to do with or for the client (whether the client is a single individual, a community or an organisation). Is your aim to ensure that your client complies with your programme and changes behaviour, as is the case with a social marketing approach? Or is it to enable your client to make an informed choice and have the skills and confidence to carry that choice through into action, whatever that choice may be?

For example, a health promoter is working with a client whose sexual behaviour is such that there is a serious risk of catching sexually transmitted infections including HIV. If the aim is compliance, it is more likely that the health promoter will be persuasive, will stress the risks to the client and will consider the session a failure if the client does not choose to behave differently. If, on the other hand, the health promoter's aim is to enable the client to make an informed choice, the health promoter will ensure that the client understands the facts and the risks, will encourage and support the client and accept that if the client chooses not to change their behaviour then this choice will be respected. It would not be interpreted as a failure because the client made an informed choice.

The same issues arise with health promotion and public health interventions on a larger scale. For example, is the aim of a campaign to change diets and to promote the consumption of five pieces of fruit or vegetables a day (NHS Choices 2016), to persuade people to a particular point of view or to give them the information on which to make up their own minds? This is a difficult question. Most health promoters are doing their jobs because they believe that the action they are advocating is in the best interests of individuals and of society as a whole, and their actions are backed by evidence. It raises the question about how far to go in imposing your own values and ideas of what are appropriate lifestyle choices on other people. In the case of the five-a-day campaign, there is also the ethical issue of food poverty (see the Food Ethics Council website in the references at the end of the chapter).

ANALYSING AIMS AND VALUES: FIVE APPROACHES

There is no consensus on what is the right aim for health promotion and public health practice or the right approach or set of activities. Health promoters need to work out for themselves which aim and which activities they use, in accordance with professional codes of conduct (if they exist), professional values and an assessment of the clients' needs.

Different approaches to promoting health are useful tools of analysis, which can help you to clarify your own aims and values. A framework of five approaches is suggested with the values implicit in any particular approach identified.

1. The Medical Approach

The aim is freedom from medically defined disease and disability such as infectious diseases, cancers and heart disease. The approach involves medical intervention to prevent or ameliorate ill health, possibly using a persuasive or paternalistic method: persuading, for example, parents to bring their children for immunisation (PHE 2016a) and men over 50 to be screened for cholesterol and high blood pressure and to comply with prescribed medication (Maningat et al 2013). This approach values preventive medical measures and the medical profession's responsibility to ensure that patients comply with recommended procedures.

2. The Behaviour-Change Approach

The aim is to change people's individual attitudes and behaviours so that they adopt what is deemed a healthy lifestyle. Examples include supporting people in stopping smoking through smoking cessation programmes (NICE 2013), encouraging people to be more physically active through exercise prescription or referral schemes (Campbell et al 2015) and changing people's lifestyle and exercise levels through the Change4Life initiative (NHS 2016). See also NICE lifestyle and wellbeing website pages referenced at the end of the chapter for evidence on the behavioural change approach.

Health promoters and public health practitioners using this approach will be convinced that a lifestyle change is in the best interests of their clients and will see it as their responsibility to encourage as many people as possible to adopt the healthy lifestyle they advocate. Health-related social marketing fits into this approach when the aim is to change behaviour.

3. The Educational Approach

The aim is to give information, ensure knowledge and understanding of health issues and to enable the skills required to make well-informed decisions. Information about health is presented, and people are helped to explore their values and attitudes, develop appropriate skills and to make their own decisions. Help in carrying out those decisions and adopting new health practices may also be offered. School-sponsored personal, social, economic and health education (PSHE) programmes, whilst nonstatutory in the UK, emphasise helping pupils to learn the skills of healthy living, not merely to acquire knowledge (PSHE 2016).

Those favouring this approach will value the educational process, will respect individuals' right to choose, and will see it as their responsibility to raise with clients the health issues which they think will be in the clients' best interests.

4. The Client-Centred Approach

The aim is to work in partnership with clients to help them identify what they want to know about and take action on, and make their own decisions and choices according to their own interests and values. The health promoter's role is to act as a facilitator, helping people to identify their concerns and gain the knowledge and skills they require to make changes happen. Self-empowerment (or community empowerment; Tengland 2012) of the client is seen as central. Clients are valued as equals who have knowledge, skills and abilities to contribute and who have an absolute right to control their own health destinies.

5. The Societal-Change Approach

The aim is to effect changes on the physical, social and economic environment to make it more conducive to good health. The focus is on changing society, not on changing the behaviour of individuals.

Those using this approach will value their democratic right to change society and will be committed to putting health on the political agenda at all levels and to the importance of shaping the socioeconomic and health environment rather than shaping the individual lives of the people who live in it (see Frieden 2010 for an interesting framework for public health which puts action targeting socioeconomic factors as the most important).

Table 4.1 summarises and illustrates these five approaches to health promotion and public health practice. An important point to note is that some of these approaches can be used together. For example, a client-centred approach may also use educational processes and a comprehensive health promotion strategy to deal with a public health problem. (See Box 4.1 for examples of using approaches in practice.) Exercise 4.2 is designed to enable you to think through the aims and values of your health promotion practice.

TABLE 4.1				
Five Approaches to Health Promotion – Summary and Example				
	Aim	Health Promotion Activity	Important Values	Example – smoking
Medical	Freedom from medically defined disease and disability	Promotion of medical intervention to prevent or ameliorate ill health	Patient compliance with preventive medical procedures	Aim – freedom from lung disease, heart disease and other smoking-related disorders Activity – encourage people to seek early detection and treatment of smoking-related disorders
Behaviour change	Individual behaviour conducive to freedom from disease	Attitude and behaviour change to encourage adoption of 'healthier' lifestyle	Healthy lifestyle as defined by health promoter	Aim – behaviour changes from smoking to not smoking Activity – persuasive education to prevent nonsmokers from starting and to persuade smokers to stop
Educational	Individuals with knowledge and understanding enabling well-informed decisions to be made and acted upon	Information about cause and effects of health-demoting factors. Exploration of values and attitudes. Development of skills required for healthy living	Individual right of free choice. Health promoter's responsibility to identify educational content	Aim – clients will have understanding of the effects of smoking on health. They will make a decision whether or not to smoke and act on the decision Activity – giving information to clients about the effects of smoking. Helping them to explore their own values and attitudes and come to a decision. Helping them to learn how to stop smoking if they want to
Client-centred	Working with clients on their own terms	Working with health issues, choices and actions that clients identify. Empowering the client	Clients as equals. Clients' rights to set agenda. Self-empowerment of clients	Anti-smoking issue is considered only if clients identify it as a concern. Clients identify what, if anything, they want to know and do about it
Societal change	Physical and social environment that enables choice of healthier lifestyle	Political/social action to change physical/social/economic environment	Right and need to make environment health enhancing	Aim – make smoking socially unacceptable so it is easier not to smoke than to smoke Activity – no-smoking policy in all public places. Cigarette sales less accessible, especially to children, promotion of nonsmoking as social norm. Banning tobacco advertising and sports' sponsorship

BOX 4.1
APPROACHES A AND B

APPROACH A

Jill is a hospital nurse running a programme of rehabilitation for patients who have had heart attacks. She decides that she is working with an educational approach, aiming for her patients to make informed decisions and have knowledge about taking exercise and modifying their diet and other risk factors like smoking. She accepts that some patients will choose not to do so. She thinks that sometimes she may be working in a behaviour change model, because she sincerely believes that her patients would be better off if they changed their behaviour, and she finds that she sometimes really wants to persuade them. In the end, she decides that it is their choice and their life and that she will not pressure them into doing what they do not want to do. Jill is aware, though, that some of her colleagues (who favour the behaviour change approach) think she should be tougher and shock patients into complying by horror stories of what may happen to them if they do not adjust their lifestyles.

APPROACH B

Terry is a community health worker based in a deprived housing estate. Facilities for recreation, exercise, and buying good food, among other things, are poor. He decides that he is working with a mixture of client-centred and societal change approaches, because people in the community have identified that they want a better diet, and he is helping them to set up a food cooperative and to help each other to learn new cooking skills. He is also helping them to lobby their local councillor for better green spaces on the estate where the children can play.

EXERCISE 4.2
Identifying Your Health Promotion and Public Health Practice Aims and Values

Select two or three specific health promotion activities you are engaged in or have been engaged in such as a group health education programme, a social media campaign, a patient education scheme, an immunisation programme, a one-to-one meeting with a client, a community activity or working on a health policy. Select different kinds of activities if you can or use Case Studies 4.1 and 4.2.

CASE STUDY 4.1
Ethical issues relating to drug education in schools

A group of local people, led by a woman whose son died of a heroin overdose, has got together because they are concerned about drug misuse in the neighbourhood. They are afraid for the safety of their teenagers and younger children: drugs seem to be an established part of the teenage social scene, are easily available in the neighbourhood, and needles and syringes are found in local alleyways.

The group has decided that the best way to combat drugs is to go into local schools and scare the children off drugs with horror stories of bad 'trips' and addiction. They have recruited a former drug addict who is prepared to tell his story. They have asked the school nurse to help by providing supplies of leaflets and supporting them in their approach to the schools.

The school nurse believes that the shock-horror approach the group proposes has been shown by drug education research to be ineffective. At best it will do no good, and at worst it could glamorise the drug scene and a make a hero out of the ex-addict. She believes that the local schools' approach is best: education on the facts of drug taking and how to minimise harm from taking drugs, coupled with building up self-esteem, social skills and confidence for young people to deal with drug situations. The parents think this is inadequate and believe that their idea for a hard-hitting approach will work for their children:

- Identify the ethical issues in this situation.
- What do you think the school nurse should do and why?

CASE STUDY 4.2
Ethical Issues relating to funding public health research

An environmental health officer (EHO) wants to undertake some research into the impact of air pollution on asthma rates in a neighbourhood that straddles a main road. Town planning colleagues have told the EHO that they expect this road to become even busier soon because it will become the feeder road to a new bypass leading to a massive new out-of-town office development. The EHO has a well worked-out research proposal and the cooperation of local general practitioners (GPs) which will enable him to see if there is any correlation between traffic flow, air pollution levels and asthma rates. If he can show a correlation, it will help to put health issues on the agenda of the council's planning committee so that the health impact of planning decisions will be taken into account in future.

He needs to secure a research grant to pay for the additional pollution measurements and traffic flow counts and to collect and process the data from the GPs. If he does not start within the next month, he will miss the chance to collect vital baseline measurements before the expected increase in traffic when the bypass opens.

Despite applications to many sources, the only offer of research money he has received has come from a research trust which specialises in the impact of environmental pollution on respiratory disease. It is funded primarily by the tobacco industry. The trust assures the EHO that that they will not interfere with the research in any way and the grant will be given with 'no strings attached'. The EHO is unhappy about accepting money from the tobacco industry, but this is now his only chance to get the research under way.

■ Identify the ethical issues in this situation.
■ What do you think the EHO should do and why?

With reference to Table 4.1, identify which approach you are using for each activity (you may find that you will identify more than one approach).

For each activity, define the aim and the important values implicit in your work. You may find it helpful to look at Case Studies 4.1 and 4.2.

Discuss your findings with a partner or in a small group.

ETHICAL DILEMMAS

The following are some of the more common ethical dilemmas that health promoters and others working in public health may encounter.

Bottom Up or Top Down?

There is a key issue of control and power at the heart of health promotion and public health practice: Who decides what health issue to target and how? Who sets the agenda? Is it bottom up, set by people who themselves identify issues they perceive as relevant? Or is it top down, set by health promoters who often have the power (supported by government policy) and the resources to impose strategies? There is a spectrum of possible modes of interventions, from those that eliminate choice and remove freedom to those that just involve information giving (see Fig. 4.1). The interplay and interaction between individuals, communities and the wider population is important and central to deciding on whether a top-down or bottom-up approach is used. One of the difficulties in applying ethical principles when promoting health is the tension between the individual and population. Decisions have to be taken about when an individual's rights should be overridden in the interests of the greater good. Is it ever an ethical choice to initiate public health action that ultimately leads to an infringement of individual liberty to achieve overall health gain within the population?

There is also a danger that local populations can be manipulated into changing their agenda to match that of the health promoter or public health practitioner. Community development approaches should be about empowering the public to work on their own agendas of health issues, even if these are radically different from the priorities of those working for health in a professional capacity who may have to confront contradictions between citizen involvement and evidence-based

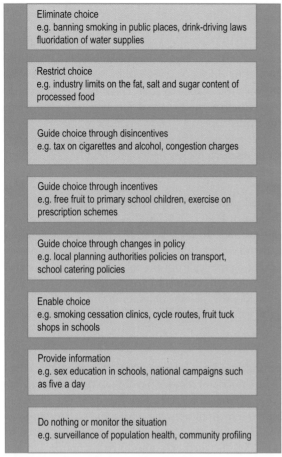

Eliminate choice
e.g. banning smoking in public places, drink-driving laws fluoridation of water supplies

Restrict choice
e.g. industry limits on the fat, salt and sugar content of processed food

Guide choice through disincentives
e.g. tax on cigarettes and alcohol, congestion charges

Guide choice through incentives
e.g. free fruit to primary school children, exercise on prescription schemes

Guide choice through changes in policy
e.g. local planning authorities policies on transport, school catering policies

Enable choice
e.g. smoking cessation clinics, cycle routes, fruit tuck shops in schools

Provide information
e.g. sex education in schools, national campaigns such as five a day

Do nothing or monitor the situation
e.g. surveillance of population health, community profiling

FIG. 4.1 ■ Public health intervention ladder, with examples. *(Source: Nuffield Council on Bioethics-Full report Public health: ethical issues (2007): http://nuffieldbioethics.org/wp-content/uploads/2014/07/Public-health-ethical-issues.pdf)*

practice (South 2014). Health promoters and public health practitioners raise awareness of health issues; they provide information about them and, in doing so, create demand for change. So where does this process differ from manipulating the community into wanting what the health promoters wanted in the first place? (See Chapter 15.)

Just Widening the Inequalities?

As discussed in Chapter 1, there are wide differences in the health status of different groups of people; generally those in poorer social and economic circumstances are the least healthy with a widening

gap between the health status of rich and poor (Marmot 2016).

There is a danger that health promotion and public health activities only reach the people who have the resources and education to make use of health information and take health action. Those who are trapped in poor financial circumstances are often less likely to be in a position to change their lifestyle, to have the health literacy to fully understand the health messages, to effectively access health services or to have the other competencies necessary to lobby for social or political changes. There is clearly a need to be sensitive to this.

Some ways of working with those most in need, and often hardest to reach, are discussed in Chapter 15.

Efforts to change people's physical environments to improve health may have negative outcomes. Health impact assessment of a housing and community regeneration programme highlighted both positive and negative potential health and wellbeing outcomes (Byrne et al 2014).

The Health Promoter and Public Health Practitioner: A Shining Example?

Consider the cases of an overweight dietitian, a public health practitioner who consumes alcohol over the safe limits and a health visitor who smokes. All three are in a position where they need to address these issues as part of their work and may be asked for advice which they clearly do not follow themselves.

Few health promoters would claim that they are perfect examples of healthy living, but we suggest that they have a responsibility to consider their own health and think of ways in which it could be improved and in which they could contribute to a healthier environment. Health promoters are teaching by example, and the examples previously discussed convey silent messages that it is okay to be overweight, to smoke or to risk health by overconsuming alcohol. It is probably best to be open and honest in situations where health promoters' own lifestyles are at odds with the health-promoting ways they are advocating. Personal experience can also be turned to good advantage. For example, if the dietitian has a constant struggle to control her own weight, she can use that experience to develop a greater understanding of her clients' difficulties.

Facts, Fads or Fashions?

A concern for the public is that health advice changes. A difficulty is that research continuously turns up new evidence. At what point do you decide that the evidence is sufficiently convincing to begin publicising a new message or to campaign to change an aspect of health policy or legislation? If you have insufficient knowledge or experience to judge questions that may be medically or technically complex, on what basis do you make your decision? Is it more ethical to discuss the conflicting views openly and just air the debate more widely?

See Chapter 11 for an overview of the mass media and the social media influence on public health.

Health At Any Cost?

What being healthy means to different people is discussed in Chapter 1.

In their enthusiasm for improving health, there is a danger that health promoters and public health practitioners might lose sight that health means different things to different people and is shaped by their various values and experiences. Health may become a stereotyped image of the health promoter's own idea of perfection, leading to a prescription of what people should and should not do. This is clearly contrary to the concept that health promotion is about enabling people to increase control over their health and improve it in ways they see as appropriate.

Health Information: An Insensitive Blunderbuss?

Health promoters should be sensitive to the social, ethnic, economic and cultural background of the individuals and communities with which they work. Health information and large-scale health promotion programmes which portray only white Caucasians, are available only in the English language, or assume a common set of values are unethical.

Empower the People?

Health promotion and public health requires special competencies, some of which are the subject of this book. It is all or part of the work of very many professions including health, education and community work.

Health promoters from this wide range of disciplinary backgrounds, if they are to empower people to take more control over their own health, need to seek to share their knowledge and experience with lay people, to learn from them and to see them and other workers as valued partners in the promotion of health.

Health for Sale?

With a scarcity of resources available for health promotion and public health and in a climate of market economy and income generation, commercial companies now sponsor some health-promotion activities. One pitfall is the issue of perceived endorsement of products. For example, an NHS organisation could be seen as promoting the use of vitamins if it accepted sponsorship of appointment cards printed with the name of the sponsoring vitamin manufacturer.

There is also a move to involve commercial companies in promoting products in a way that also promotes health. For example, food manufacturers may be involved in special promotions for lower fat products. There are dangers here. The most obvious one being that the interests of the company may not be in harmony with those of the health promoter who will be perceived as endorsing the product. There is also a possibility that the independent credibility of the health promoter is compromised.

Another pitfall is that promoting individual and population health, which should be a fundamental part of health prevention and promotion services, is seen as a potential moneymaker. Basic services such as health information materials, health teaching and giving advice to commercial companies on health for employees become subject to charges.

Individual Freedom or Community Health?

Promoting health can be seen as paternalistic, interfering with personal liberty and freedom. Some might hold the view that doing nothing is the most morally acceptable option as it gives individuals the greatest freedom. However, this does not redress the distribution of power in society, which may limit the ability of individuals (particularly vulnerable groups) to act autonomously. Health-promotion principles address this by empowering individuals and communities to increase control over factors that affect their health and wellbeing. However, the interplay and interaction between individuals, communities, and the wider populations is important. One of the difficulties in applying ethical principles in health promotion is the tension between the individual and population. In what instances should an individual's rights be overridden in the interests of the greater good? When should society step in and save us from ourselves? Our apparently insatiable appetites for smoking, drinking and eating are resulting in a growth in noncommunicable diseases which are putting a strain on health and social care budgets, and some lifestyle choices may present a health risk to others such as drinking and driving or smoking in a home where there are children. Where and how should we draw the line between individual freedom and public health? When do we reach the point where the consequences are such a drain on the national purse that we can no longer afford the luxury of letting people have the freedom to make health-damaging lifestyle choices? (The Moral Maze 2014; see also McCarteny and Capwell 2016 for a discussion of a range of ethical issues linked to dealing with obesity.)

BEHAVIOUR CHANGE AND NUDGING, AN ETHICAL APPROACH?

Promoting health often focuses on the behavioural change approach previously outlined and in Chapter 14. Is this ethical, and is nudging ethically more acceptable than other forms of behavioural change interventions? It has been argued that a nudging intervention must not restrict choice. It must be in the interests of the person being nudged; it should involve a change in the architecture or environment of the choice; and it should exploit a mechanism of less than fully deliberative choice. But is nudging manipulation, and is manipulation ethically acceptable? Should governments seek to change the culture of society? Is it legitimate for the government to nudge social norms which were already changing as in the case of binge drinking? See the Science and Technology Select Committee House

of Lords (2011) for a full discussion of the ethics of public health behaviour change approaches including nudging.

MAKING ETHICAL DECISIONS

Areas of ethical concern have been raised that do not present easy resolutions or answers. Beauchamp and Childress (2001) offer four ethical principles which can act as a guide to ethical practice:

Respect for autonomy. Respecting the decision-making capacities of autonomous persons and enabling individuals to make reasoned informed choices. Are there groups in society who might be seen as incapable of autonomy such as people with learning disabilities, young children or prisoners? And, if so, will this affect your health promotion or public health practice approach? If an individual makes a choice that you consider harmful, the dilemma may be how to respect that person's autonomy while doing good and avoiding harm. The key question is: By what right am I intervening, and how do I justify the action I am taking?

Beneficence. This considers the balancing of benefits of an intervention against the risks and costs; the health promoter should act in a way that benefits the client.

Nonmaleficence. Avoiding the causation of harm; the health promoter should not harm the client. The harm should not be disproportionate to the benefits of intervention. Victim-blaming would be considered harm as would stigma. It may not always be possible to simultaneously do good and avoid harm. For example, a mass media campaign showing the dangers of drink driving may have the effect of reducing the rates of drink driving but may also impact negatively on those who have been convicted of drink driving by labelling them and/or increasing their feelings of guilt. You will be able to think of other examples.

Justice. This involves distributing benefits, risks and costs fairly; the notion that clients in similar positions should be treated in a similar manner. Health promotion involves difficult decisions in the dividing of time and resources between individuals and communities, and between high-risk groups and whole populations. How do you balance general campaigns on healthy eating for the whole population with targeted interventions such as setting up a food cooperative in a deprived area?

The principles provide a framework for consistent moral decision making, but health promotion and public health interventions can encapsulate complex and sometimes conflicting choices. Because of this, ethics is a core public health competency, and its importance is being increasingly recognised. Questions regarding the justification of paternalistic interventions, fair distribution of health and responsibility for health are prominent (Blackster 2014; FPH 2016a). Some of the previous examples are taken from SFHP/SHEPS Cymru (2009). The sets of questions in Box 4.2 draw on the four ethical principles previously outlined and are designed for you to think about intervention ethics.

These questions are designed to help you to think through health promotion and public health actions in terms of the ethical implications of practice.

Exercise 4.3 and Exercise 4.4 (which uses Fig. 4.1) are designed to help you to think about intervention ethics. Please also refer to Fig. 4.2 which provides an overview of ethical ways of working that highlight goals and principles.

EXERCISE 4.3

Ethical Decisions in Health Promotion

Look again at Case Studies 4.1 and 4.2. You may find it helpful to use the questions in Box 4.2 on making ethical decisions to identify the issues relevant to each situation and to decide what you would do.

BOX 4.2
SOME ETHICAL QUESTIONS ON HEALTH PROMOTION AND PUBLIC HEALTH PRACTICE INTERVENTIONS

1. To what extent can the public good or the public interest justify state interventions that impose limits upon the freedom of individuals in terms of lifestyle choices?
2. What role should the law, both regulatory and fiscal measures, play in regulating health risks?
3. Should governments actively aim to change our preferences about such things as food, smoking or physical exercise?
4. To what extent do individuals have moral obligations to contribute to protecting the community or the public good?
5. When is it appropriate to concentrate resources on prevention rather than cure?
6. Given the fact that we cannot protect population groups from all harm, what sorts of harm provide a justification for public health action?
7. What limits do we wish to place upon public health activities?
8. How do we ensure that the interests of individuals are not set aside or forgotten in the pursuit of population health benefits?
9. What should be the balance between individual and government responsibility for heath?
10. Should medical treatment by refused to those who are obese?

EXERCISE 4.4

Ladder of Health Promotion Action

Work in small groups of three or four. Consider the health promotion intervention ladder in Fig. 4.1 and discuss the following:

■ The ethical issues that might be relevant to each rung of the ladder
■ Are there modes of intervention that you would reject on ethical grounds?

TOWARDS AN ETHICAL CODE OF PRACTICE

Many professions have codes of practice, which are broad principles and guidelines on how professionals should and should not act. They reflect the values accepted as underpinning ethical practice. Health promoters from different professional backgrounds should ensure they are familiar with the codes of practice of their own professional bodies and also be familiar with the ethical standards embedded in the Faculty of Public Health's Good Public Health Practice Framework (2016b) and Public Health England's Public Health Skills and Knowledge Framework (2016b). For further reading on ethics and the promotion of health see Carter et al (2012) and Holland (2014).

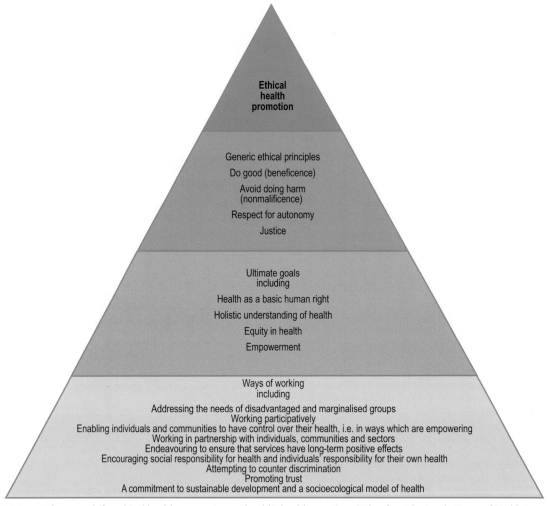

FIG. 4.2 ■ A framework for ethical health promotion and public health practice. *(Taken from Shaping the Future of Health Promotion (SFHP) and Society of Health Education and Promotion Specialists (SHEPS) Cymru 2009. Reproduced with permission.)*

PRACTICE POINTS

- In choosing approaches to health promotion and public health practice, take account of the different aims and values they reflect.
- Remember that ethical issues and dilemmas are inherent in promoting health and you need to think through the process of how you will make ethical decisions.
- Be familiar with the code of professional practice of any profession to which you belong.

- Good practice in health promotion and public health involves working to the specific values and principles of practice.

REFERENCES

Beauchamp TL, Childress JF 2001 Principles of biomedical ethics, 5th edn. Oxford, Oxford University Press.
Blacksher E 2014 Public health ethics. Ethics in medicine, University of Washington School of Medicine. https://depts.washington.edu/bioethx/topics/public.html.

Byrne E, Elliott E, Green L, Lester J 2014 Housing and Health Evidence Review for Health Impact Assessment (HIA). Cardiff, Wales Health Impact Assessment Support Unit (WHIASU).

Campbell F, Holmes M, Everson-Hock E, et al 2015 A systematic review and economic evaluation of exercise referral schemes in primary care: A short report. Health Technology Assessment 19(60).

Carter SM, Cribb A, Allegrante P 2012 How to think about health promotion ethics. Public Health Reviews 34(1):122–145.

Dawson A, Verwejj M (Eds) 2009 Ethics, prevention, and public health. Issues in biomedical ethics. Oxford, Oxford University Press.

Faculty of Public Health 2016a Public health ethics in practice. http://www.fph.org.uk/events/public_health_ethics_in_practice.

Faculty of Public Health 2016b Good public health practice framework. http://www.fph.org.uk/uploads/Good%20Public%20Health%20Practice%20Framework_%202016_Final.pdf.

Frieden TR 2010 A framework for public health action: The Health Impact Pyramid. American Journal of Public Health 100(4):590–595.

Holland S 2014 Public health ethics, 2nd edn. Cambridge, Polity Press.

Kumar J 2011 Responses to health promotion campaigns: Resistance, denial, and othering. Critical Public Health 21(1):105–117.

Lambie-Mumford H, Crossley D, Jensen E, Verbeke M, Dowler E 2014 Household Food Security in the UK: A review of food aid. Food Ethics Council and Warwick University.

Maningat P, Gordon BR, Breslow JL 2013 How Do We Improve Patient Compliance and Adherence to Long-Term Statin Therapy? Current Atherosclerosis Reports 15:291. http://dx.doi.org/10.1007/s11883-012-0291-7.

Marmot M 2016 Health inequalities and the causes of the causes. 57th Boyer Lecture Series Episode 1. http://www.abc.net.au/radionational/programs/boyerlectures/.

Mays D, Stephen E, Gilman SE et al 2014 Parental smoking exposure and adolescent smoking trajectories. Pediatrics 133(6):983–991.

McCartney M Capewell S 2016 Is obesity really the new smoking. Radio 4 in four. http://www.bbc.co.uk/programmes/p047t7v6.

McDaid D, Oliver A, Murkur S 2014 What do we know about the strengths and weakness of different policy mechanisms to influence health behaviour in the population? European Observatory on Health Systems and Policies. http://www.euro.who.int/__data/assets/pdf_file/0003/270138/PS15-web.pdf.

Nagler RH 2014 Adverse outcomes associated with media exposure to contradictory nutrition messages. Journal of Health Communication 19(1):24–40.

National Institute for Health and Clinical Excellence 2013 Public health guidance PH10: Stop smoking services. https://www.nice.org.uk/guidance/ph10/chapter/4-Recommendations.

NHS 2016 Change4life. http://www.nhs.uk/change4life/Pages/change-for-life.aspx.

NHS Choices 2016 5 a day.

Personal, Social and Health Education Association 2016 PSHE Association programme of study for PSHE education (Key Stages 1–4). https://www.pshe-association.org.uk/curriculum-and-resources/resources/pshe-association-programme-study-pshe-education.

Public Health England 2016a Immunisation. https://www.gov.uk/government/collections/immunisation#history.

Public Health England 2016b Public health skills and knowledge framework. https://www.gov.uk/government/uploads/system/uploads/attachment_data/file/545012/Public_Health_Skills_and_Knowledge_Framework_2016.pdf.

Science and Technology Select Committee House of Lords 2011 Behaviour Change 2nd Report of Session 2010–12 HL Paper 179. London, The Stationery Office.

Shaping the Future of Health Promotion and Society of Health Education and Promotion Specialists Cymru 2009 A framework for ethical health promotion (draft). London, Royal Society for Public Health and SHEPS Wales.

South J 2014 Health promotion by communities and in communities: Current issues for research and practice. Scandinavian Journal of Public Health 42, 82–87.

Sperlich S, Maina MN 2014 Are single mothers' higher smoking rates mediated by dysfunctional coping styles? BMC Womens Health 14, 124. http://dx.doi.org/10.1186/1472-6874-14-124.

Tengland P 2012 Behavior change or empowerment: On the ethics of health-promotion strategies. Public Health Ethics 5(2):140–153.

The Moral Maze. 2014 Public health vs individual freedom. http://www.bbc.co.uk/programmes/b03tt510.

WEBSITES

Food Ethics Council for details on food poverty in the UK. http://www.foodethicscouncil.org/society/food-poverty.html.

NICE webpages for lifestyle and wellbeing. https://www.nice.org.uk/guidance/lifestyle-and-wellbeing.

Nuffield Council on Bioethics – exploring ethical issues in biology and medicine. http://nuffieldbioethics.org/.

FACEBOOK

Nuffield Council on Bioethics https://www.facebook.com/nuffieldbioethics.

BLOG

Nuffield Council on Bioethics http://nuffieldbioethics.org/blog/.

YOUTUBE

Nuffield Council on Bioethics, selection of videos on ethical issues https://www.youtube.com/user/NuffieldBioethics.

BBC IPLAYER

Is obesity the new smoking? http://www.bbc.co.uk/programmes/p047t7v6.

PART 2

Planning and Managing Health Promotion and Public Health Practice

PART SUMMARY

Part 2 aims to provide guidance on how you can:

- plan and evaluate your health promotion and public health practice work using a basic framework
- identify the views and needs of the clients/users/receivers of health promotion and set priorities for your work
- link your work to the efforts of colleagues and to local and national strategies
- use an evidence-based approach through using published research, doing your own research when necessary and auditing your work, thus ensuring that your efforts are effective and provide value for money
- organise yourself and manage your work to be effective and efficient
- develop competencies to work more effectively with colleagues and people from other organisations

Chapter 5 sets out a seven-stage planning and evaluation framework, which will help you to clarify what you are trying to achieve, what you are going to do and how you will know whether you are succeeding. The meaning of terms such as aims, objectives and targets are discussed, and there is guidance on how to specify them.

Chapter 6 explains how to identify need and describes the sources of information you require to establish the needs of a community, a group or an individual. Guidelines are provided on how to gather and apply information to assess needs and set priorities.

Chapter 7 provides an overview of the knowledge and skills required to plan health promotion and public health practice activities effectively including how to find and use published research. Guidance is included on how you can contribute to national and local public health strategic plans and complement what other people are doing. Evidence-informed practice is discussed and advice offered on how you can carry out small-scale research, audit your activities and ensure value for money. The chapter includes the key steps required to undertake a health impact assessment.

Chapter 8 focuses on how you can develop the competencies to manage yourself and your work effectively including managing information, writing reports, using time effectively, planning project work, managing change and working for quality.

Chapter 9 is about how to work with other people including communicating with colleagues, coordination and teamwork, participating in meetings and working in partnerships with other organisations.

5

PLANNING AND EVALUATING HEALTH PROMOTION AND PUBLIC HEALTH INTERVENTIONS

CHAPTER CONTENTS

SUMMARY

This chapter presents an outline of a planning and evaluation cycle for use in the everyday work of public health practitioners and health promoters. It involves seven stages which include the measurement and specification of needs and priorities, the setting of aims and objectives, decisions on the best way of achieving aims, the identification of resources, the planning of evaluation methods, and the establishment of an action plan followed by an intervention. Examples are given of aims, objectives, and action plans, and exercises are provided on setting aims and objectives and using the planning framework to turn ideas into action.

This chapter is about planning and evaluation at the level of your daily work in health promotion and public health practice. It provides a basic framework for you to use to plan and evaluate your projects and activities whether you work with clients on a one-to-one or group basis or undertake specific projects or programmes.

THE PLANNING PROCESS

Planning is a process that, at its very simplest, should give you the answers to three questions:

1. **What am I trying to achieve?** This question is concerned with identifying needs and priorities, then with being clear about your specific aims and objectives.
2. **What am I going to do?** This can be helpfully broken down into smaller steps:
   - Select the best approach to achieving your aims using evidence.
   - Identify the resources you are going to use.
   - Set a clear action plan of who does what and when.
3. **How will I know whether I have been successful?** This question highlights the importance of evaluation and the integral part it plays in planning health promotion and public health interventions. It should not be an afterthought or left too late to capture the information you need.

The planning process has been put together in the seven-stage flowchart in Fig. 5.1. The arrows on the flowchart lead you around in a circle. This is because, as you carry out your plan and evaluation, you will probably find things that make you rethink and change your original ideas. For example, things you might want to change could include working on a need you found you had overlooked; scaling down your objectives because they were too ambitious; changing the health educational resources or social media posts because you found that they were not as useful or effective as you had hoped; or, on the basis of new evidence, completely rethinking your strategy. The direction of the arrows in the flowchart is anticlockwise, but in reality planning is not always an orderly process. You may actually start at Stage 6 with a basic idea of a health-promotion intervention. Thinking more about it may lead you to clarify exactly what your aims are (Stage 2). Next, you might think about what resources you are going to need (Stage 4) and realise that you do not have enough time or money to do what you had in mind, so you go back to Stage 2 and modify your aims. Then you think about the best way of achieving your aims (Stage 3) and work out an action plan (Stage 6) with milestones. After that, you start to think seriously about how you will know whether you are successful (Stage 5), and you put your evaluation plans into your action plan (Stage 6 again). In effect, you are continually reviewing and improving your plan, using the framework appropriately to help you keep on course.

Planning takes place at many levels. If you are embarking on a major national public health intervention, you will need to take time to plan it in depth and in detail. If you are simply planning a short one-to-one session with a client, you will still need to plan and go through all the stages, but the process might be quick and may not even be written down.

For example, a chiropodist seeing a client with a foot care problem may identify that the client needs knowledge and skills in cutting toenails correctly. They decide that their aim is to give the patient basic information and training on this. They will know if they have been successful by examining the client's feet and by getting feedback about how they managed next time they see them. They identify an information leaflet that they can give the patient as reinforcement. They decide on an action plan of explanation and demonstration, and then get the patient to practise. They review the patient's toenail cutting skills next time they see them, reinforcing or correcting as necessary. All this planning takes place inside the chiropodist's head and is an integral part of his or her everyday professional practice.

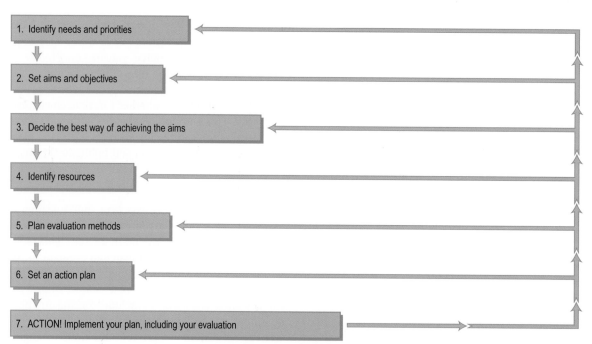

FIG. 5.1 ■ A framework for planning and evaluating health promotion and public health practice interventions and projects.

THE PLANNING FRAMEWORK

Stage 1: Identify Needs and Priorities

How do you determine what health promotion is needed? If you think you already know, what are you basing your judgement on? Who has identified the need: you, your clients, the local health and wellbeing board, or national policy directives? Identifying need is a complex process, which is looked at in depth in the next chapter. (See Chapter 6.)

You may have a long list of public health needs you have to respond to professionally such as those set out in the Public Health Outcomes Framework (PHOF; see Department of Health (DoH) 2016 and the PHOF website in the references at the end of the chapter) or in your local health and wellbeing strategy, so another issue is how to establish your priorities. Again, this is discussed in detail in the next chapter, but an important point is that you must have a clear view of which needs you are responding to and why, and what your priorities are.

Stage 2: Set Aims and Objectives

People use a range of words to describe statements about what they are trying to achieve such as aims, objectives, targets, goals, mission, purpose, result, product, and outcomes. It can be helpful to think of them as forming a hierarchy as in Fig. 5.2. At the top of the hierarchy are words that tell you why your job exists such as your job purpose or remit, or your overall mission. In the middle of the hierarchy are words that describe what you are trying to do in general terms such as your goals or aims. At the bottom of the hierarchy are words that describe in specific detail what you are trying to do such as targets or objectives.

It is worth noting that objectives can be of different kinds. Health objectives are usually expressed as the outcome or end state to be achieved in terms of health status such as reduced rates of illness or death. However, in health promotion and public health practice, work objectives are often expressed in terms of steps along the way towards an ultimate improvement in the health of individuals, groups, or populations such as increasing exercise levels or reduction in body mass index (BMI) or numbers of people who quit smoking.

In health education, educational objectives are framed in terms of the knowledge, attitudes or behaviour to be exhibited by the individual or group. Objectives can also be in terms of other kinds of changes, for example, a change in health policy (introducing a healthy eating policy in the workplace) or health-promotion practice (providing health information in minority ethnic languages). (See the following section on setting health-education objectives.)

The term 'target' is often used in public health and health promotion. Targets usually specify how the achievement of an objective will be measured, in terms of quantity, quality and time (the date by which the objective will be achieved). So a health target can be defined as a measurable improvement in health status by a given date that achieves a health objective. This is the approach used in national strategies for health such as the strategy for public health in England Healthy Lives Healthy People (DoH 2010) and the Public Health Outcome Framework which uses indicators to map progress (Public Health England (PHE) 2016). For evidence to inform the setting of goals/aims/objective, see, as an example, PHE publications such as Sugar reduction: The evidence for action (PHE 2015).

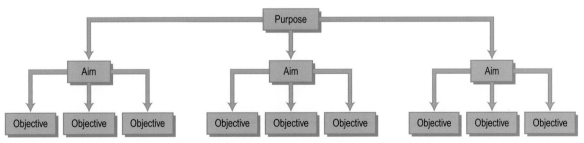

FIG. 5.2 ■ A hierarchy of aims.

Objectives are framed as health objectives, and the targets are framed as health targets (changes in rates of death or illness by a specific date), behaviour targets (such as changes in population rates of smoking or drinking by a specific date) or progress measures (such as the number of people attending a smoking cessation service and the number setting a date when they plan to stop smoking).

When you plan health promotion and public health initiatives, you need to set aims, objectives and targets or goals and outcomes.

Your aims (or aim, as there does not have to be more than one) are broad statements of what you are trying to achieve. Your objectives are much more specific, and setting these is a critical stage in the planning process.

Objectives are the desired end state (or result or outcome) to be achieved within a specified time period. They are not tasks or activities. Objectives should be as follows:

- **Challenging.** The objective should provide you with a health promotion/public health challenge in relation to what needs to be achieved.
- **Attainable.** On the other hand, it should be both realistic and achievable within the constraints of your professional role.
- **Relevant.** It should be consistent with the aims of the organisation and with the overall purpose/remit of your job.
- **Measurable.** You should try to identify objectives that are measurable, for example, specifying quantity, quality, and a time when they will be achieved. For instance (using the example in Exercise 5.1), an objective of 'to improve access to health information through the use of videos and social media…' has been achieved by working out the appropriate number of videos and languages and then specifying the target as 'to have videos covering five different health topics in three different languages…'

It is sometimes difficult to distinguish between aims, objectives and action plans. For example, a dietician who wants to improve the information they give to obese patients may describe their aim as 'to produce an information leaflet', but this is also their objective and their action plan. The answer is to think it through

further and ask: Why produce a leaflet? What am I aiming to achieve by producing the leaflet? It then becomes clearer that the aim is to improve patient compliance with dietary treatment, and one of the objectives is to improve patients' understanding of their dietary instructions. The action is to produce the leaflet. The importance of actually thinking through your aims and objectives in this way is that it helps you to be absolutely clear about *why* you are doing something, not just *what* you are doing. Failure to think through this stage means that health promoters waste time and energy proceeding with what seems like a good idea only to realise, too late, that what they are doing is not actually achieving what they want.

Setting Health Educational Objectives

If your health-promotion activity is based on a health-education approach (as it often is if you are a health trainer or a PSHE teacher, for example), it is useful to plan in terms of *educational* objectives (see Chapter 3 for more information on the role of health trainers and PSHE teachers).

Educationalists traditionally think of objectives (sometimes called learning outcomes) in terms of what the clients will gain. Furthermore, the objectives are considered to be of three kinds: what the health educator would like the clients to *know*, *feel* and *do* as a result of the education. In the language of the educationalist, these may be referred to as cognitive, affective and behavioural objectives.

Objectives About 'Knowing'. These are concerned with giving information, explaining it and ensuring that the client understands it, thus increasing the client's knowledge, for example, explaining the weight loss advantages of increasing exercise levels to someone who is obese. Here, the objective would be to develop an understanding of the value of exercise in the client with regard to their weight loss programme to enable them to make informed choices in terms of their weight loss strategies.

Objectives About 'Feeling'. These objectives are concerned with attitudes, beliefs, values and opinions. These are complex psychological concepts, but the important feature to note is that they are all concerned with how people feel. Objectives about feelings are about clarifying, forming or changing attitudes, beliefs, values or opinions. In the previous example, when the health promoter is educating a client about exercise and weight loss, in addition to the knowledge objective, there could be an objective about helping the client to explore their attitude towards exercise and any values, beliefs or opinions that might be forming a barrier to increasing exercise levels.

Objectives About 'Doing'. These objectives are concerned with a client's skills and actions. For example, teaching a routine of aerobic or yoga exercises has the objective that clients acquire practical skills and are able to do exercise-related specific tasks.

In the health-education approach to health promotion and public health, a combination of the knowing, feeling or doing educational objectives is usually required. For example, when a health visitor is advising a parent about feeding their toddler, they may be planning to achieve the following objectives within three home visits:

- The objective of ensuring that the parent knows which foods constitute a healthy eating

programme for their child and which are best given in restricted amounts.
- The objective of relieving the parents' anxiety that their healthy child's food fads may cause serious ill health.
- The objective that the parent learns what to do at meal times when the child has a tantrum about eating.

To summarise the key points about setting aims and objectives:

- The focus is on what you are trying to achieve.
- Be as specific as possible. Avoid vague or subjective notions of what you want to achieve.
- Express your objectives in ways that can be measured. How much? How many? When?
- Do not get bogged down in terminology. It does not matter whether you talk about goals, aims, objectives, targets or outcomes. The key principle is to be very clear about what you are trying to achieve.

To practise setting aims and objectives, undertake Exercise 5.1 and Exercise 5.2.

EXERCISE 5.2
Setting Aims and Objectives

Yewtree Scheme

The three practices at Yewtree Health Centre have agreed to establish physical activity assessment sessions, backed up by a display in the shared waiting area, with the long-term aim of reducing the incidence of coronary heart disease in the practice populations.
  The detailed objectives are:

1. to raise the users' awareness of the link between inadequate exercise and coronary heart disease, and the part which individuals can play in reducing their own vulnerability to the disease
2. to assess and advise about individuals' physical fitness levels and help them to prepare an appropriate exercise action programme based on those results
3. to monitor and evaluate, on a continuing basis, the effectiveness of the fitness testing in respect of the resources involved and the reduction in vulnerability to heart disease.

Ask yourself the following questions:

1. Do the objectives match the characteristics of objectives previously described? Are they challenging, attainable, as measurable as possible and relevant?
2. How would you suggest changing the objectives?

Stage 3: Decide the Best Way of Achieving the Aims

Occasionally, there might be only one possible way of accomplishing your aims and objectives. Usually, however, there will be a range of options. In Case Study 5.1, Jim has a number of options about how to achieve his objective of increasing the sun safety measures being taken by the school and the children. He could write to the schools or to parents of school-age children; he could hand out leaflets at school gates; he could lobby parents to take up the cause; he could find out if there are any school governors' meetings and ask to speak at them; he could conduct a sun safety campaign in the local media; he could write an article on the issue of sun safety in school playgrounds for the education journals that teachers read; or he could try to meet each Head Teacher face-to-face. Or he could do two or more of these together.

CASE STUDY 5.1

Jim is an environmental health officer. His project is to tackle sun safety in schools. This fits in with the overall purpose of his job which is to ensure safer environments. Jim works out that his *aim* is to work with local schools to set up a scheme that will result in sun safety measures being taken by the school and the children. He researches the subject in detail, looking at the results achieved from similar projects and working out how much time and money it is likely to take. He then decides that it is reasonable to set his *objective* as follows:

- Within 6 months to have raised awareness of the feasibility and advantages of developing shaded play areas with 10 primary schools and worked with at least five to set up shaded areas.

Health promoters such as Jim in this Case Study and Sue in Case Study 5.2 are faced with the problem of how to identify the best strategy for achieving their objectives. Factors to consider include:

- which methods are the most appropriate and effective in meeting your aims and objectives?
- which methods will be most acceptable to the individual or population group?
- which methods will be easiest?
- which methods are cheapest?
- which methods do you find comfortable to use?

CASE STUDY 5.2

Sue is a nurse specialising in coronary care. Her project is to run patient education programmes so that discharged patients know how to look after themselves. This fits in with the overall purpose of her job, which is to care for patients while they are in hospital and maximise their chances of a healthy life following discharge.

Sue decides that her *aim* is that patients will have participated in a cardiac rehabilitation programme for post-heart attack patients. Her *objectives* are:

- that every patient, before leaving the hospital, knows what they are advised to do about diet, exercise, smoking and stress control
- that every patient will be confident and competent to put this advice into practice
- that every patient and his or her carers and relatives will have had an opportunity to discuss questions and anxieties with a qualified member of the staff.

Sue's programme is a continuous course of group sessions each week with each session focusing on a specific issue. So each individual session also has a set of objectives. Objectives for the session on 'Eating well when you go home', for example, include the following:

- Patients will understand the basic principles of a healthy diet: low fat, low salt, low sugar, and high fibre.
- Patients will know which foods they can eat in unlimited amounts, which they should restrict, and which they should avoid.
- Patients will know what their ideal weight should be.
- Patients who are overweight will have devised a personal weight loss plan.

There is more about evidence for success, cost-effectiveness and value for money in Chapter 7, and Part 3 of this book covers how to use these methods to develop the necessary competency.

Looking at the first of these questions about which methods are most appropriate and effective for your aims, there is an accumulated body of evidence that helps identify effective methods for particular aims at the National Institute for Health and Care Excellence (NICE 2016) and at the Cochrane Database of Systematic

Reviews or the Cochrane Library (see website references at the end of the chapter). Table 5.1 identifies the range of aims, grouped into categories, and the appropriate and effective methods for achieving them. This provides a general guideline which may have exceptions.

TABLE 5.1	
Aims and Methods in Health Promotion and Public Health Practice	
Aim	Appropriate Method
Health awareness goal Raising awareness, or consciousness, of health issues	Talks Group work Mass media and social media Displays and exhibitions Campaigns (which could include the mass media and social media)
Improving knowledge Providing information	One-to-one teaching Displays and exhibitions Written materials Mass media and social media Campaigns Group teaching
Self-empowering Improving self-awareness, self-esteem, decision making	Group work Practising decision making Values clarification Social skills training Simulation, gaming, and role play Assertiveness training Counselling
Changing attitudes and behaviour Changing the lifestyles of individuals	Group work Skills training Self-help groups and peer support One-to-one advice and instruction Group or individual therapy Nudging Written material, social media, YouTube Social marketing approach
Societal/ environmental change Changing the physical or social environment	Positive action for under-served groups Lobbying for fiscal and legislative change Pressure and campaign groups, e.g. 38 Degrees Community development Community-based work Advocacy schemes Environmental and social measures Planning and policy making Organisational change Enforcement of laws and regulations

You may have decided on more than one of these categories of aims. For example, the inputs that contribute towards changing the behaviour of individuals can be complemented by societal changes, so that, together, they are more effective than either intervention alone by creating synergy. So, for example, to reduce the over-consumption of alcohol by young people, you could:

■ provide health education about alcohol as part of schools' personal, social, health and economic education programmes

■ provide educational rehabilitation programmes for young drink-drive offenders

■ work with young people to promote the social acceptability of consuming nonalcoholic drinks

■ lobby for an increase in alcohol taxation (a unit price) or for increasing the age at which young people can buy alcohol or for changes to the labelling of alcoholic drinks

■ work with alcohol companies in terms of promoting sensible drinking.

The example in Fig. 5.3 shows a range of aims and methods that might be used to promote healthy eating. A health promoter or public health practitioner may not use all these at any one time, but they are given here to illustrate the range of possibilities.

Stage 4: Identify Resources

What resources are you going to use? You have to establish what resources you are going to need and what are already available, what additional resources you are going to have to acquire and whether you will need extra funding. A number of different kinds of resources can be identified.

Professional Input

Your experience, knowledge, skills, time, enthusiasm and energy are vital resources. It helps identify all the other professional and lay people with something to offer. This may include colleagues and others in your professional networks (see Exercise 3.2 in Chapter 3) with relevant expertise who can advise and help you make your plans, clerical and secretarial staff who can help with administration, technicians, graphic designers, and web designers and artists who can help with exhibitions, displays, teaching/publicity materials and internet-based resources.

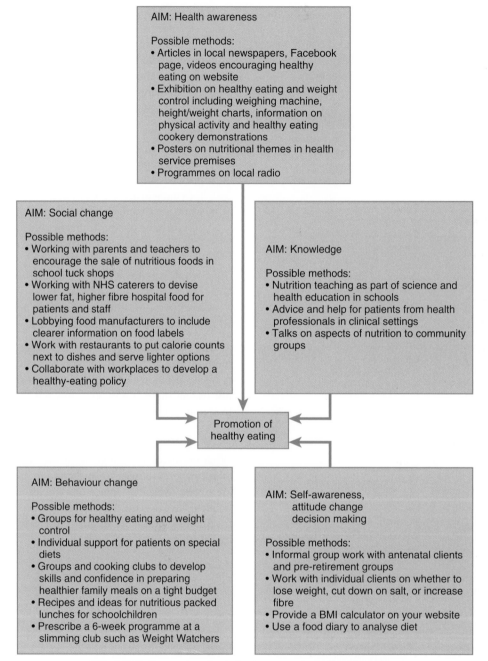

FIG. 5.3 ■ Aims and methods for the promotion of healthy eating.

Your Client or Client/Target Group

These are another key resource. Clients may have knowledge, skills, enthusiasm, energy and time, which can be used and built upon. In a group, clients can share their knowledge and previous experience and,

in this way, help each other to learn and change. An ex-client can be a very valuable resource too. For example, someone who has successfully lost weight, an ex-smoker or a person who has undergone a particular health-related experience can be a great help to clients who are grappling with similar problems and experiences.

People Who Influence Your Client or Client Group

These may include clients' relatives, friends, volunteers, patients' associations and self-help groups. It may also be possible to harness the help of significant people in the community who are regarded as opinion leaders or trendsetters such as political figures, religious leaders or media celebrities.

Existing Policies and Public Health Strategies

National and local policies and strategies for public health are useful to locate in terms of the work that you are planning. If, for example, you are planning to develop an intervention to help prevent the spread of sexually transmitted infections and HIV and reduce unwanted pregnancies, find out if there is already a policy on promoting sexual health in your area. Also find out whether your work fits into *A Framework for Sexual Health Improvement in England* (DoH 2013) and use the associated NICE guidance such as Preventing sexually transmitted infections and under-18 conceptions overview (NICE 2016).

Existing Facilities and Services

Find out what relevant local facilities already exist and whether they are fully utilised, for example, sports centres offering facilities for exercise and local classes or groups on cooking for healthy eating.

Material Resources

These might include leaflets, posters and display/publicity materials, or, if you are planning health promotion involving group work, you need resources such as rooms, space, seats, audiovisual equipment and teaching/learning materials.

Media Resources

Multimedia resources can include Facebook, blogs, Twitter, Instagram and YouTube on a wide range of health-related topics including those provided by statutory public health agencies such as the DoH and PHE. There is a wide assortment of media resources available on the internet, but it might be that your public health project would lend itself to the development of a new Facebook page, YouTube presentation

or blog, for example, in which case you will need resources for these.

Stage 5: Plan Evaluation Methods

How will you measure success and know whether your health promotion and public health practice is successful? Sophisticated methods are required to evaluate large-scale health promotion interventions. However, this should not deter health promoters; less complex methods of evaluating the everyday practice of health promotion can, and should, be used routinely.

What is Meant by Evaluation?

Evaluation is about making a judgement about the value of a public health or health promotion intervention, whether it is, for example, a health-education programme, a community project or an awareness-raising campaign to change local policy. Evaluation is crucial for ongoing quality improvement in your practice and involves the process of assessing *what* has been achieved and *how* it has been achieved. It means looking critically at the activity or programme, working out what were its strengths and its weaknesses, and how it could be improved.

The judgement can be about the *outcome* (what has been achieved) and whether you achieved the objectives which you set. So, for example, you should judge whether people understood the recommended limits for alcohol consumption as a result of your sensible drinking education, whether people in a particular community became more articulate about their health needs as a result of your community empowerment work or whether you achieved media coverage for your health campaign.

Judgements should also be about the *process* (how it has been achieved) and the cost benefit, for example, whether the most appropriate methods were used, whether they were used in the most effective way and whether they gave value for money. So, for example, you could consider whether the video-based discussion you used in your teaching programme was the best teaching method to use, whether the community development approach you chose was the most appropriate one in the circumstances, or whether you would have achieved more public awareness with less money if you had opted for a media stunt with possible free news coverage rather than an expensive advertising and leaflet campaign (see Pettman et al 2012 for a discussion on the complexities of public health practice evaluation).

Key terms often used in discussions about evaluation are defined in the Glossary at the end of this book.

Why Evaluate?

You need to be clear about why you are evaluating your work because this will affect the way you do it and the amount of effort you put in. Some reasons could be the following:

- To improve your own practice: Next time you deliver a similar intervention, you will build on your successes and learn from any mistakes.
- To help other people to improve their public health practice: If you disseminate your evaluation, it can help others improve their practice as well. It is vital to publicise failures as well as successes.
- To justify the use of the resources that went into the intervention and to provide evidence to support the case for doing this type of health-promoting intervention in the future.
- To give you the satisfaction of knowing how useful or effective your work has been; in other words, for your own job satisfaction.
- To identify any unplanned or unexpected outcomes that could be important. For example, a publicity campaign to deter young people from taking drugs could have the opposite effect by unwittingly glamorising drug-taking and making it appear to be a more common activity than it really is.

Who is the Evaluation For?

Who will be using your evaluation data? The answer to this affects what questions you ask, how much depth and detail you go into and how you present the information.

If you are solely assessing how well a health-promotion intervention went for your own benefit so you can change it appropriately next time you run a similar session, you will simply make a judgement on how you think it went based on your observation and the clients' reactions and make a few notes. But if you are writing a report for your manager or for a body that you want to fund the work, you need to think through what questions those people will expect to be answered and how much detail they will want.

For example, a group of health visitors evaluating a pilot scheme for a telephone advisory service at evenings and weekends need an evaluation report after 6 months for their manager who is funding the service. What will the manager need to know? At the very least, they will probably need a clear indication of the use made of the service. This might include how many people used it, the characteristics of the users (for example, whether they were first-time parents), how much it was used, what sort of issues people rang about, what the clients gained from it and how much it cost. It would be helpful for the health visitors to ask their manager what evaluation data will be required at the planning stage of the project so that the appropriate data can be collected from the start.

Assessing the Outcome

Looking first at outcome measures, which are called summative evaluation, you need to go back to the objectives you set and plan how you are going to determine whether you have achieved the objectives. Objectives are about the changes the intervention was designed to achieve and might have included changes in people's knowledge or behaviour or changes in policies or ways of working. Long-term health promotion projects may also have objectives about changes in health status. The following lists indicate the kinds of changes that may be reflected in your objectives and what methods you might use to assess or measure those changes.

Changes in Health Awareness Can Be Assessed By:

- measuring the interest shown by consumers, for example, how many people took up offers of leaflets, how many people enquired about preventive services, or how many people visited a website, friended or shared a Facebook page or retweeted.
- monitoring changes in demand for health-related services such as smoking cessation.
- analysis of media coverage of the public health issue, if it is a national campaign.
- questionnaires, interviews, focus group discussion or observation with individuals or groups.

Changes in Knowledge or Attitude Can Be Assessed By:

- observing changes in what clients say and do: Does this show a change in understanding and attitude?
- interviews and discussions involving question-and-answer between health promoter and clients.
- discussion and observation on how clients apply knowledge to real-life situations and how they solve problems.
- observing how clients demonstrate their knowledge of newly acquired skills.
- written tests or questionnaires that require clients to answer questions about what they know. The results can be compared with those of tests taken before the health intervention or from a comparable group that has not received the health promotion.

Behaviour Change Can Be Assessed By:

- observing clients' behaviour.
- recording behaviour. This could be based on records such as numbers attending a smoking cessation clinic or clients keeping a diary which is used at the end to assess behaviour change. It could be a periodical inventory such as a follow-up questionnaire or interview to check on smoking habits 6 and 12 months after attending the smoking cessation clinic. Records of client behaviour can be compared with those of comparable groups in other areas or with national average figures.

Policy Changes Can Be Assessed By:

- policy statements and implementation such as increased introduction of healthy eating choices in workplaces and schools.
- legislative changes such as increased restriction on smoking in cars where there are children as passengers; the introduction of a sugar tax.
- increases in the availability of health-promoting products, facilities and services such as exercise prescription schemes.

- changes in procedures or organisation such as more time being given to patient education or GP Brief Interventions.

Changes to the Physical Environment Can Be Assessed By:

- measuring changes in such things as air quality, traffic or pedestrian flows, the number of bike lanes or the amount of open green space available to the public within a defined area.

Changes in Health Status Can Be Assessed By:

- keeping records of simple health indicators such as weight, blood pressure rates, pulse rates on standard exercise or cholesterol levels.
- health surveys to identify larger scale changes in health behaviour or self-reported health status.
- analysis of trends in routine health statistics such as infant mortality rates or hospital admission rates.

It will be seen from this list that common evaluative methods are the generation of data from observation, holding discussions and distributing questionnaires and data analysis of health and other records.

Assessing the Process

Assessing intervention processes, often referred to as process formative evaluation, is an important but complex aspect of a comprehensive evaluation of health promotion and public health activities. For example, attempts to tackle problems such as smoking and obesity increasingly use multifaceted interventions that comprise multiple interacting components (Moore et al 2015). These types of interventions require a systematic approach to designing and conducting the process evaluations, drawing on clear descriptions and identification of key process questions. This involves examining what went on during the process of implementation and making judgements about effectiveness and efficiency. Was it done as cheaply and quickly as possible? Was the quality as good as you wished? Were the appropriate methods and materials used? You may, for instance, achieve your objectives but in a time-consuming, costly or inefficient way. So it is important to evaluate the process and identify whether you have achieved your desired outcome. Formative evaluation can be ongoing so that changes can be made to the intervention if it is found not to be working while it is in the process of delivery.

How are you going to assess the process? There are key aspects to process evaluation which involve measuring the input, self-evaluation by asking yourself questions and getting feedback from other people.

Measuring the Input. This is essential if you are going to make judgements about whether the outcome was worthwhile. You need to record everything that went into your health promotion or public health intervention in terms of time, money and materials. Then, you can make an informed judgement about cost–benefit and whether the outcome justified the cost.

Self-evaluation. Ask yourself 'What did I do well?', 'What would I like to change?' and 'How could I improve that next time?' All kinds of health promotion and public health interventions can be subjected to process evaluation, whether it is a one-to-one health-education intervention with a client, facilitating a self-help group, undertaking community empowerment work, developing and implementing a health policy or lobbying for organisational and structural changes.

An important point to note about self-evaluation is the need for a balanced objective critique which highlights both the positive and the negative aspects. Identify the things that have worked and look for constructive ways of moving forward with things that could be improved.

Feedback From Other People. Giving and receiving feedback is an essential skill for every health promoter. Getting feedback from a trusted colleague on your intervention is a valuable form of peer evaluation. Asking for and getting feedback from your manager should be part of the regular monitoring of your performance. (See the section in Chapter 10 on asking questions and getting feedback.)

Obtaining feedback from the clients or users themselves should also be part of assessing the process of every intervention. The important thing is to encourage a nonjudgemental atmosphere of openness and honesty. It can be done in many ways; simply observing clients and users accurately is an important tool. Do they look anxious or relaxed? Do they look interested and alert or bored and detached? You can also ask for feedback in such ways as a suggestions box, through noting any spontaneous verbal feedback you receive or through asking questions.

Stage 6: Set an Action Plan

Now that you know:

- what you are trying to achieve and have identified the best way to go about it
- how to evaluate it
- what resources you need

you can get down to planning in detail exactly what you are going to do. This means writing a detailed statement of who will do what, with what resources, and by when.

It is helpful, especially if you are tackling a large project, to break down your plan into smaller, manageable elements. One way of doing this is by thinking in terms of *key events*. Draw up a schedule showing the key events that are planned to happen at particular points in time. The schedule should specify deadlines that must be met by the people involved. Another way of breaking down a large project is by *milestone* planning. This is different from key events planning: instead of listing events, it lists a series of significant dates at fixed intervals (the milestones) and shows what must have happened by each of them. Box 5.1 illustrates both types of action plans. See also PHE (2014) for an example of an action plan.

For more discussion about the skills of project management, see Chapter 8, section on managing project work.

Stage 7: Action!

This is the stage in which you deliver your health-promoting intervention, remembering to evaluate the process as you go along.

Exercise 5.3 gives you the opportunity to apply this planning framework.

Be aware that when you are thinking about one section of the planning framework, it may have

BOX 5.1
ACTION PLANS

A **key events plan** drawn up by a public health practitioner who plans to set up an interactive multimedia health stall in a local supermarket to promote sensible drinking over the Christmas period could look like this:

1. *Discuss with my manager* at June meeting.
2. *Identify support from colleagues* by July.
3. *Approach supermarket manager*; by August agree to space and times.
4. *Convene planning group* of colleagues in August to sort out who will do what and when, evaluate plans and identify the resources required.
5. Planning phase, September to November including resource development.
6. *Set up first stall* in late November.

A brief **milestone plan** for the early stages of setting up a community health project could be like this in a framework of 3-monthly 'milestones':

January to March 2017	Steering group agrees job description for community health worker. Job advertised.
By end of June 2017	Interviews; appointment made. Community worker takes up post.
By end of September 2017	Community worker induction programme completed.
By end of December 2017	First progress report to Steering Group.

EXERCISE 5.3

Ideas Into Action: Planning a Health Promotion and Public Health Practice Intervention

Work alone or in a small group.

Think of an area of health promotion or public health practice where there is an identified need and within the remit of your job to meet that need. It could be an established area of work such as antenatal education, smoking cessation, teaching food hygiene, or an area of new work you would like to tackle such as an intervention to prevent obesity in children. If you are not currently in a job which involves health promotion or public health, think of a health-related project you would like to tackle in your personal life or a project for any voluntary/community group you are associated with, or just imagine what you would like to do if you had the opportunity (see the WHO website in the following references for programme and project ideas).

Work through the following stages of the planning cycle. Start by writing each of the following headings at the top of a separate large sheet of paper or word document, and then work through them:

1. **Aims and objectives**
   Ask yourself 'What am I trying to achieve?' Identify your broad aim or aims, then be more specific and identify your objectives.
2. **The best way of achieving my aims**
   Think of all the ways in which you could achieve your aims and identify the best way.
3. **Resources**
   Identify the resources you already have available and any extra ones you will need.
4. **Evaluation**
   Ask yourself 'How will I know if I am succeeding?' Identify how you will evaluate both the process and outcome of your work.
5. **Action plan**
   Identify who will do what, with what resources, and by when. Set milestones, if appropriate.

implications for the others, so you may find yourself going back to modify and refine what you have already written.

To summarise, the planning process consists of a series of stages which enable you to more systematically organise your health promotion and public health practice work by focusing on key questions around What? Why? When? Who? Where? and How?

Useful additional reading to support planning is Eldredge et al (2016) who propose an intervention mapping approach, and for some theoretical and practice insights into evaluation of complex health interventions, see Bell and Aggleton (2016). NICE provides excellent guidance on planning for behavioural change interventions based on a series of principles. The social context principle is an important one for those planning behavioural change interventions (refer to the website reference at the end of the chapter). Finally, the National Social Marketing Centre also provides a planning model and tools for planning behavioural change interventions. Their website is also referenced at the end of this chapter.

PRACTICE POINTS

- Health promotion and public health practice interventions benefit from being planned and evaluated in a systematic way.
- A planning cycle should ensure that needs and priorities are identified, aims and objectives are clearly set and methods for achieving aims and objectives are carefully considered in the context of available resources.
- Evaluation is an important component of the planning process, and evaluation methods should be formative, measuring the process, and summative, measuring the outcome of the intervention.

REFERENCES

Bell S, Aggleton P 2016 Monitoring and evaluation in health and social development: Interpretive and ethnographic perspectives. Oxford, Routledge.

Department of Health 2010 Healthy lives, healthy people. London, The Stationery Office.

Department of Health 2013 A framework for sexual health improvement in England. London, The Stationery Office.

Department of Health 2016 Improving outcomes and supporting transparency part 2: Summary technical specifications of public health indicators. London, The Stationery Office.

Eldredge LKB, Markham CM, Reiter RACE, Fernandez ME, Kook G, Parcel GAS 2016 Planning health promotion programs: An inter-

vention mapping approach, 4th edn. Jossey-Bass Public Health. http://greatist.com/live/best-health-happiness-blogs-2016.

Moore GF, Audrey S, Barker, et al 2015 Process evaluation of complex interventions: Medical Research Council guidance. British Medical Journal 350: 1258.

NICE 2016 Preventing sexually transmitted infections and under-18 conceptions overview. http://pathways.nice.org.uk/pathways/preventing-sexually-transmitted-infections-and-under-18-conceptions.

Pettman TL, Armstrong R, Doyle J, et al 2012 Strengthening evaluation to capture the breadth of public health practice: Ideal vs. real. Journal of Public Health 34(1):151–155.

Public Health England 2014 Guidance for developing a local suicide prevention action plan: Information for public health staff in local authorities. https://www.gov.uk/government/uploads/system/uploads/attachment_data/file/359993/Guidance_for_developing_a_local_suicide_prevention_action_plan__2_.pdf.

Public Health England 2015 Sugar reduction: Evidence for action. England, HSCIC.

Public Health England 2016 Public health outcomes framework. http://www.phoutcomes.info/public-health-outcomes-framework.

WEBSITES

Cochrane reviews for evidence to inform the planning of interventions. http://www.cochrane.org/reviews.

For social marketing planning models and tools. http://www.nsms.org.uk.

NICE for their Health and Lifestyle pathway and for guidance on behavioural change interventions. https://www.nice.org.uk/guidance/ph6/chapter/3-Recommendations#planning.

Programmes and projects initiated by the WHO. http://www.who.int/entity/en/.

Public Health Outcomes Framework 2016 to 2019. https://www.gov.uk/government/publications/public-health-outcomes-framework-2016-to-2019.

FACEBOOK

Public Health England's Facebook pages for updates on current initiatives and news items. www.facebook.com/PublicHealthEngland.

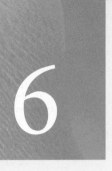

6

IDENTIFYING HEALTH PROMOTION AND PUBLIC HEALTH PRACTICE NEEDS AND PRIORITIES

CHAPTER CONTENTS

SUMMARY

This chapter begins with an analysis of the concept of need. This is accompanied by an overview of essential factors for you to consider when identifying health promotion and public health needs. These include the scope and boundaries of professional remits, the difference between reactive and proactive choices and the importance of placing the people who are the targets and users of health promotion at the centre of the needs identification process. This discussion is supplemented with an exercise on the user friendliness of services. In the next section on finding and using health information, types and sources of information are identified and exercises included on gathering and applying information. This is followed by a framework for assessing health promotion needs with a case study and an exercise. In the final section, there is a focus on priority setting with exercises on analysing the reasons for and the setting of health promotion and public health practice priorities and on setting priorities.

Many organisations at different levels have a role in identifying public health needs including those needs that can be addressed by health promotion

and public health practice interventions. These range from international agencies such as the World Health Organization (WHO), national organisations such as government departments, to organisations at local level such as local authorities or National Health Service (NHS) Trusts.

See Chapter 3 for information on the range of agencies with a public health and health promotion role, Chapters 3 and 16 for national and local health strategies, and Chapter 16 for making and implementing national and local health policies.

The focus in this chapter is on the need for interventions undertaken by health promoters and public health practitioners working with individual clients, families, groups and communities.

Identifying the people or target group who are intended to benefit from health-promotion activities is a complex process. These people may be referred to as *users*, which implies they use health-promotion services such as smoking cessation groups. In some cases, people receive help that they may or may not use, for example, receiving advice and information leaflets. Alternatively, people may be called *consumers*, *customers*, *clients* or *patients* if they are receiving their health promotion via medical services such as a coronary rehabilitation service. Positive action may be necessary to ensure that everyone has equal access to services and can benefit from them.

Going one stage further and identifying and prioritising people's needs is also a complex and difficult process. Needs may exceed the finite resources available to meet them, so difficult choices may have to be made.

Before looking further at how the needs of the users and receivers of health promotion can be met, it is worth considering what is understood by a need.

CONCEPTS OF NEED

It is useful to think of need in terms of:

- the kinds of health problems that people experience or are at risk from
- the requirements for a particular kind of health-promotion response
- the relationship between health problems and the health-promotion responses available.

Bradshaw's (1972) taxonomy of need was established many years ago, but it is still very useful in distinguishing between four different kinds of need.

1. Normative Need – Defined by the Expert

Normative need is a need defined by experts or professionals according to their own standards; falling short of those standards means that there is a need. For example, a dietitian may identify a certain level of nutritional knowledge as the desirable standard for her client and defines a need for nutrition education if her client's knowledge does not reach that standard. This normative need is based on the judgements of professional experts, which may lead to problems. One is that expert opinion may vary over what is the acceptable standard, and the values and standards of the experts may be different from those of their clients.

Some normative needs are prescribed by law such as food standards regulation with much of the detailed legislation for the UK originating in the European Union (see Food Standards Agency 2013) or by national policy and related public health outcomes framework (see, for example, Department of Health (DoH) 2012a).

2. Felt Need – Wants

Felt need is the need that people feel; it is what they *want*. For example, a pregnant woman may feel the need for (and want) information about childbirth. Felt needs may be limited or inflated by people's awareness and knowledge about what could be available; for example, people will not feel the need to know their blood cholesterol level if they have never heard that such a thing is possible or know about the potential risk of high blood cholesterol levels to health.

3. Expressed Need – Demands

Expressed need is what people say they need; it is felt need that has been turned into an expressed request or demand. Commercial weight-control groups and exercise classes are examples of expressed need; they are provided in response to demand.

Not all felt need is turned into expressed need or demand. Lack of opportunity, motivation, or assertiveness could all prevent the expression of a felt need. Lack of demand, therefore, should not be equated with lack of felt need.

Expressed needs may conflict with a professional's normative needs. For example, a patient may express a need for a course of individual professional counselling as a result of experiencing a mental health problem, but the resources may not be available for this type of health-promoting service and normative needs and priorities may be focused on other types of interventions to promote mental health.

4. Comparative Need

Comparative need for health promotion is defined by comparison between similar groups of clients, some in receipt of health promotion and some not. Those who are not are then defined as being in need. For example, if Company A has an employee health policy covering stress at work and the provision of healthy food choices in the staff canteen and Company B does not, it could be said that there is a comparative need for health promotion in Company B. This assumes that the health promotion in Company A is desirable and ideal, which of course it may not be.

NEED, DEMAND AND SUPPLY

Over time, there has been debate over need, demand, supply, and quality of health services and other public sector services that relate to health such as education. Levels and quality of service vary nationally and internationally (see Dorling 2015 for a global analysis), and in the UK between GPs and hospitals even in the same neighbourhood, resulting in what has been termed as a postcode lottery (Public Health England 2015). The need for services may be similar or different, but supply is unevenly distributed, and this results in significant health inequalities (see, for example, Hatchard (2015) in relation to mental health services, Macmillan (2014) in relation to cancer care and survival, and Stephenson (2016) reporting variation in specialist children's care provision).

If demand outstrips supply, it means that people do not always get the access or the quality of the health provision they want or that health professionals believe they need. This issue of uneven provision also applies to health promotion and public health services with an early survey showing different levels of health-promotion provision in different geographical areas in the UK (Scriven 2002). The problem of uneven provision arises because the health services and other public bodies have a finite pot of money to spend, so they have to prioritise. This results in rationing (Edwards et al 2015). To overcome some of the problems associated with rationing, adults receiving NHS Continuing Healthcare and children in receipt of continuing care have had a right to have a personal health budget. A personal health budget is an amount of money to support personally identified health and wellbeing needs, planned and agreed upon between the person and their local NHS team. The aim is to give people with long-term conditions and disabilities greater choice and control over the health care and support they receive, if they desire this (NHS Choices 2016). Measures to address the uneven supply and quality of health services have also included the development of national standards. The National Institute for Health and Care Excellence (NICE) provides the standards not only for clinical and healthcare practice but also for public health and health promotion. Quality standards set out the priority areas for quality improvement. Quality standards cover:

- areas where there is variation in care
- topics across health and social care.

Each standard contains a set of statements to help you improve quality. It also tells you how to measure progress against the statement.

The standards are developed independently in collaboration with health and social care professionals, practitioners and service users. They are based on NICE guidance and other NICE-accredited sources.

Example of a Quality Statement

Older people using home care services have a home care plan that identifies how their personal priorities and outcomes will be met, *Home care for older people, NICE quality standard* (NICE 2016a).

Anyone wanting to improve the quality of health and care services should consult the standards. For example:

- commissioners – Use the quality standards to ensure that high-quality care or services are being commissioned.
- service providers – Use the quality standards to monitor service improvements, to show that high-quality care or services are being provided and highlight areas for improvement.
- health, public health, and social care practitioners – Use audit and governance reports to demonstrate the quality of care, as described in a quality standard, or in professional development and validation.
- regulators – For example, the Care Quality Commission.

Quality standards are not mandatory. They support the UK government's vision for a health and care system focused on delivering the best possible health outcomes and are therefore important for all professionals with a public health remit.

The Health and Social Care Act (DoH 2012b) says that the Secretary of State for health, in discharging their duty to improve the quality of services, must have regard for the quality standards prepared by NICE (NICE 2016b).

IDENTIFYING HEALTH PROMOTION NEEDS

How do health promoters and public health practitioners set about identifying individual and/or group needs? There are three key areas that are useful to think about first: the scope and boundaries of your job; the balance between being reactive and proactive in your work; and the extent to which you are putting your clients first. Each of these is addressed in turn.

The Scope

For some public health practitioners and health promoters, the task of identifying needs has already taken place. For example, dental hygienists working in dental surgery with individual patients already have the clearly identified task of educating patients in oral hygiene. But they may want to think carefully about how they can make their service as person-centred and user friendly as possible. And they will certainly have to identify and respond to the individual needs of each patient.

Some professionals with a public health remit, however, have more choice and scope in the range of health-promotion activities they can undertake. Health visitors and community workers may have considerable scope, but the degree of autonomy they have will vary according to the policy of their managers and the resources available. All health promoters will need some competency in being responsive to the health promotion needs of their clients and will need to be clear about the boundaries of their work: Which health-promotion activities are within their remit to undertake and which are not (however desirable they may be)? For example, a family planning nurse may be asked to undertake sex education with young people in schools, but is this within the boundaries of her job?

Reactive or Proactive?

It is useful to make an initial distinction between being *reactive* and being *proactive* when identifying needs. Being reactive means responding or reacting to the needs and demands that other people make. Pressure from vested interest groups and the media may introduce bias into how needs are perceived and produce pressure to react. Being proactive means taking the initiative and deciding on the area of work to be done. It may include rejecting the demands of other people if these do not fit existing policies and priorities. (See Chapter 4, section on analysing your aims and values: Five approaches.)

Being reactive or proactive can be related to the approaches to health promotion, which were discussed

in Chapter 4. Using a client-directed approach means being reactive to consumers' expressed needs, whereas using a medical or behaviour change approach probably means being proactive. This is particularly true of preventive medical interventions such as immunisation campaigns. In practice, there is usually a balance to be struck between being reactive and proactive.

Putting Users' Needs First

It is important to ask the questions about whose needs should come first, the users or the providers of health promotion. There may be conflict between the two: for example, users may want a family planning service to be open on Saturdays to improve access, but providers are unable to supply this service because of difficulties in getting staff to work on weekends. However, numerous international policy directives such as the seminal *Ottawa Charter* (WHO 1986) and national public health strategies such as *Healthy Lives Healthy People* (DoH 2010) have emphasised the need for more people-centred health promotion. For example, Healthy Lives Healthy People states that a new approach is needed that empowers individuals to make healthy choices and gives communities the tools to address their own particular needs. The White Paper puts local communities at the heart of public health, ending central control and giving local government the freedom, responsibility, and funding to innovate and develop their own ways of improving public health in their area.

The core values that would be embedded in people-centred health promotion are:

- empowerment
- participation
- the central role of the individuals, family, and community in any process of health development
- equity and nondiscrimination.

The implications of these values are clear. People have the right to participate in making decisions about their health and should be enabled to do so. The needs, wants, and expectations of individuals, families, and communities should be respected by health promoters and public health practitioners and influence priority setting and the delivery of health-promotion services. You can measure how user friendly your services are by undertaking Exercise 6.1.

EXERCISE 6.1

Using Services That Promote Health or Prevent Ill Health: User Views

Find out about some services available locally, designed for the public, that aim to promote health and wellbeing or prevent ill health. The public library, NHS trust, or local council, for example, may be able to provide information about what services are available. These could include swimming facilities, exercise classes, weight support, or smoking cessation classes, or be part of the services, campaigns, or activities of your local public health departments.

Select one of these that are appropriate and acceptable to you, and visit it. Make notes about what happens and how the service was responsive to its users.

See also the section on working for quality in Chapter 8 for information on quality in health promotion and public health services.

■ Is it easy to find out that the service exists?

■ Is it easy to locate with clear signposting where needed?

■ Is public transport easily available? Is there easy access for parking your car?

■ Are the times convenient to you?

■ If there is a charge for the service? Is it affordable and a good value for money?

■ How are you welcomed? Are you given all the information you need? Do you feel at ease? Are the health promoters or public health practitioners friendly?

■ What do you think about the environment? Is it safe, clean and comfortable?

■ What do you think about the quality of the service you received? Do you have any ideas about how it could be improved? Will you use this service again?

■ What have you learned as a service user which you can now apply to health promotion and public health practice?

These values suggest that key characteristics of people-centred health promotion and public health practice might include the following:

For individuals, communities, and population groups:

■ Access to clear, concise and intelligible health information and education that increase health literacy and enable needs to be expressed.

■ Equitable access to health including treatments and psychosocial support.

■ Development of personal skills which allow control over health and engagement with healthcare systems: Communication, mutual collaboration and respect, goal setting, decision making, problem solving and self-care.

■ Supported involvement in health decision making including health policy.

For health promotion and public health practitioners and specialists:

■ Holistic understanding and approach to health improvement.

■ Respect for people and their decisions.

■ Recognition of the needs of people seeking to improve their health.

■ Professional and personal skills to meet these needs: Competence in promoting health, communication, mutual collaboration and respect, empathy, responsiveness, and sensitivity.

■ Commitment and adherence to quality, evidence-informed decision making, and practice and ethical practice.

■ Team work, collaboration and partnership across organisations and professional disciplines and with clients.

Source: Adjusted from http://www.wpro.who.int.

Let us now return to the central question: How are needs for health promotion and public health practice identified?

FINDING AND USING INFORMATION

The starting point for defining health promotion and public health practice needs is information of various kinds from a range of sources. If you are gathering information on a local area for the first time, it would be helpful to share the work and the findings with colleagues. For example, health visitors may have done a neighbourhood profile as part of their training; the public health department in the local authority (LA) will probably have health data on the local population. Gathering and updating all these different kinds of information is an ongoing project for every health promoter, and sharing the task is a more efficient use of time. Working with colleagues needs to be done in conjunction with establishing links with local people to ensure the active participation of users and receivers.

There are a number of different kinds of information you can access when identifying need.

Epidemiological Data

Epidemiology is the key quantitative discipline that underpins public health. It is the study of the distribution and determinants of disease in communities. Epidemiological data indicate how many people are affected by a health problem, how many people die from a particular health problem, and who are most at risk within sex, age, ethnic, socioeconomic, occupational or geographical groupings or perhaps by taking account of lifestyle factors such as smoking or physical activity levels or personal characteristics such as weight.

Detailed discussion of the sources and limitations of epidemiological data is outside the scope of this book, but for texts on epidemiology see, for example, Friis and Sellars (2013) and Katz et al (2013). The important point to make here is that epidemiological data provide essential information on the health of the population, the causes and risk factors related to ill health, and, in doing this, highlights the potential for prevention and health promotion.

Mortality and morbidity data are collected nationally, and some data are also available on a regional and local basis. Mortality data are concerned with causes of death, whereas morbidity data are concerned with types of illness and disability. Mortality data are derived from death certificates; morbidity data are derived from a wide range of sources including medical records, sickness absence certificates, child health records, returns of notifiable diseases, disability registers, and many others. In addition, the Office for National Statistics (ONS) is the UK's largest independent producer of official statistics and the recognised national statistical institute for the UK. It is responsible for collecting and publishing statistics related to the economy, population (and population health), and society at national, regional and local levels (see ONS 2016). Other health surveys carried out for research purposes by, for example, university research centres provide a considerable amount of health statistics and information (see, for example, the global health research unit, Imperial College London 2016).

Your local NHS organisation, such as a Trust, and the LA will have information about the local population including mortality and morbidity data (such as hospital admission rates for particular conditions). This may be broken down to the level of the population of smaller areas such as electoral wards. It might be helpful to compare data for the whole population and electoral ward data (for a neighbourhood) on, for example:

- the major causes of mortality
- the key causes of childhood admission to hospital
- the main conditions for which adults are admitted to hospital.

In England, the area Health and Wellbeing Boards (and their equivalent in other countries) will also have assessed the health and wellbeing needs of people in LA districts (adults, young people and children) through a Joint Strategic Needs Assessment process. The data from this will have been used to produce a Joint Health and Wellbeing Strategy which will have set out the priorities for action based on the health and wellbeing needs identified.

Exercise 6.2 is designed to enable you to find out about local health information.

EXERCISE 6.2
Gathering Local Public Health Information

Undertake an internet search of your local NHS organisations, such as your local Trust and LA (or equivalent in Scotland, Wales and Northern Ireland), for reports or data on the health status of your local population. Some local data may also be available on national websites such as Department of Health Office of National Statistics (see websites at the end of the chapter). Browse through the data and see if you can find out the following for your local population:

- What are the major causes of death?
- What are the major reasons for people to be admitted to hospital?
- What are the major risk factors for ill health? For example, is there information on what percentage of people smoke in your local population or are living in poverty?
- How many people have had communicable diseases (diseases caught from other people) such as measles or sexually transmitted infections?
- Which neighbourhoods or communities have the poorest health? How is health being measured?
- What is the Joint Health and Wellbeing Strategy (or equivalent) for your area?
- What steps are being taken to achieve the local health and wellbeing strategy and prevent ill health and promote good health?

Can you find information on anything else to help you in your health promotion and public health work?

Lifestyle Data

An increasing amount of information about people's health-related behaviour and lifestyles such as physical activity, sexual behaviour, smoking and drinking is available on a national basis from survey data. See, for example, the Schools and Students Health Education Unit (HEU) surveys (http://www.sheu.org.uk) which have up-to-date data on the lifestyle of young people at school. There are active surveys that date back to 1977 and therefore act as valuable benchmarks. You may also find that a local authority or regional NHS organisation has done a lifestyle survey of your local population and published the findings (see, for a good example, Porter 2016).

Socioeconomic Data

The planning or information departments of local councils should be able to help with information about housing, employment, social class and social/leisure/recreation/shopping facilities. Many produce summaries of census data. It might be helpful to compare district/borough/city and electoral ward data on social and economic factors such as:

- unemployment
- household amenities
- income
- ethnicity.

It is advisable to ask for figures that are as full and recent as possible. Much information is obtained from the national census, which takes place every 10 years. Information from the analysis of the data is available at the ONS. The ONS has an online facility which will allow you to search for detailed information online (http://www.neighbourhood.statistics.gov.uk).

By setting illness data alongside social and economic data, you may be able to see patterns that might inform your needs identification and priority setting process. You may want, for example, to determine if areas where people with less financial and other resources live are also likely to be the areas of poorest health. For international comparisons, statistics can be gleaned from, for example, the World Health Organization global observatory (WHO 2016).

Professional Views

The views of the wider public health workforce reflect experience and perceptions accumulated over the years, which would be foolish to ignore. What do other professionals in your geographical area such as teachers, youth workers, social workers, GPs, health visitors, district nurses, environmental health officers, police officers, community workers and religious leaders consider the major health concerns?

Public Views

Public sector organisations are now charged with the responsibility of seeking the views of the communities that they serve, but some organisations have developed good practice in this area over a number of years. Try contacting the local government in your area for information on this type of work such as Citizens' Panels, which are representative samples of residents who give their views on local services, priorities, and plans (for an example of the work of Citizens' Panels, see Scottish Government (2016) or perhaps look at your own local council website).

There is more about research methods for finding out people's views in Chapter 7, section on doing your own small-scale research.

There are several methods of obtaining the views of the public, from informal discussions/interviews to large-scale surveys using questionnaires or in-depth interview techniques. Identifying priority groups and thinking clearly about them will influence the choice of methods used to contact and involve them.

It is best to start with the characteristics of the groups and then design the best approach. For instance, how large are the relevant groups? Do they have particular age, class or ethnic structures? What makes it a group (geography, membership, current use of services and facilities)? Are the members of the group mobile? Do they have easy access to transport? What times of day are they likely to be available for meetings? Be absolutely clear about what sort of relationship you are proposing to have with local groups and individuals. For example, if you plan simply to establish consultation mechanisms, there may be hostility if local people have played a much stronger partnership role in the past. Public consultation and involvement are discussed in detail in Chapter 15.

The groups involved may include local Health Watch (see Healthwatch England 2016 and Case Study 6.1) and patient advice and liaison services (PALS; http://www.pals.nhs.uk), local voluntary organisations, and community groups such as self-help groups, black and minority ethnic groups, pensioners' clubs, tenants' associations, and a variety of local advisory groups or planning subcommittees, in addition to groups of key clients such as parents. Gathering views informally is useful, but there are problems in ensuring accuracy and that subjective information is representative. However, these subjective data can usefully feed into the wider picture.

You might want to consider undertaking some first-hand research but first think about how much time and money it will take. Will the results justify the costs? If you still think it is worth doing, who could do it? If it is very small scale, you could perhaps undertake it yourself, maybe in collaboration with some colleagues.

Local and National Media and Social Media

The opinions and data collected from local and national media will provide you with a picture at a particular point in time. Monitoring radio, TV, newspapers, webpages, Twitter and Facebook pages (particularly those focusing on specific community issues) will give a view of any major needs in the community. All this adds to the profile of needs you are building up, providing a basis for planning health promotion and public health action.

CASE STUDY 6.1
Seeking Out Men's Views in Blackburn

The staff at Healthwatch Blackburn with Darwen are always thinking of new ways they can find out the views of different sections of their community. In 2015, they decided they needed a new approach to increase the number of men they engaged with.

They embarked on a tour of local pubs and clubs to hear about men's views and experiences of health and care. They raised awareness with beer mats and used pub quizzes and informal interviews to speak to more than 185 men.

What they heard informed eight recommendations for improvements to services. To share their findings, the local Healthwatch held a pub quiz at a local working men's club and invited health professionals as well as men from the local community.

Source: Healthwatch England (2016)

ASSESSING HEALTH PROMOTION AND PUBLIC HEALTH PRACTICE NEEDS

The assessment of health promotion and public health needs can be approached systematically by asking a series of key questions. The answers will help you to decide whether you should respond to a particular need, and if so, how.

1. What TYPE of Need Is It?

Is this a normative, felt, expressed or comparative health need?

In a sex education class in a school, for example, what kind of need is being met: the **normative needs** decided by the school nurse or the personal, social and health education (PSHE) teaching team or the school governors; or the **felt or expressed needs** of the school pupils or their parents; or the **comparative needs** decided after comparing the PSHE curriculum in other schools; or for example, when teenage pregnancy rates in a local area are compared to national figures and suggest a need for more work on contraception?

2. Who Decided That There Is a Need?

Whose decision is it: The health promoter/public health practitioner, the individual or target group, or both?

Sometimes the answer to this question is not immediately obvious, because the need has emerged after discussion between the health promoter/public health practitioner and their clients. People do not always know what they need or want, because their awareness and knowledge of the possibilities are limited. The health promoter may help by raising awareness and knowledge of health issues; in this way, he or she may create a demand (an expressed need) for health promotion. For example, the public's demand for nonsmoking in restaurants came only after health promoters had raised awareness of the hazards of passive smoking, which motivated people to express their need for a smoke-free environment in eateries. An ideal situation is when there is a synergy between client's, health promoter's and public health practitioner's needs.

3. What are the Grounds for Deciding That There Is a Need?

Is there any evidence of need in the form of objective data? If local data are not available, has the information been collected in other localities and is it reasonable to assume that the same conditions will apply? Be aware that gathering data can be a delaying tactic to avoid doing something about an obvious problem. For example, surveys have shown that elderly people without cars find it difficult to get to hospitals if public transport is poor. It is reasonable to assume that this applies in most localities with poor public transport. So, collect information only if the answer to a question is really not known. Have the views of the clients been sought? Do they see this as a need?

4. What are the Aims and the Appropriate Response to the Need?

See the section on setting aims and objectives in Chapter 5 for a more detailed look at setting aims and objectives and identifying appropriate ways of achieving them.

Health promotion and public health cannot solve all problems or meet all health needs. You should be clear on what the need is, then what your aims are for meeting that need, then the appropriate way to meet it. For example, there may be an identified normative need to increase the uptake of immunisation and aim to achieve an 80% uptake rate. You then have to decide the appropriate way to achieve your aim. It would be all too easy in this case to say that there is a need for a health education campaign to get parents to have their children immunised because messages about attending immunisation clinics may be seen to be the answer. But this may make no difference because the appropriate response is to educate the health professionals who are being too cautious and withholding immunisation wrongly when a child has only a mild contraindication, or to move the time and/or location of the clinics so that working parents, and those without cars, are able to bring their children.

Case Study 6.2 is an example of how need for health promotion and public health practice is assessed, applying the four assessment questions.

CASE STUDY 6.2

Eat 4 Health

Case study prepared by Leena Sankla, Solutions4Health, Reading, Berkshire, UK.

BACKGROUND

Levels of obesity in Western Berkshire are higher than the national average and are a cause for concern as a number of severe and chronic medical conditions are associated with overweight and obesity including type 2 diabetes, hypertension, coronary heart disease, stroke, osteoarthritis and some cancers (West Berkshire JSNA (**Joint Strategic Needs Assessment**) 2015).

Body Mass Index (BMI) is a strong predictor of premature mortality among adults. Overall moderate obesity (BMI 30 to 35 kg/m2) was found to reduce life expectancy by an average of 3 years. While morbid obesity (40 to 50 kg/m2) reduces life expectancy by 8 to 10 years, research shows that 19% of adults in Reading (Reading JSNA 2016), 18.5% of adults in West Berkshire (West Berkshire JSNA 2015)

and 19.7% of adults in Wokingham (Wokingham JSNA 2012) are obese, whereas 55.3% of adults in Reading, 65.5% of adults in West Berkshire and 57.4% of adults in Wokingham are overweight.

Levels of physical activity are closely linked to the prevalence of obesity with fewer people taking enough exercise to maintain a healthy weight. Research shows that 56.6% of adults in Reading, 55.4% of adults in West Berkshire and 62.3% of adults in Wokingham are physically active.

WHAT TYPE OF NEED IS IT?

Assist residents of West Berkshire to access a community-based weight-management programme and achieve long-term weight loss. The underlying principles of the programme are based on NICE guidelines including principle of behavioural change and self-management.

Continued on following page

Eat 4 Health (Continued)

WHO DECIDED THERE IS A NEED?

The local public health specialists and practitioners acting on national policy directives decided there was a need for this initiative. The main aims and outcomes of national policy directives were as follows:

- To decrease the percentage of adults who are overweight or obese in West Berkshire
- To help adults who have a BMI >25 to decrease their weight to become a healthy weight and maintain their weight
- To increase the percentage of adults eating a healthy diet
- To increase the percentage of adults being moderately physically active for 30 minutes per day on most days of the week
- To decrease the rates of coronary heart disease, stroke, diabetes, hypertension, osteoarthritis and some cancers in West Berkshire

WHAT ARE THE GROUNDS FOR DECIDING THERE IS A NEED?

The grounds for deciding that there was a need to provide weight-management programmes across West Berkshire was the above average overweight and obesity levels across the area and low uptake of physical activity.

WHAT ARE THE AIMS AND APPROPRIATE RESPONSE TO THE NEED?

The aim and appropriate response is to provide an accessible tier 2 lifestyle adult weight-management programme service for overweight and obese adults aged 16 and over within the locality, which forms an integral part of the weight management care pathway.

The Eat 4 Health programme is adapted to ensure it is appropriate for different cultures. Courses are delivered in many different languages including English, Urdu, Hindu and Nepalese ensuring the service is provided to groups that are usually hard to reach. Eat 4 Health have also developed different resources including recipes, snacking and cooking guidance specific to different cultures and traditions to support participants in making changes towards a healthier diet. Eat 4 Health target local high footfall events including local Caribbean and Diwali events to increase accessibility for hard-to-reach groups.

The team have been active in taking the Eat 4 Health programme into the heart of the community through provision of sessions and outreach in some of the most deprived areas in West Berkshire.

Courses are held in a range of different locations, including evenings to increase accessibility.

Target outreach has been held in a number of different surgery waiting rooms across GP surgeries in West Berkshire. This is a great opportunity to engage with patients at a time when they are receptive to bettering their health.

Training is delivered to local GP surgery staff to ensure they have appropriate knowledge of Eat 4 Health services in their local area. The training session also equips practice staff with the skills to raise the issue of weight with patients and motivate them to join a local service.

Monthly newsletters are distributed to GP practices across Berkshire to increase interest and maintain engagement.

SETTING HEALTH PROMOTION AND PUBLIC HEALTH PRIORITIES

You may have a large number of needs that you feel should be met, but there are always constraints on resources such as time and finance. Concentrating effort on priority areas is essential to ensure quality and effectiveness.

Before attempting to set priorities, it is helpful to analyse current practice and recognise the wide range of criteria that will affect decisions about health-promotion interventions. Undertaking Exercises 6.3 and 6.4 enables you to focus on these factors.

The need to prioritise is vital, but one difficult issue to consider is how to approach work with people

---

EXERCISE 6.3

Analysing the Reasons for Health Promotion and Public Health Practitioner Priorities

Identify a health promotion activity that has a high priority in your work. This could be work that you undertake with a number of clients (such as a smoking cessation programme) or just one (for example, a health visitor talking to a mother about maintaining breastfeeding); it could be part of your usual work or a special event such as a campaign. It will be especially helpful for the purposes of this exercise if you can identify an area of work that has recently become a priority.

Now work through the following tasks.

1. Identify who it was who decided that this work should take priority (e.g. You? Your manager(s)? Your clients? All three?).

2. List all the possible reasons why this work has priority; include the reasons that you are sure about as well as any that are speculation.

Your reasons could include any of the following and probably many more:

  ■ I feel that it is an important public health issue.
  ■ It is the established public health priority of senior managers.
  ■ We have always had it as a priority and see no reason to change.
  ■ There was pressure from the public.
  ■ It was in response to a public health crisis.
  ■ There is new evidence of need.
  ■ There is evidence that the work has been effective in a similar area.
  ■ It was the current national/local theme (e.g. No Smoking Day; https://nosmokingday.org.uk/).
  ■ We had a new staff member with special expertise, which we wanted to use.
  ■ We had to economise and be more efficient.
  ■ It was politically expedient.
  ■ There was a change in national public health policy or local public health strategy.

3. Identify what you think the most important reasons are. Do you think that they are sound reasons for setting priorities?

---

whose health experience is poor. It is automatic to consider that these people should be top priority, but it is important to consider whether focusing all health promotion effort on those most at risk will, in the end, be of greatest benefit.

When reducing the incidence of coronary heart disease, for example, two broad approaches can be used: the *high-risk* and the *whole population* approaches. The high-risk approach identifies people particularly at risk, such as smokers, people who are obese or who have high blood pressure, and develops interventions with these people to change lifestyle factors and treat their raised blood pressure, for example. But there may be poor return for effort, as these groups could include addictive smokers with poor diets who have no intention of changing or people so overwhelmed with social and/or psychological issues in their lives that tackling smoking and eating habits is too difficult, even if they would like to make changes.

The whole population approach works at community rather than individual level, with, for example, strategies to improve access to cheap healthy food, increase skills and confidence in producing healthy meals for families, and community development approaches to build up social support. At the same time, supporting changes at a wider population level, such as reducing the underage sales of cigarettes, and lobbying for increased income support, could result in better health gain across whole populations.

Generally, both approaches need to be taken (not necessarily by the same health promoters), as they complement each other. This is why developing partnership working is so important as it allows different aspects of the same issue to be addressed by the health promoters who are best placed to tackle a particular aspect at a particular time, thus achieving greater impact.

There can be no exact method for setting priorities because they ultimately depend upon the normative judgements and the available resources of the health promoters involved. But it may be helpful to work through the checklist in Exercise 6.4.

1. Health promotion issues, approaches, and activities

Do you define your priorities in terms of:

- issues that have an influence on health (the wider determinants such as poverty, unemployment, racism, ageism, inequalities)?
- health-promotion approaches (such as medical, behaviour change, social marketing, educational, client-centred, societal/environmental change)?
- health-promotion activities (preventive health services, community-based work, organisational development, economic and regulatory activities, environmental measures, health education programmes, healthy public policies)?
- health problems (such as heart disease, food poisoning, cancers, HIV/AIDS, obesity, mental illness)?

Why?

2. Consumer/target groups

Who are the people your health promotion/public health practice is aimed at?

- Policy makers and planners?
- Individual clients or service users?
- Families?
- Selected target groups?
- The whole community? If so, how do you define your community? Why?

3. Age groups

Do you define your target groups further in terms of age: children, young people, older people, etc.? Why?

4. At-risk groups

- Do you define your target groups further in terms of high-risk categories such as smokers, people with high blood pressure, the unemployed, or those living on low incomes? If so, why? Have you examined the evidence leading to the identification of these at-risk groups?
- If your group includes people with highest health needs, for example, people living in areas of social deprivation with many health and social needs, do you know whether there is evidence that work focusing on specific issues will be successful? Would you get more health gain for your effort if you focused on whole populations rather than those most in need?

5. Effectiveness

- Have you any evidence that health promotion in your priority areas is likely to be effective?

See Chapter 7 for information on how to collect evidence.

- Have you any evidence that it will provide value for money?
- How could such evidence be collected?

6. Feasibility

- Is it feasible for you to spend time with your priority groups?
- Do you have access to these groups?
- Do you have credibility with these groups?
- Do you have the skills and resources to work with these groups?

7. Working with others

- Do you know what work is already being done with your target groups, by other health promoters/public health practitioners, community groups and voluntary organisations?
- Are you sure that your work will complement other public health activities that are going on and not be seen as duplication or interference?
- Does your work fit in with existing local and national public health strategies and plans for health promotion?
- Are there any local partnership groups already set up to address the needs of your target group?

8. Ethics

- Are there ethical aspects to your work which you need to consider?
- Is your work ethically acceptable to you?
- Will it be acceptable to your consumer groups?
- Will it be congruent with their values?
- How may the desired outcome affect their lives?

9. Add anything else you feel it is important to consider.

Now identify your top priority and add any other priorities.

PRACTICE POINTS

- You will have some scope for making choices about the range of health promotion and public health activities you undertake. These choices must be based on a careful assessment of public health needs. The starting point is to undertake a needs identification process.

- The views of users and receivers of services are paramount, therefore developing skills in gathering information directly from them is especially important.

- You can assess public health needs systematically by asking four key questions: What kind of need is it? Who decided that there was a need? What is the evidence for deciding that there is a need? What is the appropriate response to the need?

- Health promoters and public health practitioners have a duty to reassess priorities regularly through analysing, whether your activities are targeted effectively, are feasible, complement the work of other practitioners and are acceptable to local people.

- Priorities depend ultimately on the normative judgments of those involved. Best practice involves in-depth discussion on priority setting with other health promotion and public health practitioners and local people.

REFERENCES

Bradshaw, JR (1972). A taxonomy of social need in McLachlan, G. (ed), Problems and Progress in Medical Care. Oxford: Oxford University Press.

Department of Health 2010 Healthy Lives Healthy People: Our strategy for public health in England. London, The Stationery Office.

Department of Health 2012a The Public Health Outcomes Framework for England, 2013–2016. London, The Stationery Office.

Department of Health 2012b Health and Social Care Act. London, The Stationery Office. https://www.gov.uk/government/uploads/system/uploads/attachment_data/file/138257/A1.-Factsheet-Overview-240412.pdf.

Dorling D 2015 Unequal Health: The scandal of our time. Bristol, Policy Press.

Edwards N, Crump H, Dayan M 2015 Rationing in the NHS London. London, Nuffield Trust.

Food Standards Agency 2013 The food safety and hygiene (England) regulations 2013. http://www.legislation.gov.uk/uksi/2013/2996/made/data.pdf.

Friis, R, & Sellers, TA 2013 Epidemiology for public health. Practice Burlington Jones and Bartlett. Burlington: MA.

Hatchard S 2015 Postcode lottery for mental health talking therapies, BBC. http://www.bbc.co.uk/news/health-34583155.

Healthwatch England 2016 Making your voice count. London, Healthwatch England.

Imperial College London 2016 Institute for Global Health Innovation—Research centres. https://www.imperial.ac.uk/global-health-innovation/our-research/our-research-centres/.

Katz, Dl, Wild, D, Elmore, JG et al 2013 Jekel's epidemiology, biostatistics, preventive medicine, and public health (4th edn). London: Elsevier.

Macmillan 2014 6,000 cancer patients dying needlessly under a year due to postcode lottery. http://www.macmillan.org.uk/aboutus/news/latest_news/6,000cancerpatientsdyingneedlesslyunderayearduetopostcodelottery.aspx.

NHS Choices 2016 Personal health budgets. http://www.nhs.uk/choiceintheNHS/Yourchoices/personal-health-budgets/Pages/about-personal-health-budgets.aspx.

NICE 2016a Home care for older people, NICE quality standard [QS123] June 2016. https://www.nice.org.uk/guidance/qs123.

NICE 2016b Standards and Indicators. https://www.nice.org.uk/standards-and-indicators.

Office for National Statistics 2016 General Health in England and Wales: 2011 and comparison with 2001. https://www.ons.gov.uk/peoplepopulationandcommunity/healthandsocialcare/healthandwellbeing/articles/generalhealthinenglandandwales/2013-01-30.

Porter M 2016 Hull's Adult Health and Lifestyle Survey 2014. Public Health Sciences, Hull City Council. http://www.hullpublichealth.org/assets/PrevalenceSurveyMainReport2014v2.pdf.

Public Health England 2015 The NHS Atlas on Variations in Healthcare PHE. 2015. http://www.rightcare.nhs.uk/atlas/RC_nhsAtlas3_HIGH_150915.pdf.

Reading JSNA 2016. http://www.reading.gov.uk/article/9534/Obesity---adult-and-child.

Scriven A 2002 Report of the survey into the impact of recent national health policies on specialist health promotion services in England. London, Brunel University.

Scottish Government 2016 Citizens Panels. http://www.gov.scot/Topics/Built-Environment/regeneration/engage/HowToGuide/CitizensPanels.

Stephenson J 2016 Charity nurses warn of 'postcode lottery' in specialist children's care. Nursing Times 23 May 2016. http://www.nursingtimes.net/news/workforce/specialist-childrens-nurses-warn-of-postcode-lottery/7004943.article?blocktitle=Today%27s-headlines&contentID=19152.

West Berkshire JSNA 2015. http://info.westberks.gov.uk/CHttpHandler.ashx?id=37366&p=0.

Wokingham JSNA 2012. http://jsna.wokingham.gov.uk/living-and-working-well/overweight-and-obese-adults/.

World Health Organization 1986 The Ottawa charter for health promotion. Geneva, WHO.

World Health Organization 2016 World Health Statistics 2016: Monitoring health for the SDGs. Geneva, WHO.

WEBSITES

NICE for evidence and advice on what interventions works. http://www.nice.org.uk.

Office of National Statistics, for a wide range of people, population and community data. https://www.ons.gov.uk/peoplepopulationandcommunity.

An example of a PALs website. http://www.surreyandsussex.nhs.uk/patients-visitors/pals/.

SHEU lifestyle survey results. http://sheu.org.uk/content/page/lifestyle-surveys.

For local health and social statistics. http://www.neighbourhood.statistics.gov.uk.

WHO Global Health Observatory for international comparison data. http://www.who.int/gho/en/.

FACEBOOK

ONS for up to date notifications on national health and wellbeing statistics. https://www.facebook.com/ONS.

TWITTER

ONS notification of data and discussion of national (England and Wales) health statistics. https://twitter.com/ONS.

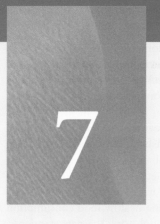

7

EVIDENCE AND RESEARCH FOR HEALTH PROMOTION AND PUBLIC HEALTH PRACTICE

CHAPTER CONTENTS

SUMMARY

This chapter covers particular aspects of knowledge and skills that enable you to draw on evidence, undertake research and use various techniques to inform and prioritise your health promotion and public health practice work. These include basing your work on evidence of effectiveness, using published research, doing your own small-scale research, getting value for money, audit and health impact assessment (HIA).

EVIDENCE-INFORMED HEALTH PROMOTION AND PUBLIC HEALTH PRACTICE

Evidence underpins international, national and local public health strategies and policies that health promoters and public health practitioners act on. Many of these policies charge those with a responsibility for promoting health to adopt an evidence informed approach to their work. For example, the national strategy in England, Healthy Lives, Healthy People White Paper, recommends interventions based on the evi-

dence of what works (DoH 2012). Health promoters and public health practitioners are therefore required to know how to access, assess and apply the evidence to practice.

This requires competencies in:

- critically appraising primary and secondary research
- knowledge of the hierarchy of evidence
- assessment of evidence of effectiveness of services, programmes and interventions, which impact on health
- conducting a literature review, which includes the use of electronic databases, defining a search strategy and summarizing results
- applying research evidence, evidence of effectiveness, outcome measures, evaluation and audit to influence public health programme interventions, services or development of practice guidelines
- interpreting and balancing evidence of effectiveness from a range of sources to inform decision making.

An evidence-informed approach provides a defence against the indiscriminate use of practices in situations which have no research-based legitimacy. Evidence-based health promotion and public health practice requires a culture where you openly share your experience and write up and publish or write a report on your work, which enables others to learn from your successes and failures. It uses the skills of reflective practice, thinking about what you do and questioning whether it is the right approach and offers value for money.

What Health Promotion and Public Health Interventions Work?

There can be a gap between evidence and practice. It is not always easy for health promoters and public health practitioners to keep up-to-date with new research findings or to apply research findings in their own particular situation. Attention needs to be given to how research findings can best influence and also emerge from practice, and the processes of disseminating and implementing health promotion and public health research. There are many published research studies that help to show which health promotion interventions work best. These are easily accessible on the internet at such sites as Cochrane (http://www.cochrane.org) and the main evidence-based internet site for health promotion and public health in England, the National Institute for Health and Care (NICE; http://www.nice.org.uk). In addition to Cochrane and NICE, Strategic Health Asset Planning and Evaluation (SHAPE) links national datasets for public health and maps local populations by medical conditions, age, socioeconomic and public health factors. SHAPE also enables interactive investigations by Local Area Teams, Providing Trusts, Clinical Commissioning Groups (CCGs), GP practices and Local Authorities and supports key policy initiatives such as Quality Innovation Productivity Prevention (QIPP) and Transforming Community Services (see SHAPE 2016).

In addition to online evidence websites, there are also many tools and models online to help you engage in an evidence-informed approach. For an example of one model, see Fig. 7.1 and its explanatory notes, and then undertake Exercise 7.1 to research further models.

Promoting health is complex and it is sometimes difficult to provide evidence of effectiveness for single interventions. This is because it often is not one intervention that produces results but a combination of public health activities of which you may be involved in just one. An example of this complexity is preventing childhood obesity, where the evidence is that a multifaceted approach is the most effective. A combination of interventions which range from working with the parents to develop healthy eating behaviour, including eating as a family, reducing television time and focusing on healthy nutrition; increasing exercise and improving children's emotional wellbeing (see Brown et al 2013 and Chapter 6 in Townsend and Scriven 2014 for an overview of evidence-informed approaches to combatting obesity); and ensuring healthy food consumption while children are at school using the new standards, which cover all food sold or served in schools in England (Department for Education 2015).

Research shows that for many health promotion issues, particularly around tackling the social determinants and inequalities in health, a more comprehensive, integrated approach that focuses both on attitudes and behaviours and changes to such things as the environment and legislative and fiscal policies is the most effective (see, for example, Jackson et al 2013 arguing for a comprehensive health-promotion approach to tackling the social determinants of health in the Americas).

Evidence may also not exist. The particular piece of work you plan to undertake may not have been done before, and indeed the particular set of circumstances in which you are working may be unique. So the best that can be done is to be aware of what the published research in related areas of work tells you, and to reflect on how what was learned might apply to your circumstances. Where evidence is not available, it is vital to ensure that you evaluate your work to add to the evidence base by drawing the evidence from your practice and disseminating the results.

It also helps to think carefully about what constitutes evidence in public health. Public health evidence often derives from cross-sectional studies, quasi-experimental studies and intervention evaluations rather than the gold standard of randomized controlled trials often used in clinical medicine. Study designs in public health sometimes lack a comparison group, and the interpretation of study results may have to account for different types of variables. As already pointed out, public health interventions are seldom a single intervention and are often alongside large-scale environmental or policy changes (Jacobs et al 2012). Evidence can also be drawn informally, with the views of local people and your own experience also constituting evidence. Your job as a health promoter or public health practitioner is to use your judgement to decide whether the evidence available applies to your clients and circumstances and, if so, how. GPs, for example, may quote a number of factors which they believe provide evidence that health promotion is effective including changes in the health or health behaviour of their patients over time.

However, formal sources of evidence are generally regarded as the most reliable, so you should plan carefully and evaluate or audit what you do. In this way you will be building up your own body of knowledge about what is effective.

Audit is discussed later in this chapter.

Finally, it is also important to bear in mind that your decision about whether to do a particular piece of health promotion work should also be based on ethical considerations. You could decide that it is your responsibility to intervene, even though you have little or no information about what might work. Health promotion is driven by both values and evidence, which are often intertwined. So there are two key questions: 'Do we think this ought to be done?' And 'Will it work?'

See Chapter 4 for more about values and ethics in health promotion.

Evidence-Informed Health Promotion and Public Health Practice

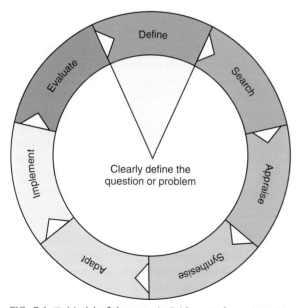

FIG. 7.1 ■ Model of the steps in Evidence-Informed Health Promotion and Public Health Practice. *(Source: National Collaborating Centre for Methods and Tools (NCCMT) 2016) the upside down writing in the synthesise and adapt sections of this figure*

Notes on Fig. 7.1 – The 7 Stage Model of Evidence-Informed Health Promotion and Public Health Practice

Stage 1. Define – Clearly define the issue or problem.

"Who is my target group? What is the issue we are dealing with? What interventions are we considering? What specifically are we trying to change or understand?"

The more specific you are in framing the question, the easier it will be to search for relevant information. Quantitative questions about the effectiveness of a possible intervention should include four elements: Population, Intervention, Comparison and Outcome (PICO). Quantitative questions about exposure should include: Population, Exposure, Comparison and Outcome (PECO). Qualitative questions should identify Population and Situation (PS).

Stage 2. Search – Efficiently search for research evidence.

"Where should I look to find the best available research evidence to address the issue?"

Your search strategy should first aim to locate the strongest quality and most relevant evidence. When searching for quantitative evidence (e.g. effectiveness of an intervention, health effects, cost effectiveness, etc.) some study designs (such as randomized trials or cohort studies) are considered stronger than others. It is important that the research design is the most appropriate to answer the question being asked.

Stage 3. Appraise – Critically and efficiently appraise the research sources.

"Were the methods used in this study good enough for me to be confident in the findings?"

Different types of public health questions will require distinct research designs. Critical appraisal tools can be applied to assess quality and relevance of each type of research question.

Stage 4. Synthesise – Interpret information and/or form recommendations for practice based on the relevant literature found.

"What does the research evidence tell me about the issue?"

Decipher the 'actionable messages' (i.e. clear recommendations or actions for practice) from the research evidence that you have reviewed. Base recommendations on the highest quality and most synthesized research evidence available.

Stage 5. Adapt – Adapt the information to a local context.

"Can I use this research with my client, community or population?"

Having developed 'actionable messages', you can now tailor those messages to ensure their relevance and suitability for the local community.

Stage 6. Implement – Decide whether (and plan how) to implement the adapted evidence in practice or policy.

"How will I use the research evidence in my practice?"

The implementation plan uses the adapted research evidence to create a tangible plan of action to create a change in practice, policy or to deliver a new programme. This step focuses on identifying how to use the adapted evidence in your local setting.

Stage 7. Evaluate – Assess the effectiveness of the implementation efforts.

"Did we do what we planned to do? Did we achieve what we expected?"

Evaluate the intervention (programme evaluation) if applicable and the implementation strategies (the knowledge translation strategy).

Source: NCCMT 2016

> ### EXERCISE 7.1
>
> Consider the model and the explanatory notes of the steps in evidence-informed health promotion and public health practice outlined in Fig. 7.1. Is this a suitable model for use in your health promoting practice? Undertake a search of the internet for other evidence-informed practice models and compare the one in Fig. 7.1 to these and to the planning model, Fig. 5.1, in Chapter 5. What are the similarities? What are the differences? Which is the best for your practice?

JUDGING THE COST EFFECTIVENESS OF PUBLIC HEALTH INTERVENTIONS

In addition to assessing the evidence, it is important to judge cost effectiveness. The funds available for prevention are limited and finite. As an example, local authorities in England are given a ring-fenced public health budget. So any spending in this area needs to be clearly justified on cost-effectiveness grounds. This says investment in public health should be based on the best available evidence of effectiveness from a range of sources. As a health promoter and public health practitioner, therefore, you need to think not only about evidence but also the question of whether you are getting value for money. Using robust methods to identify and interpret evidence, along with clear and transparent processes, will enable you to provide effective and cost-effective health promotion and public health interventions and services.

NICE (2016a) use a number of ways of assessing the cost effectiveness of public health promotion interventions:

Cost–Utility Analysis

Up to 2012, cost–utility analysis was NICE's main method of determining the cost effectiveness of public health interventions (NICE 2009). This method considers someone's quality of life and the length of life they will gain as a result of an intervention. The health benefits are expressed as quality-adjusted life years (QALYs). Generally, NICE considers that interventions costing the National Health System (NHS) less than £20,000 per QALY gained are cost effective. Those costing between £20,000 and £30,000 per QALY gained may also be deemed cost effective, if certain conditions are satisfied (for further details of this, see NICE 2012). NICE does not accept or reject interventions on cost-effectiveness grounds alone, but assessing effectiveness and cost effectiveness is an integral part of the way they develop guidance. Health promoters and public health practitioners are recommended to use the NICE guidance when planning interventions.

Cost–Consequences and Cost–Benefit Analyses

NICE now places more emphasis on cost–consequences and cost–benefit analyses when assessing public health interventions (NICE 2012). This dual approach aims to ensure all relevant benefits (health, non-health and community benefits) are taken into account. The idea is to help local authorities (and other organisations interested in improving people's health) better judge whether or not a public health intervention represents value for money. Cost-utility analysis is also used, when needed, to make comparisons with previous economic analyses, as well as to compare treatment and prevention programmes. It is important to note that it may take several years before the health benefits of some public health interventions start to have an impact, although the costs may need to be incurred in advance. Such interventions may be cost effective or even cost saving over the medium to long term and so would be recommended for funding on that basis, using the cost effectiveness threshold. However, they may not be deemed to be value for money in the short term in a simple return on investment analysis (cost savings minus cost of intervention). Where possible, NICE will report on costs and benefits over the short, medium and long term (NICE 2016a). See Case Study 7.1 for an example of cost effectiveness applied to a smoking cessation intervention.

AUDIT

Results of audits provide valuable evidence. Audit is the systematic examination of the operations of a service, followed by the implementation of recommendations to improve quality. Basically, an audit will scrutinise how the service carries out each stage of the planning/evaluation cycle, which are described in Chapter 5.

CASE STUDY 7.1

Smoking Cessation Interventions: Bury – A Case Study in Cost Effectiveness

To illustrate the costs of smoking and the savings that can be achieved by tackling tobacco use, NICE ran an analysis for Bury Metropolitan Borough Council using NICE's Return on Investment Tobacco Model (NICE 2016b). This tool was developed to help local decision making on tobacco control.

Bury has an adult population of around 141,000. Roughly 23% smoke and 33% are ex-smokers. The model estimated the total annual cost of smoking at £10.7 million, broken down as follows:

- Business – £3.7 million
- NHS – £6.8 million
- Second-hand smoke – £110,000.

Investing £751,692 in smoking cessation interventions for 1 year (equivalent to current practice) would achieve estimated gross savings of £321,579 overall in the first 2 years (this does not include the cost of implementation). Cost savings were broken down as follows:

Sector	Item	Number of events saved	Cost saving (£)
Business	Days lost from smoking (excludes smoking breaks)	1272	113,162
NHS	GP and other consultations, hospital admissions and prescriptions	2135	205,004

Sector	Item	Number of events saved	Cost saving (£)
	Passive smoking-related treatment	148	3322

The proposed package of interventions was compared with a range of background activities to combat tobacco use. The following are a selection of the outputs calculated using the tobacco return on investment tool.

Taking implementation into account, it was estimated that the package would:

- lead to a return of 63p, £1.46, £2.82 and £9.35 over 2 years, 5 years, 10 years and a lifetime respectively for each pound spent on the package of interventions. (This takes both NHS savings and the value of health gains into account.)
- cost an additional £21, £19, £15 and £1 per smoker over 2 years, 5 years, 10 years and a lifetime respectively after deducting the costs of the package. (Only NHS savings are considered here.)
- cost an additional £9 per smoker over 2 years but lead to a saving of £11, £43 and £199 per smoker over 5 years, 10 years and a lifetime respectively, net of the costs of the package. (This takes both NHS savings and the value of the health gains into account.)
- cost an additional £34,199 per QALY gained over 2 years, £12,574 per QALY gained over 5 years, £5040 per QALY gained over 10 years and £80 per QALY gained over a lifetime.

Source: NICE 2016c

Strengths and weaknesses will be revealed, and ways of overcoming weaknesses will be identified. Audit can involve either an internal review by the people responsible for delivering a service or scrutiny by an independent external auditor. For examples of audits relevant to health promotion and public health practice, such as the national audit of cardiac rehabilitation or patient's experience of diabetes services, see NHS Digital (2016).

You may wish to undertake your own audit of the service or intervention you are providing. The example of an audit cycle in Fig. 7.2 starts with the specification of standards or criteria, followed by the collection of data, the assessment of performance and the identification of the need for change and implementing the improvements.

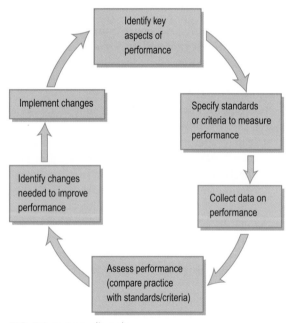

FIG. 7.2 ■ An audit cycle.

It is in the nature of cycles that you can, in practice, start anywhere. So you might start with collecting data on performance, assess performance and recommend the need to specify standards. The difficulty with auditing health promotion practice is that it is often embedded in other work. For example, audit of health promotion in clinical settings, such as cardiac rehabilitation, may involve scrutinising issues about relationships and communication,

all of which are vital to the quality of health promotion work but may not relate specifically to clinical audit. It is important to note that in the specifying of standards to measure performance these may be specified in legislation, such as those currently in England, with standards published as per Health and Social Care 2012, Section 250 (http://www.legislation.gov.uk/ukpga/2012/7/contents). For further reading on quality standards, see Chapter 8, section on working for quality.

Many of the tools described in the section on research in this chapter can also be used in audit. So, for example, you could use a telephone survey after discharge to collect data on performance to study the satisfaction of patients with health information and health education they received as inpatients. When telephoning patients, you would need to reassure them that participation in the survey is voluntary, and that their comments would be completely confidential. An example of the sort of questions you might ask are set out later in the chapter in Box 7.2.

Audit, Research and Evaluation

Audit, research and evaluation are complementary activities. Research is concerned with generating new knowledge and new approaches, which can be applied beyond the specific context of the research study (see Case Study 7.1 for an example of research designed to inform alcohol interventions). Evaluation involves making a judgement about one specific intervention, campaign or project, which is the focus of its concern. Audit seeks to improve the performance of a continuing service, such as an environmental health service or a midwifery service, through reviewing its practice. All three are crucial to the pursuit of evidence-informed health promotion and public health practice.

You should not need to do a detailed evaluation of everything you do, because you may be basing what you do on techniques and materials that have already been evaluated by others and form part of the published evidence. What you *should* do is to audit your health promotion practices regularly to check whether what you have planned and the techniques you have chosen are working properly. If you need further training in how to carry out an audit of your health promotion practice, it would be worth finding out about local opportunities for training in clinical audit as the basic concepts can be applied to health promotion and public health. Another area to pursue could be training related to measuring and improving quality or quality assurance. Quality cycles and audit cycles are very closely related, and the purpose of audit is to improve quality. You could also discuss local arrangements for performance appraisal with your manager (mechanisms for checking on and improving the performance of staff), professional development plans and supervision, because these are all related to audit.

See the section on working for quality in Chapter 8.

HEALTH IMPACT ASSESSMENT

Chadderton et al 2012 (citing Elliott et al 2010) define a HIA as a process through which different kinds of evidence, interests, values and meanings are brought into dialogue between relevant stakeholders (which might include politicians, health professionals and the general public) to understand and anticipate the effects of a proposed change on health and health inequalities in a given population. HIA recognises that social, economic and environmental factors, as well as genetic make-up and health care, make a difference to people's health. It is a systematic way of assessing what difference a policy, programme or project (often about social, economic or environmental factors) makes to people's health. For example, it has been used when public sector organisations have wanted to understand the effect of public health policies on transport, air quality, economic development, regeneration or housing.

The assessment can be carried out before, during or after a policy is implemented, but ideally it is done before so that the findings can inform decisions about whether and how to implement the policy. Key steps are to:

- select and analyse policies, programmes or projects for assessment
- profile the population who are likely to be affected and their characteristics
- identify the potential health impacts by getting information from the range of people who have an interest in the policy or who are likely to be affected by it
- evaluate the importance, scale and likelihood of the potential impacts
- report on and make recommendations for managing the impacts.

The World Health Organization (2016a) offer advice and tools on conducting HIAs and point out while there is no single agreed-upon method for undertaking HIA, from the many HIA guidance documents produced in WHO regions, a general pattern has emerged amongst methods and there is much overlap between them. Guidance documents often break HIA into four, five or six stages (WHO 2016b). The stages are outlined in Fig. 7.3.

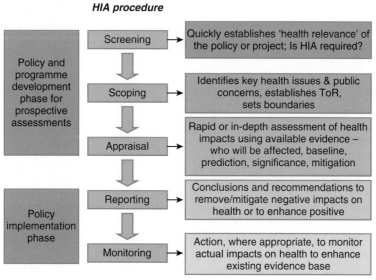

HIA procedure

FIG. 7.3 ■ Model of a HIA procedure from the World Health Organization. *(Source: WHO 2016a)*

The WHO argue that one of the key values of HIA is the ethical use of evidence and recommend that a wide variety of evidence should be collected and assessed, using appropriate and effective methods. This evidence will then provide the basis for evidence-informed advice to decision-makers, who can then make decisions based on the best available evidence before them. HIA considers several types of evidence, going beyond published reviews and grey literature to include the knowledge of stakeholders who are involved in or affected by a proposal (see WHO 2016b for more details on the type of evidence that can be drawn on for undertaking HIAs).

USING PUBLISHED RESEARCH

Health promoters and public health practitioners need to be well informed about health research and also how to *use* their knowledge of research findings to improve their practice. Familiarity with research findings can also give you arguments on which to base a case for more, different or better health promotion. Keeping abreast of current research evidence should be part of your everyday working practice.

How to Search the Literature

You may sometimes wish to find out about research on a particular topic, perhaps because you are proposing to introduce new health promotion work and want to know what has been shown to work best. For example, imagine you are a nurse working in cancer care and you are considering introducing a counselling service for women who are undergoing mastectomy (surgery to remove a breast, usually because of breast cancer). You want to know if research shows what the health promotion needs of these women are and how best to meet them. Where do you start?

First, you need to establish a research question. It pays to take time to discuss this with colleagues and you could also discuss it with someone who has recently had a mastectomy. What did she find helpful, and what was unhelpful?

Once you are clear about what you want to find out, list no more than six key words that feature in your question. The cancer care nurse might include the words 'mastectomy', 'needs' and 'counselling' in her list. Then write words that mean the same thing, or are similar in meaning, by each key word. For example, you might put 'breast removal' as an alternative to 'mastectomy' and 'advice' as an alternative to 'counselling'. These key words and their synonyms/alternatives will be helpful when you go to the library or search on the internet (for excellent guides to doing your literature search and finding information online, see Aveyard (2014) and Machi and McEvoy (2016)). In addition, many journal articles include a list of key words after the title, which will help you to know whether the article is likely to be of interest to you. When you have found a few references, you can start by reading the most recent one. This will provide you with more references. Once you are underway, the next problem is to avoid being swamped by information. Here again, your key words should be useful in stopping you from being side-tracked and in keeping your research question in mind.

It is important to keep records of what you read. There are many reference management software packages designed to help you store and retrieve references (see https://en.wikipedia.org/wiki/Comparison_of_reference_management_softwarehttp://en.wikipedia.org for a comparison of the different reference management software). For a book, you need to record:

- author's (or editor's) surname and initials
- year published
- title and subtitle
- edition, if not the first
- chapter, or numbers of pages, if you are only going to refer to part of the book
- place of publication
- publisher.

For articles in journals, you need to record:

- author's surname and initials
- year of publication
- title and subtitles of article
- journal title
- volume and part numbers
- the inclusive page numbers of the article
- date of publication.

If you are gathering research evidence that will be used to inform a health promotion decision or action, then the first thing you need to know when reading an article is whether it is a report of actual research or just a knowledgeable account of facts and opinions. The *abstract*, the summary paragraph at the start of an article, will quickly inform you why a study was done and the main findings. Research reports usually have the following format:

- Introduction – background to the study
- Literature review – critical summary of previous and related research
- Method – a description of how the study was carried out
- Results – the findings of the study
- Discussion – a discussion of the findings
- Conclusions – the implications of the findings
- References – all the studies and books referred to in the article.

You need to read research articles critically, using the following questions:

When was the research carried out? Although the article is recent, it could be reporting on research that was carried out some years previously and has been superseded by more up-to-date research.

Why was the research undertaken? Do you see the need for this research? Will it contribute new knowledge on the subject? Will this knowledge be useful in practice?

How was the research carried out? Did it use methods and tools that were likely to provide answers to the questions posed by the researchers? What type of research was carried out? For example, if the researchers wanted to find out what works in changing the behaviour of sedentary people with angina to cause them to take more exercise, then *experimental research* would be required. This is research that establishes a relationship between cause and effect, often through studying subgroups of people, where the *experimental* subgroup experiences the intervention under consideration and the *control* subgroup does not. Another type of research is *action research*. This is used to find out exactly how to implement changes, or solve problems, in a specific situation through watching and documenting in a systematic manner how the changes are introduced. (See Bowling (2014) for an excellent and detailed overview of research methods and methodological considerations in health research.)

Does the researcher draw reasonable conclusions from the results? This can be a difficult question to answer, especially if, for example, it is quantitative research and you are unfamiliar with statistics. If you are

not sure that you understand, it is important that you read more on critiquing research, particularly if you are going to be implementing the findings. (See Harris 2013 and Greenhalgh 2014 for more detail on critiquing research articles.)

How could or should this research affect health promotion practice or policy? Even if the research was not carried out in your specialty or particular area of work, it could have implications for them. For example, findings about how best to communicate with patients who are very anxious after a heart attack could be used to help improve communication with patients who have cancer.

Through asking these, and other, questions you should be able to come to a judgement about whether a piece of research is reliable. It should have:

- been carried out by competent researchers
- used an appropriate research design
- contained sound baseline data
- used a research instrument (such as a questionnaire) that has been piloted (tried and tested first to identify and correct any problems) and validated (tested to show that it really does measure what it was supposed to measure).

Some articles will have already critiqued the research for you in the form of 1) systematic reviews (see, as an example, De Kleijn et al (2015) for a systematic review of school-based smoking prevention interventions) or 2) meta-analysis (see Saba et al (2015) for a meta-analysis of smoking cessation interventions in community pharmacists). A systematic review answers a defined research question by collecting and summarising all empirical evidence that fits pre-specified eligibility criteria. A meta-analysis is the use of statistical methods to summarise the results of these studies. In both cases, articles that present systematic reviews or meta-analysis provide excellent sources of evidence on which to base public health practice and health promotion interventions.

DOING YOUR OWN SMALL-SCALE RESEARCH

While you can improve your effectiveness through examining research findings and considering whether and how they apply to your work, in certain situations you may wish to carry out research yourself. For example, you and a group of colleagues may have uncovered an unmet public health promotion need and you have agreed on funding for a study to look in more detail at the need and how it could best be met.

What is defined as *research* here is a planned, systematic gathering of information for the purpose of increasing the total body of knowledge. If you are inexperienced, it is important for you to read extensively and try to elicit help from an experienced researcher. The following information should help to guide you in your reading and also introduce you to the process of undertaking small-scale research.

The research process involves carrying out some specific tasks, which are set out in Box 7.1. Although the tasks will tend to be carried out in the sequence set out in the box, this is not always the case; for example, you may write parts of the research report incrementally as you go through each research task. You may have a much clearer idea about the purpose of the research *after* you have read the literature on other investigations in your area of interest.

BOX 7.1
RESEARCH TASKS

---

1. Define the purpose of the research (and set a research question, if appropriate).
2. Review the literature.
3. Plan the study and the method(s) of investigation.
4. Test the method by carrying out a pilot study.
5. Collect the information or data.
6. Analyse the information or data.
7. Draw objective conclusions based on the findings of the analysis.
8. Compile the research report.

The most important task in this list is the first one, as the kind of question you want to answer will form the basis of the whole project. For example, suppose you set the question 'What is the best way to encourage a group of university undergraduate students to engage in safer sex practices and to use condoms?' This question is concerned with ways of motivating and perhaps changing attitudes to encourage health-enhancing behaviour. The experts in this field are psychologists, so it is to the body of psychological research literature that you will turn to for soundly based principles. However,

you may instead be concerned to know which of a number of alternative effective ways to motivate students to use more condoms is best value for money. If so, you will want to look at cost-effectiveness studies and make use of the work of health economists. It is vital that you are clear about the practical reasons for engaging in this research. If you are very sure about why you are doing it, who will use the findings and for what purposes, then you are likely to come up with some useful answers. If you are distracted by interesting but irrelevant information, your research could be confused and therefore flawed.

Time spent on task 3, planning, is a good investment. If you are going to apply for funding, your planning must include investigating sources of funding and the particular interests of different potential funders. Many tasks can take longer than the initial estimate and you will need to allow plenty of time for consulting people; for example, to arrange interviews if this is part of the research. Ethical issues and the need to apply for permission from ethical committees if you are using human subjects must also be taken into account. Ethics committees in the NHS will evaluate the research proposal and will require additional information about issues such as confidentiality (for an example of an ethical framework for research, see Academy of Social Sciences, 2016). Facebook also has a page on research ethics which will give you up-to-date posts on research ethics issues. See the Facebook section in the references at the end of the chapter.

You will also need to consider ways of collecting the information you need. Any information collected needs to be *valid* and *reliable*. *Validity* means actually measuring what you purport to measure. For example, if you are attempting to measure the success of health education in encouraging a group of people to take more physical exercise, a valid measure would be directly to observe whether or not they spend more time on physical activities. Asking them to complete a written questionnaire may not give valid responses because research shows that people often respond to questions and questionnaires in ways they think the experts want them to. *Reliability* means that if the research is repeated using the same research instruments, it will give the same results (for details of how to test reliability and validity in social and health sciences research, see Bolarinwa 2015).

Basic Tools of Research

There are a number of basic tools used in health promotion research.

Questionnaires

These are useful when you want to collect information from relatively large numbers of people. Questionnaires should be kept as simple as possible, but this does not mean that they are easy to design. A great deal of care is needed in the formulation of questions to ensure that valid conclusions can be drawn from the answers. Questionnaires are most useful for collecting information that is quantifiable, such as factual knowledge. Advantages of questionnaires include: they can be answered anonymously and respondents may therefore be more truthful, and they can be given to a whole group of people at the same time, thereby using the respondents' and researcher's time effectively.

The questionnaire should always first be piloted on a small sample of people from the group for which it is intended. You will then be able to identify and redesign any questions that have been misinterpreted.

The response rate to questionnaires can be low, and you may need to think about the implications of this; for example, will the results really reflect the views of the target population? Also, some people may not want to complete the questionnaire and, even if they fill one in, they may do so casually without giving it careful thought.

You need to consider right from the start how the information collected will be analysed. Decisions about whether computer software programmes, such as the statistical programme SPSS (see Cunningham and Aldrich 2011), will be needed to analyse the information may affect the design of the questionnaire. Consultation with a statistician and/or an experienced researcher may be helpful at this point.

You have to put a lot of thought into the design of quantitative questionnaires by clarifying closed questions with defined ways of responding (such as tick boxes), so that they will give accurate results. Qualitative questionnaires with open questions can be more complicated to analyse.

Using online survey tools speeds up the process of generating data from questionnaires. For an excellent example of an online tool, see Survey Monkey (2016).

See Chapter 10, section on asking questions and getting feedback, for more about open and closed questions.

Personal Interviews

With face-to-face interviews, you can develop rapport and encourage people to talk more openly. You may find out things that you did not think to ask about but which are very relevant. The main advantage of personal interviews is that there is more scope for initiative by the interviewee. For example, the interviewee can seek clarification and may be able to express views and opinions more easily verbally than in writing. The disadvantage is that, unless you are very skilled, you may bias the response, that is, you may get the responses you want to get or expect to get. For example, asking 'You do feel better, don't you?' biases the answer towards 'Yes', whereas 'Do you feel better?' removes some of this bias.

Interviews can be one-to-one or with groups, face-to-face or by telephone. They can be organised through using pre-prepared questions (a *structured interview*) or allowed to flow more freely. At one extreme, you could design an interview schedule that looks like a questionnaire; at the other extreme, you might simply have three or four broad headings which you wish to discuss (a *semistructured interview*). Box 7.2 is an example of a telephone interview schedule. Special interview groups, such as focus groups, concentrate on a particular issue through focusing on pre-determined questions (see Bowling 2014 for more details on survey design, interviewing and conducting focus groups).

BOX 7.2

CLIENT SATISFACTION WITH A SMOKING CESSATION PROGRAMME: TELEPHONE SURVEY SCHEDULE

- Did the brochure on Quitting Smoking provide the information you were seeking?
- Do you now feel you have sufficient information to enable you to quit smoking?
- Were you able to discuss the barriers you feel will inhibit you from quitting?
- Who did you prefer to discuss things with? *Prompt: Was it the smoking cessation advisor or members of the group?*
- What else might the smoking cessation programme have offered that would have supported you in your efforts to quit smoking? *Prompt: Nicotine patches?*

Participant and Non-participant Observation

Observation can include observing behaviour, such as how well a person performs an exercise routine, and physiological observations, such as monitoring weight. *Participant observation* happens when the researcher is also actively involved in what is being observed, such as actively contributing to discussions in a meeting. *Non-participant observation* means that the researcher takes no part in what is being observed.

Advantages of participant observation are that the researcher may be more aware of what is going on including less tangible things such as the mood of a group of people. However, the researcher could have difficulty in making objective observations and may find it difficult to record what is happening, so that information could be lost. The nonparticipant researcher may find it easier to make objective observations and may be able to plan and record observations more easily. On the other hand, having an observer who does not participate can seem threatening; people might not open up or may not behave as they normally do. This could have a big effect on what is observed and invalidate the research (see Bowling 2014 for more details on observational methods in health research).

Sampling

If it is too expensive or time-consuming to collect information from the whole population or group you are interested in, then you need to select individuals so that you avoid getting a biased response. There are a number of sampling techniques which can be used to ensure that the sample is representative of the whole population.

Random sampling. This involves identifying people at random from the whole group. For example, imagine you are a practice nurse. Using the practice age–sex register you could decide at random on a number between 1 and 10 (say 5) and send out questionnaires to the 5th, 15th, 25th, 35th (and so on) person on the list.

Quota sampling. This uses your knowledge of a particular group to help set criteria about who to include in the sample. Criteria you might use include age, sex and ethnicity. Once the group has been divided into segments, using your criteria you can use a proportion from each segment for your sample. This ensures that people with certain characteristics are not over- or under-represented.

Convenience sampling. This means that researchers question the people they can get hold of at the time. This is biased but, accepting that it is very difficult to avoid bias altogether, it is important to decide whether the particular bias that has been introduced is acceptable. Bias should be discussed in any dissemination of the research (see Bowling 2014 for further discussion on sampling and research bias).

Case Study 7.2 provides an example of a public health research project designed to inform health promoting interventions. The summary of the research offers a clear indication of the research planning stages.

CASE STUDY 7.2

A Realist Evaluation Approach Towards Developing an Intervention to Address Harmful Drinking of 16- to 18-Year-Olds

---

Case study prepared by Michelle Hyatt, PhD research student, Southampton Solent University.

The study seeks to identify, implement and evaluate a cost-effective and sustainable intervention that will address harmful drinking of 16- to 18-year-olds in the city of Southampton (UK) and explore the social norms that reinforce hazardous drinking.

Background: Binge drinking or heavy episodic drinking is defined as drinking with a primary intention of becoming intoxicated in a short period of time, and it is becoming an increasing social norm

for young people (Litt & Stock 2011; Nicholls 2012). This is a co-funded study with Southampton Solent University and Southampton City Council in response to the individual and societal consequences of binge drinking with young people in Southampton. Between 2009 and 2015, alcohol-related hospital admissions in Southampton increased by 53% (Public Health England 2016). Furthermore, a UK government report highlighted that 1 in 10 boys and around 1 in 8 girls aged 15 to 16 years have unsafe sex after drinking alcohol (NI Direct Government

A Realist Evaluation Approach Towards Developing an Intervention to Address Harmful Drinking of 16- to 18-Year-Olds (Continued)

Services 2014). Other consequences of excessive alcohol use include the increased likelihood of being disorderly; more than 10,000 annual fines are issued in the UK to 16- to 19-year-olds, for being drunk and disorderly (NI Direct Government Services 2014).

Methodology: A Realistic Evaluation (Pawson & Tilley 1997) approach will be used as a methodological framework; this is an emerging theory-driven evaluation underpinned by realist inquiry. In contrast to other types of intervention evaluations where the outcomes are compared for participants who have and have not taken part (e.g. randomised controlled trials), a realistic evaluation seeks deeper insights from multiple viewpoints addressing 'what works, for whom, under what circumstances, and how' (Pawson & Tilley 1997).

The Realistic Evaluation will involve identifying the context, the mechanisms triggered and the outcome(s) of these mechanisms being triggered in a given context, in response to the intervention. Mechanism (M) involves the resources created by the intervention (e.g. incentives) and the participants' reaction to them; these can be motivating, cognitive and emotional responses. The term 'generative mechanism' (Pawson & Tilley 1997) refers to the underlying social or psychological drivers that cause the reasoning of participants, which is influenced by context. Context (C) can be seen as the backdrop or conditions of the intervention, which may change over time, for example, social (cultural/social norms, community values, social networks); economic (participants and programme); programme infrastructure (participants, staffing, geographical and historical context); political structures and other opportunities or barriers. Context impacts mechanisms; there is always an interaction between the two, and that interaction is what causes programme outcomes. Outcomes (O) from an intervention can be intended, unintended and intermediate, and they are all important in understanding how interventions work. CMO Configurations (CMOCs) are used to generate causal explanations about intervention

outcomes: context + mechanism = outcome. In summary, realism evaluates X (intervention) and alters context (C) by creating new resources, which triggers mechanism (M), producing intended and unintended outcomes (O) (e.g. behaviour change). A CMOC can explain the entire intervention and/or components of it.

Study design: The study has been designed into two phases. The first phase is to understand the intervention need. A realist synthesis and qualitative analysis will be used to develop an initial programme theory, as suggested by Pawson (2006). The programme theory will describe how an intervention is expected to lead to its outcomes. The realist synthesis will review relevant literature to provide a transferable evidence-based framework of successful interventions and how they can work. The review will include studies that can conceptually contribute to developing initial programme theories such as 'social norms and risk taking' with young people.

Qualitative data will then be collected from focus groups to understand the factors coming together to cause young people to binge drink in Southampton. Purposive sampling will be used to provide qualitative data from a wide socioeconomic background and an equal representation of males/females aged 16 to 19. This sampling will inform the programme theory by identifying 'what works, for whom, under what circumstances, and how' (Pawson & Tilley 1997).

Theories of change will be used to further inform the programme theory. The Theory of Planned Behaviour (TPB; Ajzen 1985) has been selected as it identifies social norms as a key motivator in behaviour. Social norms are also motivators towards risky behaviour and other behaviours linked to alcohol misuse (Moreira et al 2009; Neighbors et al 2007). The Action Theory Model of Consumption (ATMC; Bagozzi 2010) has also been selected as it is a micro model of consumption. Young people's drinking is regarded as consumer motivated (Brain et al 2000; Measham 2004) and furthermore the alcohol indus-

Continued on following page

CASE STUDY 7.2

A Realist Evaluation Approach Towards Developing an Intervention to Address Harmful Drinking of 16- to 18-Year-Olds (Continued)

try targets young people (McCreanor et al 2005). The initial programme theory developed in Phase 1 will provide a framework for the design of an intervention, which will be implemented to work alongside local services within Southampton.

The second phase of this study will involve the implementation and realistic evaluation of the intervention. The context, mechanisms and outcomes of the initial programme theory(s) will be refined and refuted and the intervention shaped accordingly. The final programme theory will describe the intervention in terms of 'what works, how, why, for whom, to what extent and in what circumstances' (Wong et al 2013). A final report of the intervention will detail how the programme theory was employed in the design of the intervention. This will include details on how theory constructs (mechanisms) led to the selection of specific features of the intervention and how these can be tailored to different populations (such as ages or locations) or contexts (Michie et al 2010). Furthermore, data can be drawn from the evaluation and synthesised to provide a final analysis on matters such as cost-effectiveness, lessons learnt, social return on investment and multi-criteria analysis (Kaplan 2016).

REFERENCES FOR CASE STUDY 7.2

Ajzen I 1985 From intentions to actions: A theory of planned behavior. In Kuhl J, Beckman J Eds., Action-control: From cognition to behavior (pp. 11–39). Springer, Heidelberg.

Bagozzi RP 2000 The poverty of economic explanations of consumption and an action theory alternative. Managerial and Decision Economics 21(3-4):95–109.

Brain K, Parker H, Carnwath T 2000 Drinking with design: young drinkers as psychoactive consumers. Drugs: Education, Prevention And Policy 7(1):5–20.

Kaplan J 2016 Better evaluation. http://betterevaluation.org/search/site/cost-effectiveness.

Litt DM, Stock ML 2011 Adolescent alcohol-related risk cognitions: the roles of social norms and social networking sites. Psychology of Addictive Behaviors 25(4):708.

Mccreanor T, Barnes HM, Gregory M, Kaiwai H, Borell S 2005 Consuming identities: Alcohol marketing and the commodification of youth experience. Addiction Research & Theory 13(6):579–590.

Measham F 2004 The decline of ecstasy, the rise of 'binge' drinking and the persistence of pleasure. Probation Journal 51(4):309–326.

Michie S, Prestwich A, Bruin MD 2010 Importance of the nature of comparison conditions for testing theory-based interventions: reply. Health Psychology 29(5):468–470.

Moreira MT, Smith A, Foxcroft D 2009 Social norms interventions to reduce alcohol misuse in university or college students. Cochrane Database Syst Rev 3.

Neighbors C, Lee CM, Lewis MA, Fossos N, Larimer ME 2007 Are social norms the best predictor of outcomes among heavy-drinking college students? Journal of Studies on Alcohol and Drugs 68(4):556–565.

NI Direct Government Services 2014 Young People and Alcohol: What Are The Risks? https://www.nidirect.gov.uk/articles/young-people-and-alcohol-what-are-risks.

Nicholls J 2012 Everyday, everywhere: alcohol marketing and social media – current trends. Alcohol and Alcoholism 47(4):486–493.

Pawson R 2006 A realist perspective. London, SAGE Publications.

Pawson R, Tilley N 1997 Realistic evaluation. London, SAGE Publications.

Public Health England. LAPE data_2009-10 to Q3 2015-16. http://www.lape.org.uk/data.html.

Webb T, Joseph J, Yardley L, Michie S 2010 Using the internet to promote health behavior change: a systematic review and meta-analysis of the impact of theoretical basis, use of behavior change techniques, and mode of delivery on efficacy. Journal of Medical Internet Research 12(1):e4.

Wong G, Greenhalgh T, Westhorp G, Buckingham J, Pawson R 2013 RAMESES publication standards: meta-narrative reviews. BMC Medicine 11(1):1–15.

The Research Report

See also the section on report writing in Chapter 8 and the section on written communication in Chapter 10.

The final stage of your research will be to produce a written report, which will disseminate your findings. People who read the report may be interested in assessing the validity of the findings for themselves, in repeating the research in similar circumstances and avoiding any pitfalls, or in applying the research findings in the context of commissioning or providing health promotion services. So the report should be written with the objective of helping readers to use it in these ways. You may need to consider producing more than one version of the report for different groups of readers; for example, a two-page summary for community groups and a full report for your health promotion professional and managers.

The contents of your research report may include the information set out in Box 7.3, although not every point will be applicable to a particular report, which should be written with the needs of the readers in mind.

Finally, in a field like health promotion and public health practice, interpretation of research data is a complex matter, often because of the multifaceted determinants of health and wellbeing. It is extremely important that any health promotion and public health research is methodologically sound, ethically conducted, unbiased and objective in its interpretation.

BOX 7.3
CHECKLIST OF THE CONTENTS OF A RESEARCH REPORT

- **Abstract** (concise summary of the research including key results and conclusions).
- **Background** (statement about the purpose of the research, the background, the reasons for carrying out the research and the questions to be answered).
- **Literature review** (critiquing other research in the field).
- **Methods**:
  A description of the methods used for collecting the information and the reasons for selecting these methods.
  A description of the population sample studied, the sampling methods and response rates.
  A discussion of the ethical implications.
  Data analysis methods and the reasons for selecting these methods.
  A description of the pilot study and any changes that were made as a result.
- **Results** (all appropriate data displayed clearly).
- **Discussion** (analysis of the findings, stating clearly the limitations of the study).
- **Conclusion** (with recommendations for further research).
- **References** (listing source material).

Poor research is worse than no research because it wastes resources and misleads.

PRACTICE POINTS

- It is important to identify how your health promotion and public health practice work contributes to local and national strategies. Your effectiveness depends not only on what you do but also on how well your work complements that of other health promoters and public health practitioners.
- All health promoters and public health practitioners have a duty to appraise evidence and to base their work on evidence of effectiveness where it exists.
- Doing research involves specialised skills, and you should aim to develop the appropriate competencies that the particular type of research requires.
- You need to consider whether you are getting value for money through using the ways of thinking developed in health economics.
- All health promoting and public health services should regularly undertake audit: take stock of how they operate and identify how things can be improved.
- If your work involves making or implementing policies that affect people's health, health impact assessment may be a useful tool.

REFERENCES

Academy of Social Sciences 2016 ESRC Framework for Research Ethics. https://www.acss.org.uk/news/esrc-framework-for-research-ethics/.

Aveyard H 2014 Doing a literature review in health and social care, 3rd edn. Berkshire, Open University Press.

Bolarinwa OA 2015 Principles and methods of validity and reliability testing of questionnaires used in social and health science researches. Nigerian Postgraduate Medical Journal 22(4):195–201.

Bowling A 2014 Research methods in health: investigating health and health services, 4th edn. Berkshire, Open University Press.

Brown RE, Willis AT, Aspinall N, Hunt C, George J, Rudolf M 2013 Preventing child obesity: a long-term evaluation of the HENRY approach. Community Practitioner 86(7):23–7.

Chadderton C, Elliot E, Hacking N, Shepherd M, Williams G 2012 2013 Health impact assessment in the UK planning system: the possibilities and limits of community engagement. Health Promotion International http://dx.doi.org/10.1093/heapro/das031.

Cunningham JB, Aldrich JO 2011 Using SPSS: an interactive hands-on approach. London, Sage.

De Kleijn MJ, Farmer MM, Booth M, Motala A, Smith A, Sherman S, Assendelft WJ, Shekelle P 2015 Systematic review of school-based interventions to prevent smoking for girls. Systematic Reviews 4:109.

Department for Education 2015 School food in England: departmental advice for governing bodies. London, Department for Education.

Department of Health 2012 Healthy Lives, Healthy People. London, The Stationery Office.

Elliott, E, Harrop, E, Bennett, P, Calmann, K, Curtis, S, Smith, D 2010. Contesting the Science: Public Health Knowledge and Action in Controversial Land Developments. In Bennett, P, Risk Communication in Public Health. 2nd Ed. Oxford: Oxford University Press.

Greenhalgh T 2014 How to read a paper: the basics of evidence-based medicine, 5th edn. New Jersey, Wiley-Blackwell.

Harris S 2013 How to critique journal articles in the social sciences. London, Sage.

Health and Social Care Act 2012 Section 250. http://www.legislation.gov.uk/ukpga/2012/7/contents or London, Stationery Office.

Jackson S, Birn A, Fawsett SB, Poland B, Shultz JA 2013 Synergy for health equity: integrating health promotion and social determinants of health approaches in and beyond the Americas. Rev Panam Salud Publica 34(6):473–480.

Jacobs JA, Jones E, Gabella BA, Spring B, Brownson RC 2012 Tools for implementing an evidence-based approach in public health practice. Preventing Chronic Diseases 9:110324. http://dx.doi.org/10.5888/pcd9.110324http://dx.doi.org/10.5888/pcd9.110324.

Local Government Association 2013 Money well spent? Assessing the cost effectiveness and return on investment of public health interventions. London, LGA.

Machi LA, McEvoy BT 2016 The literature review: six steps to success, 3rd edn. California, Corwin (Sage).

National Collaborating Centre for Methods and Tools McMasters University 2016 Evidence-informed public health. http://www.nccmt.ca/professional-development/eiph.

NHS Digital 2016 Statistics. https://www.gov.uk/government/statistics?departments%5B%5D=health-and-social-care-information-centre.

NICE 2009 Methods for the development of NICE public health guidance, 2nd edn. London, NICE.

NICE 2012 Methods for the development of NICE public health guidance, 3rd edn. London, NICE.

NICE 2016a NICE's approach to assessing public health interventions. https://www.nice.org.uk/advice/lgb10/chapter/judging-the-cost-effectiveness-of-public-health-activities.

NICE 2016b Tobacco return on investment tool. https://www.nice.org.uk/about/what-we-do/into-practice/return-on-investment-tools/tobacco-return-on-investment-tool.

NICE 2016c Smoking cessation interventions: Bury - a case study in cost-effectiveness. https://www.nice.org.uk/advice/lgb10/chapter/judging-the-cost-effectiveness-of-public-health-activities#smoking-cessation-interventions-bury---a-case-study-in-cost-effectiveness.

Public Health England 2016 Public health outcomes frameworks. http://www.phoutcomes.info/. Accessed 08 July 2016.

Saba M, Diep J, Saini B, Dhippayom T 2014 Meta-analysis of the effectiveness of smoking cessation interventions in community pharmacy. Journal of Clinical Pharmacy and Therapeutics 39(3):240–247.

SHAPE 2016 Who would benefit from SHAPE. https://shape.phe.org.uk/who_is_shape_for/index.asp.

Survey Monkey 2016 Likert do it yourself research surveys. https://www.surveymonkey.co.uk/mp/online-research/.

Townsend N, Scriven A 2014 Obesity. London, Churchill Livingstone.

World Health Organization 2016a Health impact assessment. http://www.who.int/hia/en/.

World Health Organization 2016b Tools and methods: how to undertake an HIA. http://www.who.int/hia/tools/en/.

WEBSITES

Cochrane – for evidence reviews and trials. http://www.cochranelibrary.com/.

NICE – for evidence recommendation and protocols for practice. http://www.nice.org.uk.

NHS Digital for information, data and IT systems for health and social care, including audit results. https://www.gov.uk/government/organisations/health-and-social-care-information-centre.

FACEBOOK

Research ethics posts. https://www.facebook.com/ResearchEthics/.

TWITTER

Official twitter feed of the NICE. https://twitter.com/NICEcomms?ref_src=twsrc%5Egoogle%7Ctwcamp%5Eserp%7Ctwgr%5Eauthor.

YOUTUBE

NICE recommendations. https://www.youtube.com/c/niceorguk/videos.

BLOGS

Public Health Matters, the official blog of Public health England, for evidence and data on health promotion and public health interventions. https://publichealthmatters.blog.gov.uk/.

8

SKILLS OF PERSONAL EFFECTIVENESS

CHAPTER CONTENTS

SUMMARY

This chapter is about developing skills to effectively manage your health promotion and public health practice work. A number of skills are covered including managing information, report writing, time management, project management, change management and finally working for quality. Case studies and practical exercises are included to illustrate and give the context in which health promotion and public health practice skills are applied.

Working effectively in health promotion and public health requires a clear view of your aims and plans and the necessary management competencies to implement your goals.

See also Chapters 5, 6 and 7 for details on planning for health promotion and public health practice.

MANAGEMENT SKILLS IN HEALTH PROMOTION AND PUBLIC HEALTH PRACTICE

It is not easy to define what management is, but in general terms it is about adopting practices which ensure

effectiveness and efficiency in your work. *Effectiveness* means producing effects and accomplishing your goals. Being efficient means producing results with little wasted effort or resources. It's the ability to carry out actions quickly. However, by being efficient, you may not necessarily be achieving effectiveness, so it is important to establish the correct balance.

A comprehensive introduction to management and project management is beyond the scope of this book, but for further details you may wish to consult Knight (2016) and Graham (2015) for a beginner's guide to project management and Broddy (2013) for a general introduction to management.

Some aspects of management have already been covered, such as setting priorities and planning. A number of other managerial skills that you will need to be effective and efficient as a health promoter and public health practitioner are outlined in this chapter. However, it is important to emphasise that possessing these skills will not automatically make you effective and efficient. Other factors also influence this including:

- how well you integrate ethical principles into your basic everyday work; how you exercise your *responsibility* as a health promoter. 'Response-ability' is your ability to choose your response and is a product of your conscious choice, based on values, rather than a reaction to your circumstances. (For further reading on ethics and values in health promotion and public health, see Chapter 4.)

■ the people you work with. Your effectiveness and efficiency are limited or enhanced by the competencies and motivation of those you work with: for example, receptionists, secretaries, colleagues and others within and outside your organisation.

■ your organisation. Both the structure and culture of your organisation will influence what you are able to achieve.

■ the wider world. The state of the economy, government legislation, the organisation of local government and the impact of social trends are just a few examples of factors in the world outside your organisation that influence how effective you can be.

This book is designed to increase your awareness of these wider influences on your work, as well as to develop your own competencies.

This chapter covers some key aspects of personal effectiveness which will help you to manage health promotion and public health practice.

MANAGING INFORMATION

Whether you keep information on computer and/or a manual filing system it is easy to be swamped by documents and papers, so keep only what is essential and cannot be kept by someone else or in another existing system.

Think about who else collects information in your workplace and how they store it. Is there a central filing system? Does it work? Which information could and should you keep centrally? Undertake Exercise 8.1 to enable you to identify what information you need to store.

Principles of Effective Information Systems

When reviewing or setting up your information system, it is useful to keep reminding yourself of three basic principles:

1. Keep it simple! Systems are only as effective as the people who put in and take out the information.

EXERCISE 8.1
What Information Do You Need To Store?

Make a list of all the types of information you collect at present (e.g. minutes of meetings, project reports) and analyse it by asking yourself the following questions about each one:

1. Do I need to keep this information?
2. How easy is it for me to find the information when I need it?
3. Could someone else, or another information system, keep the information for me?
4. Who else might need access to this information? How easy would it be for them to find it?
5. How could this information best be stored (e.g. electronic files on the organisation's website or portal)?

The simpler the system, the more likely it is that busy people will use it correctly.

2. Do not devise any more systems than are absolutely necessary.
3. Organise systems so that anyone who might want to use them can easily understand them.

WRITING REPORTS

Important information is often conveyed through written reports. For example, you are likely to need to write a report on plans for health promotion or an evaluation report on a specific project. You may need to write reports for your manager or formal reports for committees. Written reports are likely to be read when you are not there, so there is no immediate feedback about whether the key points have been understood. To reduce the danger of being misunderstood, good skills in preparing and writing reports are essential. (See Chapter 10, section on written communication skills.)

Work through the following stages each time you prepare and write a report:

Stage 1: Define the purpose

To help to clarify the purpose, complete the following sentence: 'As a result of reading this report, the reader will ...' What?

The purpose could be to inform, to influence decision making, to initiate a course of action or to persuade. Whatever it is, keep it clearly in mind throughout all the later stages.

Stage 2: Define the readers

Identify the readers and consider them at all stages. Direct the report to the needs and interests of the readers. What do they already know about the subject? How much time do they have for reading? What kind of style is appropriate, for example, formal or informal?

Stage 3: Prepare the structure

Decide on the structure of the report. A report normally contains the following sections:

- Title – this should accurately describe what the report is about.
- Origins – for example, the author's name, occupation, work base and date.
- Distribution list – it is a great help to readers if they know who else has seen the report. They may detect that someone vital has not received a copy.
- Contents list – a long report will need a contents list showing the main sections of the report and the pages on which the reader can find them. This is not necessary for short reports.
- Summary – this is vital for all except the very shortest of reports (less than a page or two). It helps the reader if the summary is easy to find at the beginning of the report. Remember that busy people will often read only the summary (and perhaps the conclusions and recommendations) or at least read the summary first to decide whether it is worth spending time reading any more. So the summary needs to set out the essence of the report clearly and concisely. It is sometimes referred to as the executive summary.
- Introduction – this sets the context for the report, for example, why the work was undertaken.
- The main body of the report – this will be the bulk of the report. You need to break up the content into sections and subsections, all with clear headings. Headings should be signposts to help the reader to see a route through the document and have an overview just by skimming through the headings. Sections need to be ordered in a way which will be logical for the reader. It may help to organise material into sections by writing all the possible headings and subheadings down,

then move them around until you are satisfied that they are in the most logical order. You could use a numbering system for each section, heading and subheading (e.g. 1, 1.1, 1.1.1).
- Conclusions – summarises the conclusions which can be clearly drawn from the information in the report.
- Recommendations – these relate to the future and summarise any changes needed.
- References – putting any references at the end makes the report easier to read.
- Appendices – a misused feature of some reports, to be avoided unless really necessary. Ask yourself 'What information will most of my readers need the first time they read this report?' If they need this information straight away, put it in the main body of the report.

Stage 4: Write the report

Tackle the various sections in the order that makes it easiest. For example, it may be easiest to write the detailed body of the report first, then summarise the information, then discuss the information, then draw your conclusions, then set out your recommendations, then write the summary of the report and lastly finish it off with the title, contents list, origin, distribution list and other essential details.

Stage 5: Review and revision

After the draft report has been produced, review it and revise as necessary. Make sure pages are numbered and check that sections and subsections are correctly numbered. It is a good idea to get a colleague to proofread the report, someone with good report writing skills who will give constructive comments.

Stage 6: Final check

Always do a final check for writing and typing errors, spelling and other mistakes. It can be helpful to ask someone who has not seen the report before to check it for typing and layout errors. For ideas on how to prepare, write and present reports, see Bowden (2011). There are also many examples of reports on health, health promotion and public health practice project on the internet. See the webpages in the references at the end of this chapter for suggestions.

1. Devise a recording format that suits you, based on the following example.

Then photocopy or print out a supply of the sheets. Use as many sheets as necessary each day. Remember to include any work you do away from your organisation, for example, at home.

If you discover that particular activities, for example, telephone interruptions, are causing a problem, then make a detailed log of what happens each time. *Do this immediately* – do not leave it until the end of the day. Keep the diary for at least a week. If none of your weeks are typical, you will need to keep the log for several weeks.

Using codes will save you time. For example, you could use M for meetings, I for interruptions, P for phone calls and IP for phone interruptions.

Time diary

Day _____   Date _____   Page no._____

Activity   Time spent   Comments

_____   _____   _____

_____   _____   _____

_____   _____   _____

2. Now analyse how you used your time.

Each week, analyse your use of time by answering the following questions:

- How did you actually use your time compared with how you planned to use it?
- How much of your time do you spend on different activities, such as dealing with emails? Does this reflect the importance of the different activities? Important activities are those that help you to achieve your objectives.
- Which jobs did not get done? Does it matter? Did you finish all the *important and urgent* jobs?
- How much time do you lose through interruptions? What sort of interruptions (e.g. email notifications)?
- How much of your time is spent on other people's work?
- Do you do the right job at the right time? Most people have a time of day when they work best. Do you use this time for your most important work?

3. Now plan how to improve your time management.

Some of the changes you could make will be obvious. For example:

- You discover that jobs started early in the morning tend to get completed quickly. So you decide in the future to do your most important work at this time.
- You note that you spend about 2.6 hours each day reading and answering emails. You decide to experiment with techniques to cut down this time. See Exercise 8.3 that follows.
- You discover that urgent jobs are generally done but important long-term projects tend to be neglected. You decide to make realistic plans to ensure that long-term projects are done.
- What else can you do?

For one week, try the following seven steps to try and cut down on email interruptions:

1. Unsubscribe from email newsletters that are not relevant to your work.
2. Turn off all email notifications.
3. Schedule a time each day for dealing with emails.
4. When sending emails, use the subject line to indicate all action required, for example, For Your Information (FYI; so people know it is information only); Action Required by...and Date or To Do By...and DATE; No Response Required (NRR; to avoid getting polite responses such as 'thank you' or 'Looks interesting').
5. Keep the emails you send really short, five sentences maximum or fewer.
6. If you don't have one, set up a logical filing system for emails.
7. Keep your inbox clean by deleting or filing all emails so you start each day with a clean inbox.

At the end of the week, assess how much time you can save by being efficient with your emails. See Kruse (2015) for more time-saving ideas for emails and time management in general.

USING TIME EFFECTIVELY

How well organised and effective are you at your work? The following paragraphs should give you some ideas about how to improve your effectiveness by looking at how you use your time. Time is an expensive resource and the one that some may find the hardest to manage. First of all, you need to know where your time goes. Exercise 8.2 and the next section are about analysing and improving the use of your time and scheduling your public health work appropriately.

Time Logs and Time Diaries

A time log involves keeping a record of how you spend your time at regular intervals, which may be as often as every 5 or 10 minutes. It is useful if you wish to know exactly how you are using your time on an activity that seems to be taking longer than you think it should and can help you to pinpoint the source of the problem. But keeping a log is time-consuming itself, so it is really worthwhile only if a particular activity is causing you problems.

If you want to know more about how you generally use your time, you can keep a time diary. This records how you have spent your time day-by-day and should take only a few minutes to fill in at the end of each day. If you have a short memory, you might find it better to fill in your diary more frequently, say at the end of the morning and at the end of the afternoon, or at any other convenient break between blocks of work.

Scheduling Your Work

See Chapter 6, section on setting health promotion and public health priorities.

Health promoters and public health practitioners can find that they have to do far more than their time permits, and that they are faced daily with too many requests and demands. This means that, first and foremost, they must be very clear about their priorities. Second, they must be assertive about saying 'no' to requests to take on nonpriority tasks. Third, they need to develop skills of organising time and scheduling work to ensure that priority work gets done.

Scheduling work into the time available involves three steps:

1. Identify how long you need to spend on a job. This depends on:

- the nature of the activity, for example, whether it is possible to reduce the time allowance without endangering people or public health outcomes
- how important the job is. If it is unimportant, it does not merit a large investment of your time. Ask yourself 'What am I employed for? Will doing this job contribute to my main aims and objectives?' If not, it is unimportant. If the job is important, it merits a large investment.

2. Identify how soon you need to have the job completed. This depends on how urgent it is. Urgent jobs are ones that have imminent deadlines. If an urgent job can be completed quickly, deal with it right away. That means it will not interfere with you getting on with the most important jobs.

3. Plan when the work will be done. This involves the following steps:

- Break the job or project down into manageable parts. If the job/project is big or complex, or parts of it are boring, try setting aside regular, small amounts of time to complete specific bits. Dividing it into manageable segments will help you to see that you are progressing.
- Estimate how long each part will take to complete. It can be difficult to estimate how long it will take you to complete a particular task, but an informed guess will at least help you to be more realistic in future. Here are some suggestions that may help:
  - Use your experience from similar jobs
  - Consult colleagues who have experience in doing the job
  - Build in some contingency time
  - Keep a note of how long the tasks actually take so that you can make a better estimate next time.
- Schedule in your diary or organiser (for example, Google Calendar) when the work will be done. You may find that you need to reschedule daily to take account of changing priorities. The important thing is to ensure that the key tasks you need to undertake are scheduled to allow enough time for their completion. There are many tools and tips on effective time management on the internet (see the webpages in the references section for examples).

MANAGING PROJECT WORK

Planning and managing a health promotion or public health project can be different from other managerial activities. You must turn something that does not yet exist into reality and control its progress so that it delivers effectively and efficiently. The most obvious thing about a health promoting project is that it has a particular (unique) purpose, which may be encapsulated in its name, such as 'Bromley Active Lifestyles Project' or 'Portsmouth Needle Exchange Project'. It is probably most useful to think of a project as an instrument of change, which, when it is successfully completed, will have made an impact as defined in its aims and objectives.

Another key aspect of projects is that they are usually time-limited; they have clearly identifiable start and finish times. Projects vary enormously in their scope. Small projects can last only a few days and involve activities by a single person; large projects can involve many people (and indeed many agencies) and last for several years.

All projects, however, have the same basic underlying structure and go through a number of stages, as set out in Box 8.1.

BOX 8.1
THE STAGES OF A HEALTH PROMOTION PUBLIC HEALTH PROJECT

1. The start is the most important stage of any project and covers areas such as setting the overall aims, gaining approval and the allocation of a budget. It will set the foundations for the lifetime of the project.
2. Specification involves defining the detailed objectives of the project (i.e. what the outcomes will be and the targets for delivering these outcomes in terms of quantity, quality and timing).
3. Design stage is when the 'what' is translated into 'how'. It may take the form of detailed plans.
4. In the implementation stage, the plans are put into operation. It is important to note that the end of implementation is not the end of the project.
5. The evaluation, review and final completion stage will be marked by delivery of the final report, which includes evaluation of the findings and the details of a post-implementation review. This review should take place some time after the end of the implementation stage, so that it is possible to include data on the long-term outcomes of the project.

These stages are, of course, very similar to the basic planning and evaluation cycle that was described in Chapter 5, and you should read the present section in conjunction with Chapter 5. The difference is that when you are delivering an on-going service, rather than a one-off project, the cycle repeats itself.

See Chapter 5, planning and evaluating health promotion and public health practice.

Because projects vary so much in terms of their scale and length of life it is particularly important that they are planned systematically. It is also vital to understand how the project contributes to the wider strategic plans of the organisation concerned.

See Chapter 7, section on linking your work into broader public health research and evidence.

Starting Health Promotion and Public Health Projects

A project will start with a proposal or written document, which can take a number of forms, such as 'terms of reference' or 'report of a feasibility study'. The key elements that must be described in this document include the following:

- Who is proposing to carry out the project, for example, a National Health Society (NHS) trust or voluntary organisation.
- Who is the purchaser or commissioner of the project, for example, the local authority.
- The aims and outcomes of the project.
- The scope of the project, for example, who will use or receive it, the setting in which it will be delivered and which departments, agencies and people will be affected.
- The costs of the project in terms of staffing, buildings, equipment and other resources.
- The project stages or milestones with timescales.
- Methods and standards: the use of any particular techniques or methods and the adoption of any recognised quality standards.
- Roles and responsibilities of participants in the project (especially important when the project is commissioned by a partnership of a number of agencies).

Detailed Planning

For anything but the very smallest of projects, you will need to develop a detailed plan of each stage immediately before you enter it. Typically, one of the last tasks in the planning of a stage will be planning the next stage. The Gantt chart, named after Henry Gantt, the man credited with its invention (http://www.ganttchart.com), is a tool to use for planning, scheduling and monitoring project tasks.

The Gantt chart is made up of a task information side (on the left) and a task bar side (on the right; see Fig. 8.1 for an example). The task information side sets out the nature of each task and the person or people responsible for it. The task bar is a line that represents the period during which the task will be carried out. The precise content of a Gantt chart should be determined by the intended use. Such a chart is easy to draw and presents the plan in a visual form, which is easily understood by most people (see http://www.ganttchart.com for examples of Gantt charts and available software).

The chart can be used at every level in the health promotion or public health project planning process, from initial outline planning down to the detailed planning of individual tasks. For complex projects, any single bar on the master chart for the whole project might have to be represented by a more detailed bar for that particular task or stage.

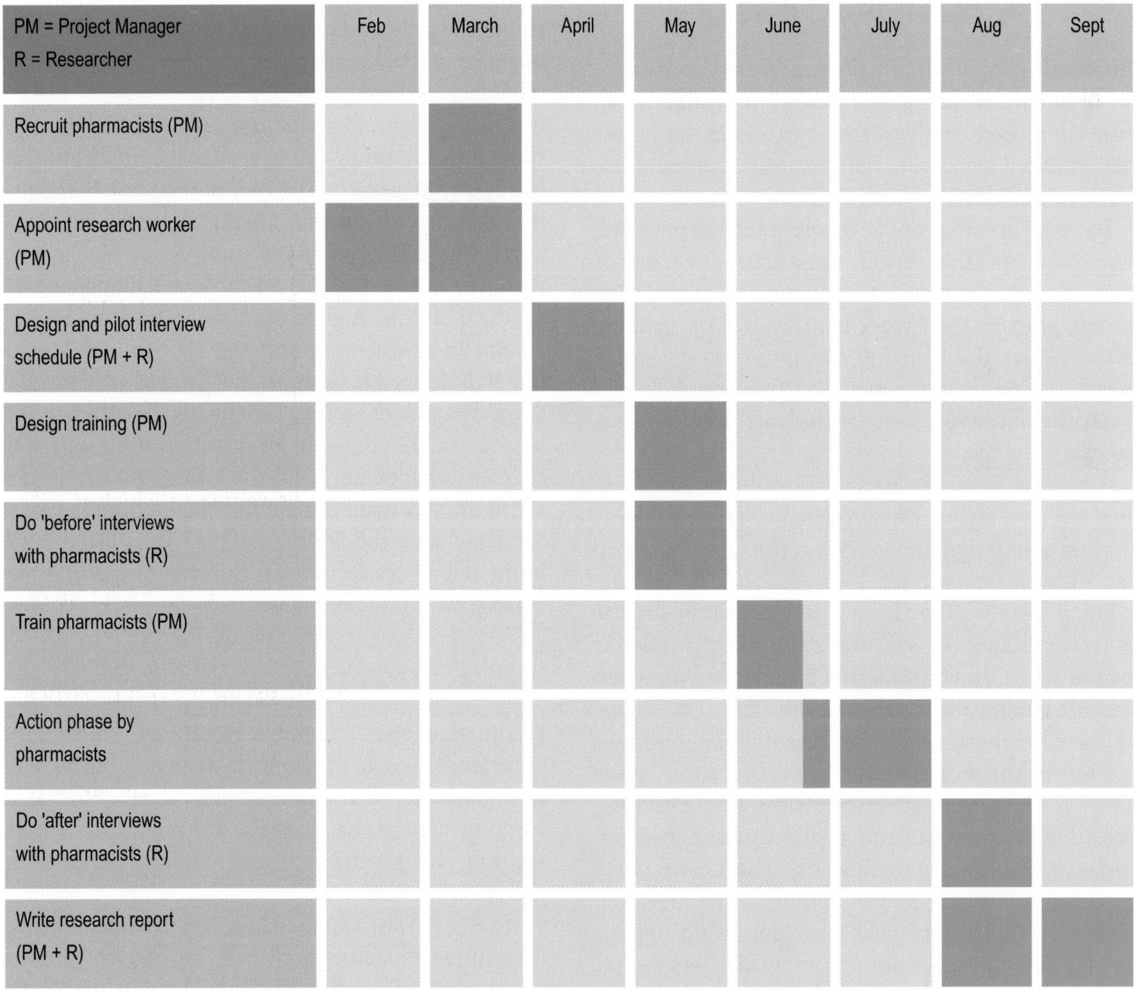

PM = Project Manager R = Researcher	Feb	March	April	May	June	July	Aug	Sept
Recruit pharmacists (PM)		■						
Appoint research worker (PM)	■							
Design and pilot interview schedule (PM + R)			■					
Design training (PM)				■				
Do 'before' interviews with pharmacists (R)				■				
Train pharmacists (PM)					■			
Action phase by pharmacists						■		
Do 'after' interviews with pharmacists (R)							■	
Write research report (PM + R)							■	■

FIG. 8.1 ■ An example of a Gantt chart (see also Case Study 8.1).

One major benefit of Gantt charts is that they highlight critical points, for example, where progress in X is dependent on Y already being completed.

Planning tools such as Gantt charts are only aids to help you to achieve your purpose. Sticking to your plan will not necessarily bring success; you may have to make adjustments because of unforeseen circumstances. However, without systematic planning you are unlikely to be able to keep your project on course at all. Case Study 8.1 describes the use of the Gantt chart in Fig. 8.1.

CASE STUDY 8.1

Using a Gantt Chart in Project Planning

This small pilot 8-month project aimed to explore the feasibility of using community pharmacists to promote physical activity with customers. Its objectives included identifying barriers and opportunities, and seeing whether training helped.

The plan was to recruit 10 volunteer pharmacists, interview them to ascertain their attitudes towards promoting physical activity with customers and their current practice then work with them in a training session. After the training, the pharmacists had a 6-week period to implement the training, followed by another interview to see if their attitudes and actions had changed.

A project manager had responsibility for planning and managing the project; a researcher was employed to design and carry out the interviews and help with the final report.

Fig. 8.1 shows the Gantt chart drawn up by the project manager. It was useful for clarifying what needed to be done and when and for seeing when possible timing difficulties could arise. For example, would pharmacists' or researchers' holidays interfere with the schedule? Were there too many tasks to be completed at one time (for example, recruiting pharmacists and appointing the research worker in February and March)? The Gantt chart also showed which stages required the research worker, so that the project manager could negotiate the appropriate numbers of hours worked at appropriate stages.

Controlling Implementation

In addition to detailed plans, a project needs to have built-in control procedures. Controlling projects is about identifying problems as soon as they arise, working out what needs to be done to ameliorate them, and then doing it. Things that need to be controlled include time, the budget (costs) and quality. Methods for control include progress reports and one-to-one and group progress meetings. Large projects will need to use all of these methods. Progress reports can sometimes be best presented in a standardised form, which compares progress with the project plan.

For more about quality, see section on working for quality later in this chapter.

Some problems will be outside the immediate control of the project. For example, a project could be influenced by the training policies of an organisation or other factors deeply embedded in the structure and culture of an organisation. In these cases, project managers should do what they can to reduce the impact of these issues on the project, but they should also remember that they have a duty to highlight these issues in reports. There are many books on project management that offer detailed advice for those managing a project for the first time. A good example is Graham (2015).

Finally, a Facebook group page can be a useful project tool if there are a team of people involved with the projects development and implementation. See the YouTube tutorial listed in the references section at the end of the chapter which demonstrates how Facebook can be used in the overall management of a public health project. See also the Facebook page and the Liquid Planner Blog in the references section which is full of useful project management tools and ideas.

MANAGING CHANGE

Health promoters and public health practitioners may experience change in two ways. One is being a part of an organisation that is undergoing change. The second way is by being a change agent, by initiating and implementing changes in health promotion or public health policy or practice.

The first way, experiencing organisational change, is common in statutory agencies as Government policy changes affect the NHS and local authorities in particular. Understanding and surviving organisational change is outside the scope of this book (see Cameron and Green 2015 for an overview). However, understanding how to implement and manage change successfully is a fundamental part of a health promoter's and public health practitioner's role.

Implementing Change

You may want to introduce a change in your public health practice, such as a different way of running health promotion programmes, introducing a health-related policy at your place of work or starting off new health promotion activities. Implementing change can be very challenging, and it will help to spend some time thinking through your strategy.

Key Factors for Successful Change

The key to gaining commitment to change, and overcoming resistance to change, lies in understanding the motivation of all the people who could be affected by the change and how they feel about it. Overall, do they feel positive or negative about the proposed change? The balance between positive and negative factors can be expressed in the change equation in Box 8.2 (Gleicher 1990) developed as a tool to help analyse the key factors involved.

BOX 8.2
THE CHANGE EQUATION

A = the individual's or group's level of dissatisfaction with things as they are now.
B = the individual's or group's shared vision of a better future.
C = the existence of an acceptable, safe first step.
D = the costs to the individual or group.
Change is likely to be viewed positively and be implemented successfully, *if:* A + B + C is greater than D.

The basis of the equation is the simple assumption that people are rarely interested in change unless the factors supporting change outweigh the costs. As a change agent, your job is either to reduce D (the perceived costs) or to increase the sum of A, B and C:

A: *Dissatisfaction with the way things are.* If you are dissatisfied, you may wrongly assume that others are too. If people are comfortable with the way things are, they are unlikely to support change.

B: *A shared vision of a better future.* If a vision of a better future does not exist or is unclear, people will not strive to achieve it. If there are several competing visions, energy will be dissipated in arguments. Few people would buy into a vision that threatens their livelihood or other cherished aspects of their lives. A vision that threatens important aspects of an individual's or a group's life is almost bound to fail.

C: *An acceptable, safe first step.* The size of the change and the risks involved can seem overwhelming. Many of us could share a common view of what better health for all would mean. But where do we begin? First steps are acceptable if they are small, are likely to be successful or, if they fail, do not cause too much damage and the situation is retrievable.

D: *The costs to the individual or group.* What is important here is how people *perceive* the costs. There will always be costs and change can be perceived as difficult or unfair. Costs can be tangible things like time, money, resources or more intangible costs like stress or loss of status (see Case Study 8.2 for an example of A–D reflected in a change in practice).

CASE STUDY 8.2

Change in a Local Health Centre

An example of significant change originating from a few people started with a physiotherapist working in a local health centre. Many of her patients were elderly and suffering from arthritis. She found that, in addition to giving instructions verbally, it was useful to write down instructions for the people she saw who needed to comply with exercises at home. She enlisted the help of a friend who was a graphic designer in designing and printing some leaflets based on her advice and instructions. A second physiotherapist had begun to collect a small library of books, such as those produced by the Arthritis and Rheumatism Council, which were left in the waiting room. A list of recommended books was added to the leaflet. Meanwhile,

Continued on following page

Change in a Local Health Centre (Continued)

the receptionist had taken another initiative. A friend had told her about a local support group for arthritis sufferers, and she pinned up a poster, giving information about it, in the waiting area.

The practice manager encouraged the staff to share their ideas. As a result, a strategy to improve the provision of information to patients was launched, and patients were asked about their needs and preferences.

Other health centres heard about the venture and expressed interest. As a result, a number of other initiatives took place to improve patient information. Plans are now underway for a Patient Education Centre to be located in the foyer of the health centre which will include a computer for online access to specific websites recommended by the practice staff.

This case study illustrates the factors in the change equation:

A. The individual's or group's level of dissatisfaction with things as they are now; two of the physiotherapists and the receptionist, and through them the practice manager, saw that there was room for improvement.

B. The individual's or group's shared vision of a better future; the idea of improved help for patients was shared and spread through an increasing number of people in the health centre and other health centres locally.

C. The existence of an acceptable, safe first step; this change was built on a number of small successes and did not present any major hurdles which could have induced resistance. If the *first step* had been to propose a Patient Education Centre, people may well have perceived major difficulties.

D. The costs to the individual or group were small in the first instance, just a little time and effort. By the time major investment was required for the Patient Education Centre, everybody was committed.

Reasons for Resistance to Change

People react differently to change. While one person may passively resist a change, another may actively try to sabotage it, whereas a third may actually embrace change. Whether you are campaigning for a change or implementing a change in policy or practice in your work, you will need to deal with the fact that many people will have reasons to resist change including the following:

Self-interest. While a change may be in the interest of most people, it may not be in everyone's best interest. For example, while most people, including some smokers, may support a no-smoking policy, others may see it as an infringement of personal liberty.

Misunderstanding. The change being proposed may be misunderstood. For example, some may think that an alcohol policy is allowing people with drinking problems to have different standards of work performance and behaviour than the rest of the workforce. Misunderstandings are particularly frequent in organisations where there is a lack of trust between the managers and the workforce.

Belief that a change is not in the interest of the people it is intended to benefit. People may believe that the costs of a change will outweigh the benefits, not only to themselves but also to others or a whole organisation. For example, people may feel that the introduction of ethnic monitoring as part of an equal opportunities policy could actually increase discrimination against black and minority ethnic groups.

Awareness of these opinions is important for the policy maker, because they may be based on knowledge of what goes on in parts of the organisation with which the policy maker has little contact. Policy formation must be based on an accurate analysis of the situation; this is particularly relevant in large organisations, such as the health service and local councils.

Low tolerance for change. People may resist change because they are anxious about new demands that will be made of them. Organisational change can require people to change too much or fail to provide them with the time and support they need.

Methods for Overcoming Resistance to Change

To overcome resistance to change, it is vital to select the best approach, or a combination of approaches, for the situation and the people involved. Five possible options are given here:

1. *Education and communication.* This involves educating people about a change before it happens and communicating with them in a variety of ways including one-to-one, group discussion and written documents. An educational and communication approach is indicated when resistance to change is based on inadequate or inaccurate information. The limitation is that it can be time-consuming, especially if a lot of people are involved.

2. *Participation and involvement.* Resistance to change may be forestalled if those initiating the change identify the people that they think will be resistant and actively involve them in the process of designing and implementing the change. The initiators of the change must genuinely be prepared to listen and learn. A token effort is liable to provoke more resistance, because people will feel let down if their contribution is not taken seriously.

Participation and involvement are necessary when full commitment to a policy change is needed to make it work; policies work when people feel ownership for them because they have been involved in their development. This approach is also useful when the initiators do not have full information about the implications of the change for certain groups of people or certain departments. It could also be the preferred option where the initiators of change have little power, because it harnesses the power of others as a force for change.

Nevertheless, this approach does have limitations. It is very time-consuming and demands a high degree of coordination. It can lead to a poor outcome if an attempt is made to accommodate everyone's needs.

3. *Facilitation and support.* This involves helping people to identify what changes are required and providing them with support to plan and manage the change themselves. This could be done, for example, by providing time for people to reflect on the situation and to identify their own objectives and how to meet them. Support could include emotional support to cope with the stress of change and the development of mentoring schemes, where more experienced people help others with their managerial or professional development. This approach works best where anxiety and fear lie at the heart of resistance. The limitation of this approach is that it too can be time-consuming and expensive (for example, if it is necessary to employ counsellors for a large workforce).

4. *Negotiation and agreement.* This involves offering incentives to actual or potential resisters, for example, through negotiating with trade unions about the effects of the change on working conditions. This is particularly appropriate when it is obvious that some people will lose out as a consequence of the changes. It can be effective if there are specific pockets of resistance but could be expensive if everyone argues that they are also losing out.

5. *Political influencing.* This approach can be useful where one or a few powerful individuals are the source of resistance. It can be relatively quick, but has the drawback that it can lead to problems in the future if people feel that they have been manipulated.

See also Chapter 16, section on the politics of influence.

WORKING FOR QUALITY

Working for quality involves examining the nature of the public health service and assessing how good it is when judged against a number of criteria.

Criteria for Quality

What are the criteria for quality in health promotion and public health practice work? The checklist in Box 8.3 may be helpful in identifying aspects of quality. The checklist can be applied to your work overall or to a particular health promotion or public health practice programme.

BOX 8.3

CHECKLIST: CRITERIA FOR QUALITY IN HEALTH PROMOTION AND PUBLIC HEALTH PRACTICE

1. **Appropriateness:** Is it relevant and acceptable to clients – the individual, group or community concerned?
2. **Effectiveness:** Does it achieve the aims and objectives you set?
3. **Social justice:** Does it produce health improvement for all concerned, not for some people at the expense of others? In other words, is it 'fair'?
4. **Equity and access:** Is it provided to all people whatever their racial, cultural or social background on the basis of equal access for equal need? (This may mean, for example, unconventional clinic times, wheelchair access, leaflets in Braille and ethnic minority languages, information on audio and video cassettes, etc.)
5. **Dignity and choice:** Does it treat all groups of people with dignity and recognise the rights of people to choose for themselves how they live their lives? Is it nonjudgemental, accepting that people have the right to withdraw from or reject health promotion if they so wish?

6. **Environment:** Does it ensure an environment conducive to people's health, safety and wellbeing? Does it recognise that people feel at home in different environments and may feel uncomfortable or intimidated in some settings? Is the social environment friendly and welcoming?
7. **Participant satisfaction:** Does it satisfy all those with an interest in the outcomes of the health promotion work, such as commissioners, managers, clients and other interest groups, acknowledging that the views of clients should be paramount?
8. **Involvement:** Does it involve all those with an interest, including clients, in planning, design and implementation? Does it avoid 'tokenism', with clients' views genuinely sought and incorporated in a non-patronising way?
9. **Efficiency:** Does it achieve the best possible use of the resources available and provide value for money?

Improving Quality

Initiatives to improve quality are usually successful if people work together to pool ideas. This could be a group of people authorised by management to examine a particular issue or problem, such as improving the quality of patient information, the way in which antenatal advice is being given to prospective parents or the way a GP practice is helping patients to stop smoking.

Sometimes such groups are called *quality circles*. These are work groups of between 3 and 12 employees who do the same (or similar) work who meet regularly to address work-related problems. The issues to tackle are selected by the group itself and the outcomes are presented to management. In many cases, the group is also involved in implementing the solutions. Management commitment to taking account of the outcomes and implementing recommended changes is crucial to success.

Typically, a quality circle will:

- begin by drawing up a list of issues for consideration, using techniques such as brainstorming
- select the issue to be addressed
- gather information about the nature of the problem, and analyse the causes
- generate a range of solutions, and establish the best options or combination of options
- prepare a report on their findings for management decision.

An example of a quality circle might be a group of nurses working in a coronary care unit looking at how to improve the quality of the patient education programmes which are run for discharged patients. The activities of such a group are described in Case Study 8.3.

CASE STUDY 8.3

Bloggsville Royal Hospital: Coronary Care Unit

IMPROVING THE QUALITY OF PATIENT EDUCATION

A group of four nurses in the coronary care unit have been meeting regularly as a quality circle and have de-

cided to investigate how to improve the quality of education for discharged patients. At present a course of six group sessions is provided for patients after discharge, and nurses take turns to organise and run the courses.

Bloggsville Royal Hospital: Coronary Care Unit (Continued)

The group first looked at the data for attendance at the group sessions. They discovered that, over the last year, 60% of discharged patients attended at least one session, but of these, only 20% attended three or more sessions.

They conducted a series of interviews with discharged patients to investigate the reasons for attendance or nonattendance and to find out patients' preferences about how they would like the education to be provided. They discovered that some patients do not like attending a group under any circumstances, and some strongly dislike coming back into the hospital environment. But some of these would like one-to-one opportunities for guidance from specialists such as a dietitian (on healthy eating), a physiotherapist (on exercise and fitness) and a psychologist (on how to stop smoking, stress management and relaxation).

Other patients would prefer to have written information, audiotapes (for relaxation and self-hypnosis) and videotapes (of appropriate exercise routines) rather than come back to the hospital. Others would like more information about community groups and facilities for exercise tailored to their needs, for example, free trials of fitness classes or swimming sessions for elderly people. Others are interested in knowing if there are self-help or voluntary groups they could join, such as clubs for people who are being rehabilitated following heart disease. Some patients, especially those who are socially isolated, have particularly valued the opportunity to meet as a group and to exchange experiences.

After analysing these findings, the group of nurses produced a report for their manager recommending that a range of educational opportunities is provided for the education of discharged patients including:

- putting patients in touch with local self-help and cardiac rehabilitation schemes
- setting up a video and audiotape library providing appropriate material for discharged patients on free loan

- offering opportunities for counselling by specialists (dietitian, physiotherapist, psychologist) before discharge
- selecting or producing appropriate written material and making it available to patients before discharge
- inviting all patients to return for an open evening with information and demonstrations about facilities and activities available locally. This would include local authority exercise and leisure facilities, alternative medicine practitioners, community and self-help groups and commercial leisure organisations.

The report includes a financial breakdown, which demonstrates that the recommendations will have additional costs, primarily related to the proposed services to be provided by the professions allied to medicine. However, savings will be made on the nursing staff time currently devoted to running the courses and through financial sponsorship of written material by approved 'ethical' commercial sponsors.

This case study shows how the quality of the patient education programme could be improved on a number of criteria:

- **Appropriateness:** Clients would find the new approach more acceptable and relevant.
- **Effectiveness:** More clients would gain from the programme.
- **Equity and access:** Clients could access advice and help in different ways, and those who disliked group meetings or found attendance difficult would have their needs met in other ways.
- **Environment:** It was recognised that some people disliked the hospital environment.
- **Participant satisfaction:** Clients and nurses would be more satisfied with the results.
- **Involvement:** Clients were involved in redesigning the programme with their views taken into account.
- **Efficiency:** It would be a better use of resources because it would reach the people intended and avoid wasting resources on a programme that reached very few.

Developing Quality Standards

It may be helpful to look at improving quality by setting specific quality standards, which are an agreed-upon level of performance either mandated by government of negotiated within available resources.

Examples of standards that relate to public health and health promotion are available on the National Institute for Health and Care Excellence website (NICE 2016). Quality standards are also available from Public Health England, such as those for NHS Health Checks (PHE 2013) and from the different professional groups who have a public health function, for example, the professional standards for public health practice for pharmacy (Royal Pharmaceutical Society 2014). The criteria listed in the following text could be used as a list of quality standards for health promotion and public health leaflets. The Accessible Information Standard (NHS England 2016) must also be followed and can be found on the Health and Social Care Information Centre website listed in the references section at the end of this chapter:

- Appropriate for achieving your health promotion and public health aims
- Content consistent with the values of health promotion
- Relevant and easily understood by the people for whom the leaflets are intended
- Developed with the involvement of the target audience to ensure it meets their needs
- Not racist or sexist
- Accurate, up-to-date information informed by evidence
- Free of inappropriate advertising.

See section on guidelines for selecting and producing health promotion resources in Chapter 11.

A further challenge is to develop standards that are *quantifiable* in some way. This is a difficult task, but you could, for example, develop a five-point scale for assessing the quality of your leaflets, so that you score them out of five for the extent to which they fulfill each quality standard. Another example could be that you decide that a quality management issue is to respond quickly to requests from your clients. You could develop this by setting a standard such as returning telephone calls within 24 hours and written requests within 3 days.

Monitoring and reviewing quality standards can involve a great deal of time and effort. The benefit comes from seeing clearly identified improvements in service.

PRACTICE POINTS

- To implement health promotion and public health practice work successfully, you need to develop management skills that include information management, report writing, time management, project management, managing change and developing quality.
- Managing information involves storing in the simplest way the paperwork and electronic files that are essential and that cannot be kept in another information-retrieval system.
- Writing a report involves being clear about the report's purpose and following a coherent and logical structure. Always get your report checked before publication.
- Managing time involves monitoring your time through using time logs and diaries and scheduling tasks appropriately.
- Project work involves detailed and systematic planning. A Gantt chart is a useful tool.
- Managing change requires an effective change strategy and is more likely to be successful if people have a shared vision and believe that the factors in favour of the change outweigh the costs.
- Working for quality is best achieved collaboratively. Management support and involvement are essential for success.

REFERENCES

Bowden J 2011 Writing a report, 9th edn. Oxfordshire, How To Books.

Broddy D 2013 Management: an introduction, 6th edn. Oxford, Pearson.

Cameron E, Green M 2015 Making sense of change management: a complete guide to the models, tools and techniques of organizational change, 4th edn. London, Kogan Page.

Gleicher D 1990 Open Business School/Institute of Health Services Management/NHS Training Authority managing health services. Milton Keynes, *The Open University Book 9*: 36–37 Managing Change.

Graham N 2015 Project management for dummies. New Jersey, John Whiley.

Knight J 2016 Project management: project management, management tips and strategies, and how to control a team to complete a project. CreateSpace Independent Publishing Platform, Amazon.

Kruse K 2015 15 Secrets successful people know about time management: the productivity habits of 7 billionaires, 13 Olympic athletes, 29 straight-A students, and 239 entrepreneurs. Philadelphia, The Kruse Group.

NHS England 2016 *Making health and social care information accessible.* https://www.england.nhs.uk/wp-content/uploads/2015/07/access-info-upd-er-july-15.pdf.

NICE 2016 *New public health quality standards announced.* https://www.nice.org.uk/news/article/new-public-health-quality-standards-announced.

Public Health England 2013 *Quality assurance standards for NHS health checks.* London, Public Health England.

Royal Pharmaceutical Society 2014 Professional standards for public health practice for pharmacy. London, The Royal Pharmaceutical Society. http://www.rpharms.com/support-pdfs/professional-standards-for-public-health.pdf.

WEBSITES

Examples of reports on public health. http://ec.europa.eu/health/mental_health/eu_compass/reports_studies/index_en.htm.

Examples of reports, such as the World Health Report. http://www.who.int/publications/en/.

Time management tools and free downloads. http://www.mytime-management.com/time-management-tools.html.

For information on quality circles. http://www.ukqcs.co.uk/five-good-reasons-to-run-a-quality-circle-programme-in-your-practice/.

Details on information standards. https://digital.nhs.uk/.

FACEBOOK

For ideas and tools on project management. https://www.facebook.com/ProjectManagementToolsThatWork/.

BLOGS

For ideas and tools on project management. https://www.liquidplanner.com/blog/.

YOUTUBE

A tutorial on how to use Facebook for project management. https://www.youtube.com/watch?v=qEpZoCHSpK0.

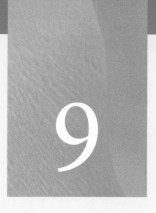

9

WORKING EFFECTIVELY
WITH OTHER PEOPLE

CHAPTER CONTENTS

SUMMARY

This chapter focuses on developing skills for working effectively with other people and organisations to plan and implement health promotion and public health practice. The following key aspects are discussed: communicating with colleagues, coordination and teamwork, participating in meetings, effective committee work and working in local public health partnerships with other agencies. Practical exercises and a case study are included.

Some health promoters and public health practitioners plan and undertake their health promotion work entirely on their own, but most are likely to be working with other people from the wide range of professional backgrounds that make up the multidisciplinary workforce with a remit for promoting health:

- Colleagues who may be peers, managers or people you manage
- Colleagues in other parts of your own organisation
- People drawn from the community and/or from different statutory and nonstatutory agencies (local, national or international) who are working with you on a health promotion activity of mutual interest and importance.

A key aspect of success will be how well you work with other people, and this chapter discusses the knowledge and skills needed for interprofessional communication and collaborative and partnership working.

COMMUNICATING WITH COLLEAGUES

Some fundamentals of effective face-to-face and written communication are dealt with in Chapter 10. While these are presented primarily with client contact in mind, they are also applicable to contact between health promotion and public health colleagues. The following factors are particularly important to ensure effective working relationships:

- Working in a team which recognises and builds on the strengths of other team members
- Actively listening to the people you are working with so that you understand clearly their opinions, ideas and feelings.

A considerable proportion of your time may be taken up by communications with working colleagues including telephone conversations, face-to-face discussions

EXERCISE 9.1
How You Communicate with Colleagues

Record all the types of communication with colleagues that you carry out over one working day by making a tally of all the occasions in four categories, as set out in the following table. Then add up your total for each category and your grand total for the day. You might like to compare your results with those of your colleagues.

	Face-to-face verbal	Telephone	Paper: Letters and memos	Electronic: email, webcam/ teleconferencing/Facebook posts
	_____	_____	_____	_____
	_____	_____	_____	_____
	_____	_____	_____	_____
	_____	_____	_____	_____
	_____	_____	_____	_____
	_____	_____	_____	_____
	_____	_____	_____	_____
	_____	_____	_____	_____
TOTALS	_____	_____	_____	_____

Think about whether there is anything you would like to change or improve; for example:

- If you spend a lot of time on the telephone, could you improve your telephone skills?
- Could you use your time more efficiently if you used less time-consuming methods of communications (for example, teleconferencing or email) instead of having meetings?
- Are there ways that you can use technology to communicate more effectively and efficiently with colleagues?
- Do you need to selectively spend more time face-to-face to understand colleagues and establish a closer working relationship?

and written communications on paper and via email. Try Exercise 9.1 to help increase your awareness of how you communicate with colleagues and how your communication might be improved.

COORDINATION AND TEAMWORK

Health promotion often involves multiagency and multidisciplinary working, therefore effective coordination and teamwork are required.

Poor coordination can result in losses in efficiency and effectiveness of programmes; it is especially difficult when big bureaucracies like the National Health Service (NHS) and local authorities are working together. There are several ways of coordinating, and it is important to use the one best suited to the situation.

Appointing a Coordinator

A potential problem for coordinators is that they may not directly manage the people they are trying to coordinate and therefore cannot control them in the same

way as a manager. They must convince people that any requests they make are legitimate. Coordinators can be at a low level in a hierarchical organisation. A diabetic nurse trying to coordinate the production of a patient information leaflet, for example, might find it difficult to obtain the commitment of a consultant. The very word *coordinator* may provoke resistance to being organised in some people.

There are several tactics that can help to overcome resistance.

Using Your Reputation

People will find it difficult to turn down any reasonable requests if your work is well known and well regarded, and you are respected by those who work with you. So you need to publicise your work and seek to establish a good reputation.

Establishing Good Relationships

Building and maintaining good relationships requires effort and is an essential investment for every coordinator.

Bargaining

It may be possible to bargain with individual people or departments: Could you offer them something in return for their cooperation?

Out-ranking

This should be used only as a last resort. It requires a senior manager from your hierarchy to request cooperation through the other person's manager. While the other tactics build trust, this one endangers it and may result in a lack of goodwill.

Discussion and Negotiation

Talking to all involved could result in clarification of responsibilities and improved mutual understanding, leading to the group giving you more legitimate authority. This could mean first discussing the issue with individuals, and later convening a meeting when you have got sufficient commitment to solving the problem. Undertake Exercise 9.2 to assess how you might improve your coordination and teamworking skills.

EXERCISE 9.2

Improving Coordination and Teamworking

In the health promotion or public health work you do that involves working with other people, can you think of any ways by which you could improve coordination and teamworking?

- What steps could you take to enhance the reputation of your health promotion work?
- With whom could you build a better relationship to improve coordination or teamwork?
- What have you got to offer if you are bargaining?
- Can you think of any health promotion activities that you undertake routinely together with other people which could be more efficient with a set procedure?
- Are there any ways by which you could develop stronger links with other staff at your level in different departments or agencies to facilitate joint working in health promotion?
- Have you any opportunities for joint objective setting or joint planning that could help to coordinate health promotion in your situation?
- Can you think of anything else? Discuss this with colleagues who are also involved in health promotion and public health

---

Policies, Procedures and Protocols

Making and implementing policies is discussed in Chapter 16.

Policies are important in coordinating health promotion and public health work. Using *set procedures* are ways of coordinating routine tasks. *Protocols* are agreed written procedures that everyone follows, ensuring that everyone carries out a particular task in the same way. For example, there may be a smoking cessation protocol in a GP surgery or health centre about how to help a patient to stop smoking. The protocol ensures that whoever is dealing with the patient (the doctor, the practice nurse, the district nurse or the health visitor) will offer the same range of help and follow the same follow-up procedures. For an excellent example of a smoking cessation protocol, see Ashcroft Surgery (2016) and for other examples of smoking cessation procedures see Public Health England (2014) and NICE (2013). There is also the National Centre for Smoking Cessation and Training (NCSCT) which not only offers guidelines on procedures but also has resources. See the NCSCT webpage under the webpages in the reference section.

Joint Planning

In this approach, the parties involved not only agree on objectives but also meet regularly to develop and implement a joint plan. This may minimise the need for one individual to be given the job of coordinator and prevent the problem of one agency or department being perceived as controlling the agenda. However, it can be very difficult to get all the people involved together on a regular basis and to ensure that communications are always clear to all those involved.

Joint Working Through Creating Teams

An autonomous team is given the authority, training, money, staff, premises and equipment to carry out the health promotion programme. There is no need for a coordinator, because the whole team is working together from the same base. Joint working of this kind is usually not suitable for short-term programmes but can be excellent for long-term projects such as those involving community development.

Creation of Lateral Relations

This type of coordination depends on strengthening relationships between individuals in broadly equivalent jobs in different departments or agencies. Setting up project teams, which are dissolved once the particular project is completed, can do this. It could also be done by forming interdepartmental or multidisciplinary teams or partnerships, which are given more authority for making decisions without having to refer them up the different hierarchies. However, this can lead to conflict with the existing vertical lines of command and works best where there are good links between the various managers.

Characteristics of Successful Teams

There are different sorts of teams. The teams of relevance here are associations of people with a common public health work purpose, for example, a primary healthcare team. Successful teams have the characteristics set out in Box 9.1. If you experience a team that does not seem to be working well, it can be helpful for the team to consider this list together to identify the roots of the difficulties (for more information on how to develop successful interdisciplinary team working, see Nancarrow et al 2013 and for general strategies for building successful teams see West 2012).

BOX 9.1
CHARACTERISTICS OF SUCCESSFUL TEAMS

- A team consists of a group of identified people.
- The team has a common purpose and shared objectives, which are known and agreed by all members.
- Members are selected because they have relevant expertise.
- Members know and agree their own role and know the roles of the other members.
- Members support each other in achieving the common purpose.
- Members trust each other, and communicate with each other in an open, honest way.
- The team has a leader, whose authority is accepted by all members.

PARTICIPATING IN MEETINGS

The detailed planning and organisation of meetings are beyond the scope of this book (see Mindtools 2016 for useful strategies for running meetings). The guidance in the following text is an aid to how to be an effective participant at meetings. As a participant, there are a number of constructive things you can do:

- Encourage the Chair into good practices; for example, ask for clarification on the purpose of the meeting, and ask for a summary of what has been agreed to at the end
- Come prepared and arrive on time
- Acknowledge the authority of the Chair
- Agree what to do about taking notes: Does each person take their own or does one person take them and circulate a copy to everyone else? Do you want detailed notes of everything you discussed or just action points?
- Actively contribute to the meeting, express your views succinctly, keep an open mind and listen to other people's opinions
- Encourage everyone to participate by referring to members' relevant experience or expertise
- Only make commitments that you are genuinely able to fulfil and make sure you fulfil them on time. Say 'no' clearly and nondefensively if you are unable or unwilling to take on a task
- Remember that discussion and debate about ideas will help decision making but personal rivalries will not.

EFFECTIVE COMMITTEE WORK

A committee is a group of people appointed for a specific purpose accountable to a larger group or organisation. Examples are the management committee of a voluntary organisation or the health committee of a local authority. There are many common routines and procedures that help facilitate committees, and it is useful to be familiar with them. The details will vary from committee to committee, although the principles remain the same. Some committees start their life with recommendations from a steering group, which include proposals for the interim committee rules. These are then approved at the first committee meeting. After review and modification, a set of rules will be agreed upon which become the accepted rules for the committee.

Officers

The officers are servants of the committee and carry out its instructions. Committees have key officers, usually the Chair, the Secretary and the Treasurer, but larger committees may have additional appointments, for example, a Minutes Secretary.

Chair

Much of the work of the Chair may be done between meetings, but it is at the meetings when the Chair is most visible and has responsibility for ensuring that the committee successfully completes its tasks. It is vital for the Chair to be heard clearly during meetings so that all the committee can be involved. Good Chairs delegate as much as possible to ensure active involvement of all members. The Chair also has the responsibility of preparing the next Chair and must ensure that opportunities are provided for the Vice Chair to develop.

Secretary

The Secretary is responsible for all the nonfinancial papers and reports, for general planning and organisation (often in collaboration with the other officers) and for seeing that the committee's work is coordinated and nothing is forgotten. Good organisation, coordination and computing skills are needed. There are a number of software programmes (such as SharePoint or BoardEffect; see websites in the reference section at the end of the chapter) that can help with this work.

The Secretary is responsible for compiling the agenda for the committee meetings. This is the list of things to be done or agreed upon during the meeting. It will often include standard items such as 'apologies for absence', 'minutes of the previous meeting', 'matters arising from the previous meeting' and 'any other business'. The important point is that the agenda acts as an advance organiser for everyone attending the meeting so that they are able to prepare. The committee members need to receive the agenda and associated papers in good time before the meeting, usually a week in advance.

The Secretary is also responsible for the final version of the minutes and for agreeing these with the Chair, even if a Minutes Secretary takes the notes at the meetings. Minutes are accurate records of the meeting and should always identify precisely who has responsibility for what action, by what date and when a report back will be made to the committee.

Treasurer

A Treasurer will only be necessary if the committee is responsible for any financial matters. Treasurers are expected to report on the financial position quickly and precisely at any time by recording and summarising every transaction so that it is easy to see the current situation. At the end of the financial year, all financial transactions are summarised in an annual statement, a clear one-page summary.

Quorum

It is unlikely that all committee members will be able to attend all meetings. The rules usually state the minimum number of members who must be present for the meeting to be considered representative of members' views and to have the authority to make decisions. This is called a quorum and is usually one-third or one-half of the total voting membership.

Committee Behaviour

Committees can be informal, but there are reasons for various formal behaviours. For example, the rule that only one person speaks at a time and is not interrupted is meant to ensure a fair hearing for everyone. The Chair should not allow a vociferous few to dominate the meeting.

The rule of everyone speaking by addressing the meeting through the Chair helps prevent a number of subdiscussions developing at the same time. On the other hand, it may seem more natural and helpful to address another committee member directly. Ultimately it is the job of the Chair to set a tone that encourages all members to participate while keeping the meeting under control.

Understanding Conflict

In itself, conflict is not bad. Conflict is inevitable at times in any group because of differences in needs, objectives or values. The results of conflict will be positive or negative depending on how it is handled. Handled well, conflict can be a creative source of new ideas and can help a group to change and develop. It can also strengthen the ability of group members to work together. Conflict is badly handled when it is either ignored so that negative feelings develop or approached on a win/lose basis rather than a compromise or a win/win position. Undertake Exercise 9.3 to assess your conflict resolution style.

EXERCISE 9.3

Your Conflict Resolution Style

When confronted with conflict in a group you work in, which of these styles do you use?

Style	Characteristic behaviour
Avoidance	Ignores the problem; avoids raising the issue; denies that there is a problem
Accommodating	Attempts to cooperate with everyone even at the expense of not meeting personal or team objectives
Win/lose	Fights to win at any cost even if it means alienating colleagues or causing the rest of the team to fail in meeting their objectives
Compromising	Suggests a compromise that would meet everyone's basic needs and maintain good relationships
Problem solving	Openly confronts the problem and encourages everyone to face the disagreements and to express fully their opinions and ideas. Searches for a new solution which meets everyone's needs as fully as possible

Review this chart with other members of groups you work in. Can you think of situations in which these different approaches to conflict resolution were used? Discuss what worked and what did not. What could have been done differently to improve the outcome?

What's your conflict resolution style?

WORKING IN PARTNERSHIP WITH OTHER ORGANISATIONS

See Chapter 3 for details on the range of public health agencies and organisations.

Health promotion programmes and projects often require people from different organisations to work together; it is an established way of working in health promotion. Health promotion partnerships may be formally structured with partners or members at different levels from chief executives to field workers. There may be a written constitution and terms of reference or arrangements may be fairly informal. They may be long term, or set up for a time-limited period to work on a specific project (see Hunter and Perkins 2014a for a detailed examination of partnership working in public health).

The main reasons for setting up local partnerships are:

- to harness a range of complementary skills and resources to work towards common public health goals
- to avoid duplication and fragmentation of effort
- to avoid gaps in public health services or programmes.

See Chapter 3, for an overview of the organisations working for public health.

Recent UK government health reforms have created the opportunity for new styles of partnerships (Local Government Association 2016). Public health work often involves health services and local authorities pooling their budgets for joint initiatives and forming partnerships for planning, commissioning and delivering services. These new-style partnerships are genuine joint enterprises with local authorities and others. However, whilst there is a long history of partnership working to deliver health improvements in England, there is little evidence to date that partnership working has led to demonstrable improvements in what really matters – health outcomes (Hayes et al 2012). Partnerships therefore have to be viewed as a means to an end, not an end in themselves. Establishing a local Health and Wellbeing Board and other partnerships, processes and planning mechanisms must have a clear focus on outcomes based on evidence of what works. The public health reforms in England have certainly created the environment necessary to facilitate that focus on a much stronger outcomes framework, a requirement for joint health and wellbeing strategies and financial rewards for achievement of health improvement through the health premium (Buck & Gregory 2013). Case Study 9.1 is an example of the focus and wide-ranging professional and community partnerships that makes up a Health and Wellbeing Board

1 HEALTH AND WELLBEING BOARD

1.1 Purpose of the Health and Wellbeing Board

The main purpose of the statutory Health and Wellbeing Board is to join-up commissioning and services across the NHS, social care, public health and voluntary sector to benefit the health and well-being of local people. The Board is working under Ways of Working (Bristol City Council 2016a).

1.2 Responsibilities of the Board

- Developing a Health and Wellbeing Strategy (HWS). This strategy sets out the core work for the Board, addressing local health and care needs as identified in the Joint Strategic Needs Assessment (JSNA).
- Investigating ways to pool budgets and share resources effectively between partners.
- Producing the JSNA. This will help steer commissioning of health services based on local health needs, data and evidence.
- A duty to consult service users and the public.
- A formal role in the annual assessment of clinical commissioning groups (GP Commissioning Consortia) and the NHS Commissioning Board.
- Being a key driver for change and a local leader across health, social care and public health services.

MEMBERSHIP OF THE BOARD

- Mayor, Co-chair of the Board
- Chair of the local Clinical Commissioning Group (CCG), Co-chair of the Board
- City Director, local City Council
- Cabinet Member for People, representative of Leader, Liberal Democrats
- Cabinet Member for City Health and Wellbeing, representative of Leader, Greens
- Representative of Leader, Conservatives
- Bristol Clinical Commissioning Group
- North and West representative, CCG
- Inner City and East representative, CCG
- Chair of GP Consortia South, Bristol CCG
- Director of Public Health, Bristol City Council
- Strategic Director, Neighbourhoods, Bristol City Council
- Strategic Director, People, Bristol City Council
- HealthWatch (Chief Executive, Carers Support Centre)
- Representative of the Voluntary and Community Sector, supported by VOSCUR (see http://www.voscur.org/)
- HealthWatch representative
- NHS England, North Somerset, Somerset and South Gloucestershire

Source: Adjusted from Bristol City Council (2016b)
See also the YouTube page in the references for OPM network discussion on health and wellbeing boards – making integration work and the OPM website in the website references for an overview of their services to health and social care.

In general, public health partnerships can take different forms and vary in terms of how closely members work together. It is useful to think of three main ways of working, spanning a range of degrees of involvement between partners: Networking – Cooperating – Joint working.

Networking

Networking means coming together with other people from different agencies, and exchanging information and ideas on activities and plans. This is useful for coordinating activities, avoiding duplication and sharing knowledge of mutual interest. Members meet and talk, but they do not actually work together. Networking has the lowest degree of involvement between organisations.

Cooperating

Cooperating means that member agencies help each other in ways that are compatible with their own goals. They meet, talk and agree to participate in each other's work when this is helpful for their own work plans. For example, in an accident prevention partnership, people who work in the accident and emergency (A&E) department of a hospital may cooperate with a local alcohol advisory service (a voluntary organisation) to ensure that patients brought in with a drink problem know that they can go to the alcohol agency for help. This cooperation helps the alcohol agency to reach needy potential clients and helps the A&E department to fulfill its role of helping patients with longer term health needs. This way of working in partnership means a moderate degree of involvement between partners.

Joint Working

Joint working means coming together to agree a mutually acceptable plan, and working together to carry it out. This necessitates a high degree of involvement between partners. For example, the police, the probation service, road safety officers from the local authority and a local alcohol advisory service may all work together to plan, implement and evaluate a joint programme of work to reduce drink-driving levels.

Partnerships can operate in one, two or all of these ways. Sometimes joint working is thought to be the most effective, but networking and cooperating can be useful when it is not always feasible or worthwhile to aim for full joint or integrated working. See Case Study 9.2 for example of nonstatutory partnerships (which include cooperation and joint working) between a national body, Public Health England, commercial and local authority partners.

CASE STUDY 9.2

Taking One You Brand Partnerships into Real Life

In March 2016 Public Health England launched One You, a nationwide campaign to address preventable disease in adults. It ran for seven weeks and was supported by TV, digital, Out of Home, PR and social media activity (Facebook and Twitter). It was amplified by nationwide partner support including new public and commercial partnerships, such as Asda, Amazon, Slimming World, BBC Get Inspired and the Ministry of Defence. Asda, for example, committed to sell more than 100,000 blood pressure monitors and perform in-store checks. A campaign principle was to involve different partners, such as 152 local authorities taking on the brand, such as One You Cornwall, to localise the campaign.

Source: Adjusted from Public Health England (2016)

For more details, see the One You webpage, Facebook and Twitter locations in the reference section at the end of the chapter.

Factors for Successful Public Health Partnership Working

Successful public health partnerships are usually the result of investing a considerable amount of resources, skill and time to enable members to work well together. Key factors for success are that:

- all partners need to be working towards a shared vision of what the partnership should achieve with an agenda and goals to which all partners concur
- there must be an agreed-upon approach. All partners need to feel a sense of ownership with no one partner dominating
- commitment from the highest level of member organisations is vital to ensure that belonging to the partnership fits in with the organisation's strategic aims and that there will be management support for input of time and other resources
- there must be commitment of sufficient time and resources and realistic expectations. Partnership working is time-consuming, and it may take months or years to develop a shared understanding and joint plans, or achieve outcomes from joint health promotion activities. There must, however, be demonstrable achievements, otherwise the partnership will be regarded as ineffective
- someone acceptable to all partners needs to take responsibility for running the partnership (for example setting up, chairing and servicing meetings) and coordinating action. A full-time coordinator can be extremely helpful
- there must be mutual respect between partners; all partners need to feel that others value their input
- working relationships need to be characterised by openness and trust. Partners need to recognise and resolve potential areas of conflict
- there must be an agreed-upon framework for reviewing the partnership, changing the way of working if necessary and even bringing it to an end if it has outlived its usefulness or is unproductive
- awareness and understanding of partner organisations should be promoted through joint

training programmes and incentives to work across organisational boundaries

▪ partnership arrangements need to be regularly reviewed and adapted to reflect the lessons learned from experience.

See also earlier sections in this chapter on coordination and teamwork.

Potential Difficulties With Public Health Partnership Working

Partnership working can result in many difficulties. Major problems are:

▪ organisational change, which blights long-term commitment and planning.
▪ competition between member agencies for funding, for example, between different voluntary organisations who are seeking funding from the same source.
▪ lack of resources, both money and person-power.
▪ lack of top-level commitment from members of the partnership.
▪ domination by an individual.
▪ an imbalance of input from different agencies, which can lead to resentment and issues about ownership of joint activities and who takes the credit for success.
▪ professional jealousy and unwillingness to share expertise and information.
▪ differences between agencies and individuals in terms of different goals and values, different organisational cultures and ways of working, different levels of expertise and experience.

It is worth bearing in mind that not all partnerships are successful. Many fade out or are wound up. Partnership working is not an end in itself; it is a means to an end, and there are circumstances where the end is better achieved by an organisation working alone.

For further reading on public health partnerships see Baggott (2013) and Hunter and Perkins (2014a and 2014b).

PRACTICE POINTS

▪ A key aspect of successfully implemented health promotion and public health programmes is how well you and other health promoters and public health practitioners work together.

▪ You need to think about how you communicate with colleagues: the channels you use, how well you use them and the quality of your professional relationships.

▪ Health promotion and public health practice often involves different professionals and disciplines working together; there is a range of ways in which you can encourage good teamwork and coordination.

▪ For effective meetings and committee work, you require knowledge of and competencies in the roles and responsibilities of committee members.

▪ Public health partnerships between two or more organisations work at varying levels of involvement with each other, from networking at a local or national level to full joint working and from local partnerships to strategic partnership. Think about the many factors that contribute to success and the potential pitfalls to avoid.

REFERENCES

Ashcroft Surgery 2016 Smoking cessation protocol. http://www.ash-croftsurgery.co.uk/smoking-cessation-protocol/.

Baggott R 2013 Partnerships for public health and well-being: policy and practice. Basingstoke, Palgrave Macmillan.

Bristol City Council 2016a Bristol health and wellbeing board ways of working (Supplement to the Terms of Reference agreed at Full Council in May 2013) https://www.bristol.gov.uk/documents/20182/138101/Agreed%20in%20July%202013%20with%20amends%20included_0_0.pdf/d81c21dd-dd0f-4607-b2c3-1f27a6596ff3.

Bristol City Council 2016b Health and wellbeing board. https://www.bristol.gov.uk/council-meetings/health-and-wellbeing-board.

Buck D, Gregory S 2013 Improving the public's health: a resource for local authorities. London, Kings Fund.

Hayes SL, Mann MK, Morgan FM, Kelly MJ, Weightman AL 2012 Collaboration between local health and local government agencies for health improvement. Cochrane Database of Systematic Reviews 10:CD007825. www.ncbi.nlm.nih.gov/pubmed/23076937

Hunter D, Perkins N 2014a Partnership working in public health (Evidence for public health practice). Bristol, Policy Press.

Hunter D, Perkins N 2014b Partnership working in public health: the implications for governance of a systems approach. Journal of Health Service Research and Policy 17(suppl 2):45–52.

Local Government Association 2016 Public health's role in local government and NHS integration. London, LGA.

MindTools 2016 Running effective meetings. https://www.mind-tools.com/CommSkll/RunningMeetings.htm.

NICE 2013 Stop smoking services. https://www.nice.org.uk/guidance/ph10?unlid=33879501620165244327.

Nancarrow S, Booth A, Ariss S, Smith T, Enderby P, Roots A 2013 Ten principles of good interdisciplinary team work. Human Resource Health 11: 19.

Public Health England 2014 Local stop smoking services: service and delivery guidelines. London, Public Health England.

Public Health England 2016 One You. https://www.nhs.uk/oneyou#VWGQC669fb3uB3MW.97.

West M 2012 Effective teamwork: practical lessons from organizational research (Psychology of work and organizations), 3rd edn. New Jersey, Wiley-Blackwell.

WEBSITES

BoardEffect. http://www.boardeffect.com/g-committee-software/?gclid=CjwKEAjwq8y8BRCstYTm8qeT9mwSJACZGjUkiwqyNvG6WXTKZ-ed2TuIII6HYG54rpozRWoWw2iWMhoCaBzw_wcB for Board Effect committee management software.

Mindtools. https://www.mindtools.com/CommSkll/RunningMeetings.htm for toolkits on leadership, communication and management skills.

National Centre for Smoking Cessation and Training. http://www.ncsct.co.uk/ for the NCSCT guidelines and resources. The webpage also includes NICE guidelines and a range of Cochrane Reviews linked to smoking cessation.

NHS England partnership pages. https://www.england.nhs.uk/ourwork/part-rel/.

One You campaign website. https://www.nhs.uk/oneyou#iMMoSvwVahrBwflc.97 and for the One You App https://www.nhs.uk/oneyou/apps#ExGv3mpqZZMjEzIh.97.

OPM. http://www.opm.co.uk/.

Sharepoint. https://products.office.com/en-us/sharepoint/collaboration for software for teamwork coordination.

FACEBOOK

Mindtools. https://www.facebook.com/mindtools for ideas and information on being more effective in management and leadership.

BLOGS

Public Health Matter – Partnership working in the North. https://publichealthmatters.blog.gov.uk/2015/02/09/partnership-working-in-the-north-2/.

One You Facebook page. https://www.facebook.com/OneYouPHE.

YOUTUBE

For information and issues linked to Health and Wellbeing Boards. https://www.youtube.com/watch?v=l4xDOB9lxQA.

TWITTER

One *You* at Twitter. https://twitter.com/OneYouPHE.

PART 3

Competencies in Health Promotion and Public Health Practice

PART SUMMARY

Part 3 aims to provide you with guidance on how to assess, develop and improve your competencies in health promotion and public health practice.

Competencies are the combinations of knowledge, attitudes and skills needed to plan, implement and evaluate health promotion and public health practice activities in a range of settings. You will also need to develop other competencies, such as communicating and educating, marketing and publicising, facilitating and networking and influencing policy and practice. Some chapters of Part 3 will be more important to some professions or disciplines than others. So you may wish to start by studying the chapters most relevant to you rather than going through them in sequence. Cross-referencing is provided to help you to identify which sections of other chapters may also be relevant to your particular needs.

In Chapter 10, the fundamentals of communication are addressed including establishing relationships and the links with promoting self-esteem and assertiveness. Four basic communication skills are identified and guidance is provided on how to improve them. Communication and language barriers, nonverbal communication and written communication are discussed.

In Chapter 11, some principles governing the choice of communication tools in health promotion are covered. The advantages and limitations of a variety of teaching and learning resources are considered and guidance provided on how to produce and use displays, written materials and statistical information. The use of mass media in health promotion is explored including practical help about working with the local press, radio and television. There is a section included on the use of information technology in health promotion.

In Chapter 12, the principles of adult learning are outlined. How you can enable people to learn and evaluate the learning outcome is described, along with guidelines on giving talks and on patient health education.

Chapter 13 covers the health promotion competencies required to work effectively with groups, covering how to lead groups and how to understand group behaviour.

Chapter 14 concentrates on how to enable people to change their behaviour towards healthier living including information on models of the process of changing health-related behaviour. Strategies that can be used, such as working with a client's own motivation and counselling to help people to make decisions are discussed alongside the principles that help with using these approaches.

In Chapter 15, the focus is community-based work in health promotion including community participation, community development and community health projects.

Chapter 16 is about how local and national policies, programmes, plans and strategies are made and how they can be influenced. The methods that health promoters can use to challenge health-damaging policies and develop, implement and evaluate public health policies are outlined including sections on the principles and the planning of campaigns.

10

FUNDAMENTALS OF COMMUNICATION IN PUBLIC HEALTH

CHAPTER CONTENTS

SUMMARY

This chapter starts with an exploration of client/professional relationships and a discussion of the links between self-esteem, self-confidence and communication, accompanied by a case study on relationship skills. Discussion on four basic communication skills (listening, helping people to talk, asking questions and getting feedback) is followed by consideration of communication and language barriers and nonverbal communication (NVC). The chapter ends with a section on written and wider forms of communication and on health literacy. Exercises are provided on overcoming communication barriers and on each basic communication skill.

See also Chapter 12, which focuses on educating for health.

Health communication is the practice of communicating promotional health information, such as in public health campaigns, health education and between health professionals and patients. The purpose of disseminating health information is to influence personal health choices by improving health literacy.

Health communication may variously seek to:

- increase audience knowledge and awareness of a health issue
- influence behaviours and attitudes towards a health issue
- demonstrate healthy practices
- demonstrate the benefits of behaviour changes to public health outcomes
- advocate a position on a health issue or policy
- increase demand or support for public health services
- argue against misconceptions about health (adjusted from Wikipedia 2016).

Effective communication in a range of contexts is core to success in health promotion and public health practice. Communication in all its forms should be clear, unambiguous and without distortion of the message. This chapter covers some of the fundamentals of relationships with clients, communication skills and barriers to effective health communication. For a more detailed coverage of spoken, written and electronic health communication, see Harvey (2012).

EXPLORING RELATIONSHIPS WITH CLIENTS

Health promoters and public health practitioners should ask themselves some fundamental questions. For example, what is your basic attitude towards the people to whom your health promotion is directed? Do you accept them on their own terms or do you judge them by your own standards? Do you aim to enable people to be independent, make their own decisions, take control of their health and solve their own health problems? Or are you actually encouraging dependency, solving their problems for them and thereby decreasing their own ability and confidence to take responsibility for their health? It may be useful to work through the following questions, thinking about how you relate to your clients.

Accepting or Judging?

Accepting people is demonstrated by:

- recognising that clients' knowledge and beliefs emerge from their life experiences, whereas your own have been modified and extended by professional education and experience
- understanding your own knowledge, beliefs, values and standards
- understanding your clients' knowledge, beliefs, values and standards from their point of view
- recognising that you and your clients may differ in your knowledge, beliefs, values and standards
- recognising that these differences do not suggest that you, the professional health promoter, are a person of greater worth than your clients.

Judging people is demonstrated by:

- equating people's intrinsic worth with their knowledge, beliefs, values, standards and behaviour. For example, saying that someone who drinks beyond safe limits is foolish both judges and condemns that person and takes no account of personal circumstances, life experience and

cultural background. Saying that drinking beyond safe levels may damage health does not judge the person in the same way
- ranking knowledge and behaviour. For example, 'I'm the expert so I know better than you' is judgemental; 'I know a considerable amount about this particular health issue' is a statement of fact. 'My standards are higher than yours' is judgemental; 'My standards are different from yours' is not.

Autonomy or Dependency?

There are a number of ways in which you can help clients to take more control over their health.

Autonomy can be enabled by:

- encouraging people to think things through and make their own health decisions, resisting the urge to dominate the decision-making process
- respecting any unusual ideas they may have.

Autonomy can be hindered if:

- you impose your own solution on your clients' health problems
- you tell them what to do because they are taking too long to think it through for themselves
- you tell them that their ideas are not good and won't work without giving an adequate explanation or an opportunity to try them out.

An aim which is compatible with health promotion principles and ethical practice is to work towards as much autonomy as possible. By doing this, you are helping people to increase control over their own health. Obviously, there are times when working towards autonomy may not be feasible. For example, it is more demanding of resources and clients may be dependent on a health promoter or public health practitioner because they are ill, uninformed or likely to put themselves or other people in danger.

A Partnership or a One-Way Process?

Do you think of yourself as working in partnership with people in pursuit of public health aims, or do you see health promotion as your sole responsibility with yourself as the expert?

A partnership means:

- there is an atmosphere of trust and openness between yourself and your clients so that they are not intimidated
- you ask people for their views and opinions, which you accept and respect even if you disagree with them
- you tell people when you learn something from them
- you use informal, participative methods when you are involved in health promotion, drawing on the experience and knowledge that clients bring with them
- you encourage clients to share their knowledge and experience with each other. People do this all the time, of course (for example, knowledge and experience are discussed between participants on a smoking cessation programme and parents in a baby clinic), but do you actively foster and encourage this?

A one-way process means:

- you do not encourage clients to ask questions and discuss health needs
- you imply that you do not expect to learn anything from your clients (and if you do learn, you don't say so)
- you do not find out people's health knowledge and experience
- you do not encourage people to learn from each other
- you use formal health promotion and public health approaches rather than participative methods.

Clients' Feelings – Positive or Negative?

A change in people's health knowledge, attitudes and actions will be helped if they feel good about themselves. It will rarely be helped if they are full of self-doubt, anxiety or guilt.

Clients will feel better about themselves if:

- you praise their progress, achievements, strengths and efforts, however small
- the consequences of unhealthy behaviour, such as smoking, are discussed without implying that the behaviour is morally bad

- time is spent exploring how to overcome difficulties, such as practical strategies to help a client stop smoking. This will help to minimise feelings of helplessness.

Clients will feel bad about themselves if:

- you ignore their strengths and concentrate on their weaknesses
- you ignore or belittle their efforts
- you attempt to motivate them by raising guilt and anxiety (such as 'if you don't stop smoking, you'll damage your baby').

To sum up, the health promotion and public health aim of enabling people to take control over and improve their health is best achieved by unconditional positive regard and working in nonjudgemental partnerships. This should seek to build on people's existing knowledge and experience, move them towards autonomy, empower them to take responsibility for their health and help them to feel positive about themselves. See NICE (2012) for evidence-informed recommendations for nonjudgemental communication in health settings.

SELF-ESTEEM, SELF-CONFIDENCE AND COMMUNICATION

The ability to communicate is closely linked to how people feel about themselves. People with low self-esteem tend to be over-critical of themselves and to underestimate their abilities. This lack of self-confidence is reflected in their ability to communicate. For example, they may lack assertiveness and thus may either fail to speak up for themselves or react with inappropriate anger and even violence (Mind 2016).

Assertiveness means saying what you think and asking for what you want openly, clearly and honestly. It does not mean being aggressive or bullying, but it is in contrast with hiding what you really feel, saying what you don't really mean or trying to manipulate people into doing what you want.

Assertiveness helps people to create win–win situations (situations where everyone involved feels that they have achieved a reasonable outcome) through direct and open communication and through avoiding aggressive behaviour (which can result in win–lose situations, where one party feels that they have won and the other party feels they have lost) or manipulation (lose–lose situations, where, for example, one party in a negotiation walks out). It builds the self-esteem of all concerned. Successful negotiation is a good example of how assertiveness can work. In a successful negotiation, both parties are more likely to come away with the following thoughts:

- This is an agreement which, while not ideal, is good enough for both of us to support.
- Both of us made some compromises and sacrifices.
- We will be able to have successful negotiations with each other in future.

Many clients with low self-esteem will need to learn how to feel better about themselves before they can communicate effectively with health promoters and public health practitioners. People with low self-esteem require key life skills to take control of their health (see Mind 2016 for communication ideas on how to improve self-esteem).

LISTENING

As a health promoter and public health practitioner, you need to develop skills of effective listening so that you can enable people to talk and identify their health needs.

Listening is an active process. It is not the same as merely hearing words. It involves a conscious effort to listen to words, to the way they are said, to be aware of the feelings shown and of attempts to hide feelings. It means taking note of the NVC and the spoken words. The listener needs to concentrate on giving the speaker full attention, being on the same level physically as the speaker and adopting a nonthreatening posture. Fig. 10.1 demonstrates that listening and hearing are not the same thing. Most people are born with the ability to hear but not with the ability to be good listeners. Hearing occurs automatically and requires no conscious effort. If the physiological elements in your ears and your brain work, then the impulses will be received. However, what you do with the impulses after you receive them belongs to the realm of listening.

Listening effectively is a deliberate process and requires that we expend energy. The greater the amount of energy we put into listening, the more effective we will be at understanding and helping others identify and meet their health needs.

Active listening requires energy and involves searching for an understanding of the underlying meaning behind the words used by the client. There are various levels of listening which require different skills and energy.

When hearing, it is easy to allow attention to wander. Some of the things you may find yourself doing instead of listening are planning what to say next, thinking about a similar experience, interrupting, agreeing or disagreeing, judging, blaming or criticising, interpreting what the speaker says, thinking about the next job to be done or just plain daydreaming.

The task of listening to help others is to encourage people to talk about their situation unhurriedly

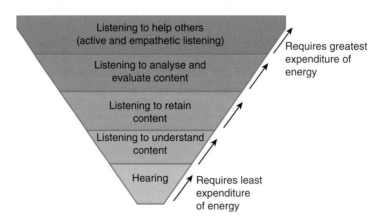

FIG. 10.1 ■ Spectrum showing the transition from hearing to listening. *(Source: Rowan (2013) citing Gamble and Gamble (2005))*

and without interruption, enabling them to express their feelings, views and opinions, and to explore their knowledge, values and attitudes. This reinforces the speakers' responsibility for themselves and is essential for helping them towards greater responsibility for their own health choices. See Gamble and Gamble (2013) for more information and ideas on effective listening. To practise listening skills, work on Exercise 10.1.

EXERCISE 10.1
Learning to Listen

Work in groups of three to six people. Appoint someone as a timekeeper.

1. Person A speaks for 2 minutes, without interruption, on a health subject of her choice to do with work or other interests (for example, sensible drinking guidelines, keeping fit and active). Everyone else in the group listens without interrupting or taking notes.

2. Person B repeats as much as she can remember without anyone else interrupting. Person B may not:
   - add anything extra to what A said
   - give interpretations (for example, 'It's obvious from what she said that ...')
   - give comments (for example, 'She's just like me ...').

3. Person A, and the rest of the group, identifies what was inaccurate, forgotten or added.

4. Repeat, with a different topic, until everyone has had a turn at being A and B.

5. Discuss the following questions:
   - What helped me to listen?
   - What helped me to remember?
   - What hindered my listening?
   - What hindered my remembering?
   - What did I learn about myself as a listener?

ENABLING PEOPLE TO TALK

The main task of the listener is to encourage and enable someone to talk. There are several useful techniques, as follows.

See also Chapter 14, section on strategies for decision making, which discusses counselling skills.

Giving an Invitation to Talk

To get someone started, it may be helpful to give out a specific invitation to talk. Examples are:

'You don't seem to be your usual self today. Is something on your mind?'

'Can we talk some more about that matter you raised briefly at yesterday's meeting?'
'You look worried – are you?'

Giving Attention

This means listening closely to what is being said and being fully aware of all the channels of communication including nonverbal behaviour. It requires effort and concentration to listen hard and give full, undivided attention.

Encouraging

This means making the occasional intervention to encourage someone to continue talking. It tells the speaker that you really are listening and want to hear more. Such interventions include noises or paralanguage like 'mm mm', words such as 'yes ...' and short phrases such as 'I see ...', 'And then ...?' or 'Go on ...'.

Another useful intervention is the repetition of a key word which the speaker has just used. For example, if the speaker says 'I am worried by my weight gain', you could repeat the word 'weight ...?'

Paraphrasing

This means responding to the speaker using your own words to state the essence of what the speaker has been saying. Use key words and phrases, for example, 'So you're not sure whether to have the baby vaccinated or not?' or 'So you are feeling unhappy because you are overweight and being unhappy triggers overeating?'

Reflecting Feelings

This involves mirroring back to the speaker, in verbal statements, the feeling he is communicating. To do this, it helps to listen for words about feelings and to observe body language. Examples are 'You seem pleased' or 'You are obviously upset about this'.

Reflecting Meanings

This means joining feelings and content in one succinct response to get a reflection of meaning:

'You feel ... because ...'
'You are ... because ...'
'You're ... about ...'

For example:

'You feel pleased about your weight loss progress.'
'You're depressed because your children have grown up and left home.'
'You're angry about all the traffic pollution on the streets of your neighbourhood.'

Summing Up

This is a brief restatement of the main content and feelings which have been expressed throughout a conversation. Check back with the speaker to ensure that the statement is accurate. For example, say 'It seems to me that the main things you've been saying are … Does that cover it?'

Exercise 10.2 gives you the opportunity to practise skills in enabling people to talk.

EXERCISE 10.2

Helping People to Talk

Work in pairs. Each person chooses a topic she feels strongly about (which might be a personal experience or topic of general concern such as sex education, traffic jams, cuts in the health service or increase in childhood obesity). Stay with the same topic for all three stages of the exercise. (The whole exercise takes about 45 minutes.)

Stage 1. Giving attention

One person speaks for 2 minutes, and the other listens, giving only nonverbal feedback. Then swap roles. After both of you have had your turn, spend 10 minutes discussing these questions:

When you were listening:
- What did you find difficult about listening?
- Did your mind wander?
- Did you maintain eye contact?
- What did you notice about the speaker's NVC?

When you were speaking:
- What did the listener do which helped you to talk?
- Did the listener do anything that made it difficult for you to talk?

Stage 2. Encouraging

One person speaks for 2 minutes. The other listens and gives encouraging interventions (such as 'mm mm'), words ('yes …') and nondirective comments ('I see …') or repeats key words. Swap roles. Then spend 5 minutes discussing these questions:

When you were listening:
- What sort of interventions did you make?
- How did you feel about making them?

When you were speaking:
- What interventions did you notice?
- Did you find them helpful?

Stage 3. Paraphrasing, reflecting back and summing up

One person speaks for 5 minutes and the other listens. The listener makes encouraging interventions as in Stage 2 but *also* paraphrases, reflects feelings and reflects meaning when she feels it is appropriate. At the end, she makes a brief statement summing up the main content and feelings of the speaker, checking with the speaker that her summing up is accurate. Exchange roles. Then spend 10 minutes discussing these questions:

When you were listening:
- What sort of interventions did you make?
- How did you feel about making them?

When you were speaking:
- What interventions did you notice?
- Did you find them helpful?

ASKING QUESTIONS AND GETTING FEEDBACK

Skillful questioning will help people to give clear, full and honest replies. It is useful to distinguish different types of questions.

Types of Questions

Closed questions are questions that require short, factual answers, often only one word. Examples are:

'What is your name?'
'Is this address correct?'
'Are you able to see me again next Tuesday?'

Closed questions are appropriate when brief, factual information is required. They are not appropriate when the aim is to encourage talking at more length. So 'Did you get on OK with your healthy eating plan last week?', which could be answered by 'yes' or 'no', is not the best way to encourage people to express their experiences of trying to change what they eat. A better question would be 'How did you get on with your healthy eating plan last week?' This is an open question.

Open questions give an opportunity for full answers. Examples are:

'How did you get on at the meeting yesterday?'
'What situations do you feel trigger overeating?'
'What do you think about trying to take a short brisk walk every day?'

Note that words like 'how', 'what', 'feel' and 'think' are useful for encouraging a full response.

Biased questions indicate the answer the questioner wants to hear or expects to hear. In other words, biased questions are likely to bias the response by leading the person who answers in a particular direction. Examples are:

'You're feeling better today, aren't you?' (This is biased because it would be easier to answer 'yes' than 'no'.)

'You have been doing what we discussed last time, haven't you?'

'Surely you aren't going to do that, are you?'

Multiple questions contain more than one question. Multiple questions are likely to confuse, because the listener will not know which question to answer and probably will not remember all of them. Examples are:

'Is this a serious problem for you – when did it start?'

'Does your store have a policy on promoting healthy foods – do you stock low-alcohol drinks and did you promote displays of low-fat products during the special campaign last September?'

'What are you going to do to get the Council to take all this rubbish away and are you going to get more bottle banks and newspaper recycling bins?'

EXERCISE 10.3
Asking Questions

Work in groups of about 10 people.

Decide on a topic on which it is easy to think of health-related questions, such as exercise levels, diet or my family.

- Person A volunteers to answer questions.
- Person B observes the length of A's response to questions.
- Person C observes A's nonverbal behaviour (body language).
- Everyone else has the task of asking questions.

First, everyone in turn asks a *closed* question on the topic.

Second, everyone in turn asks an *open* question on the topic.

Third, everyone asks *biased* questions on the topic.

After these three rounds of questions:

- Person A says how she felt about having to answer the three different kinds of questions (e.g. clear? muddled? irritated? angry? confused?).
- Person B says what she observed about the length of A's responses to the three kinds of questions.
- Person C says what she observed about A's nonverbal behaviour when answering the three different kinds of questions.

Discuss the application of what you found out to your health promotion and public health work.

'Are you sure you know what to do or would you like me to explain it again?'

Exercise 10.3 is an opportunity to practise asking appropriate questions.

Getting Feedback

After people have been given some information or have been taught a skill, it is very important to check to make sure that they really have understood what was said and remembered it, or mastered the skill. This is especially important when there is any doubt about how much has been understood, perhaps because, for example, someone is in a state of anxiety or has a limited command of English. There are two key points to note about getting feedback.

1. *It is* your *responsibility to ensure that the communication has been received and understood.* It is not the fault of the listener if they tried but did not understand.

It can be helpful to ask a question in a way which shows that it is your responsibility as a health promoter and public health practitioner to be understood. For example, say 'May I check to make sure I've covered everything – could you just recap what you understand so far?' Avoid questions, such as 'Let's see if you've learnt it yet, could you show me?' or 'I don't think you've totally understood, tell me what you think the main points are'.

2. *Ask open questions.* Closed questions such as 'Do you understand?' are not an adequate way of getting feedback. People may answer 'yes' because they are embarrassed or intimidated. Or they might just want to draw the conversation to a quick conclusion. Ask open questions, such as 'Could you please tell me what you're going to do …'

COMMUNICATION BARRIERS

As health promoters and public health practitioners, you may encounter numerous difficulties in communicating. Recognising that communication barriers exist is the necessary first stage before work can begin on tackling the problems. There are no easy solutions, but increased awareness and skill can go a long way towards improvement.

Common communication barriers may be categorised into the following six types.

1. Social and Cultural Gaps

A number of factors can cause gaps, including:

- different ethnic or social groups, which may be apparent in dress, language or accent
- different cultural or religious beliefs, for example, about hygiene, nutrition or contraception
- different values, reflected in a different emphasis on the importance of health issues
- different gender or sexual orientation, reflected in different approaches, interests or values.

2. Limited Receptiveness

You might want to communicate, but the reverse is not always true: people might not want to be communicated with. They may be unreceptive for many reasons including:

- learning difficulty or confusion
- illness, tiredness or pain
- emotional distress
- being too busy, distracted or preoccupied
- not valuing themselves or not believing that their health is important.

3. Negative Attitude to the Health Promoter and Public Health Practitioner

Some people may be resistant to you even before you have met. This may be caused by:

- previous negative experiences
- lack of trust in anyone seen as an authority figure
- lack of credibility of the health promoter (perhaps you set a poor example of good health yourself?)
- perceiving you as a threat, coming to criticise or pass judgement
- thinking that they already have the knowledge and skills
- believing that advice will be given which they cannot comply with because of financial or social constraints, or being asked to change a lifestyle or behaviour that they enjoy
- not wishing to confront issues such as personal health problems or the need to change policies and practices at an organisational level.

4. Limited Understanding and Memory

There may be difficulties because people:

- understand and/or speak little or no English

- have limited education or learning difficulties, and may be unable to read and write
- are being confronted with technical words, jargon or medical terminology that they do not understand
- have poor or failing memories and cannot remember what was discussed previously.

5. Insufficient Emphasis by the Health Promoter

Communication may fail because you do not give it sufficient time and attention. The reasons may be:

- communication was given a low priority in basic training, so it is given low priority in practice
- lack of confidence, skills and knowledge, which may be the result of inadequate training
- being too busy with other things and unable to find the time
- managers not being supportive about time spent on health promotion
- reluctance to demystify and share professionally acquired health knowledge.

6. Contradictory Messages

Communication barriers are erected when people receive different messages from different people. For example:

- different health professionals give different advice
- family, friends or neighbours contradict health promoters and public health messages or evidence
- health advice changes as evidence is updated.

To identify communication barriers in your public health work, undertake Exercise 10.4.

EXERCISE 10.4
Identifying Communication Barriers

This exercise can be done alone, but it is best carried out in pairs or small groups so that ideas can be shared.

Consider the six types of communication barriers discussed.

1. How many of them can you identify in your own health promotion and public health practice experience?
2. What other communication barriers can you add to this list?
3. What communication barriers cause you the most problems?
4. What suggestions can you make for helping to break down communication barriers? (Share examples from your own experience and make additional suggestions.)

OVERCOMING LANGUAGE BARRIERS

Language is only one facet of the gulf that may exist between people of different ethnic backgrounds. The root of communication problems may be racism. This is a huge topic, largely outside the scope of this book, but all health promoters should take part in racism awareness training when working with people from different ethnic groups (see Kale and Kumar 2012 for more about communication in multiethnic societies and how it impacts on health equity).

However, when we focus solely on the question of language barriers, learning a few essential words and phrases in the other person's language may help. Help with learning the language may be available from multicultural education centres run by local education authorities.

When faced with a language barrier, there are some useful guidelines which you can follow to help someone with limited English to understand what is being said. See Box 10.1 and Exercise 10.5.

EXERCISE 10.5

Overcoming Language Barriers

The following five extracts come from the district nurse's side of a conversation with a patient whose English is very limited.

1. 'Hello – Oh, we are looking brighter today!'
2. 'Have you been visited by the doctor today yet? Did he give you a new prescription?'
3. 'I'll see about your insulin after I've seen how your leg's getting on.'
4. 'The doctor says you should take one of these tablets three times a day ... I don't think you understand – I'll say that again ... We want you to take one of these tablets three times a day ... Oh dear ... (louder) ... DOCTOR SAYS YOU TAKE TABLET THREE TIMES A DAY.'
5. 'I'll leave this list of foods for you. There are ticks and crosses on it to show you what you can eat and what you should not eat. Do you understand? Your son can read English, can't he?'

Using the guidelines in points 1 through 8 in Box 10.1:

■ Identify what is unhelpful about the way the district nurse speaks to the patient.

■ Suggest better alternatives.

BOX 10.1
GUIDELINES FOR HEALTH PROMOTION AND PUBLIC HEALTH COMMUNICATION WITH INDIVIDUALS OR SMALL GROUPS WHO SPEAK LITTLE ENGLISH

If you are engaging in health promotion and public health with individuals or small groups who speak little English, you should attempt to find out whether a translator could be present. If you use a translator, allocate more time for the session. Give information concisely and in stages; this will allow time for the translator to explain to the clients and to translate back information from the clients. Using children or relatives to translate information to clients can be less reliable than using trained translators.

If you do not have a translator, the following points may be helpful:

1. Speak clearly and slowly, and resist raising your voice in an effort to be understood.
2. Repeat a sentence if you have not been understood using the same words. If you use different words you are likely to cause more confusion by introducing even more words which are not understood.
3. Keep it simple. Use simple words and sentences. Use active forms of verbs rather than passive forms, so say 'The nurse will see you' rather than 'You will be seen by the nurse'. Do not try to cover too much information, and stick to one topic at a time.

4. Say things in a logical sequence: the sequence in which they are going to happen. So say 'Eat first, then take the tablet' rather than 'Take the tablet after you eat'. If the listener does not pick up the word 'after' correctly, he will take the tablet first, because that is the order in which he heard the instruction.
5. Be careful of idioms, such as 'spending a penny', which may be totally incomprehensible.
6. Do not attempt to speak pidgin English. It does not help people to learn correct English and sounds patronising.
7. Use pictures, mime and simple written instructions, which may be read by relatives or friends who understand written English. Be careful of symbols on written material; ticks and crosses, for example, might not convey what you intend.
8. Check to ensure that you have been understood, but avoid asking closed questions that require a one-word answer such as 'Do you understand?' A reply of 'yes' is no guarantee that your client really has understood.

See section on asking questions and getting feedback earlier in this chapter.

NONVERBAL COMMUNICATION

Nonverbal communication (NVC) includes the ways people communicate other than by the spoken word. It is sometimes called body language. The main categories of NVC are as follows:

Bodily Contact

Bodily contact is people touching each other, how much they touch and which parts of the body are in contact. Shaking hands, holding hands or putting an arm around someone's shoulders, for example, all convey a meaning from one person to another.

Some health promoters, such as nurses, obviously touch patients frequently in the course of their work, whereas others, such as environmental health officers, would not. Touching people is governed by rules dictated by cultural expectations and taboos, and by expectations of professional distance, which may be barriers to the positive use of touch. For example, a handshake can say 'I'm glad to see you – welcome' and touching a distressed person can say 'I'm here for you'.

Proximity

Proximity is how close people are to each other. Different messages are conveyed to a patient confined to bed by someone who talks to him from 6 feet away at the foot of the bed and by someone who comes closer and sits on the bed or a chair. However, people vary in the amount of personal space they need and may feel uncomfortable when others come too close.

Orientation

How individuals position themselves in relation to other people and objects is known as orientation. A useful example is to consider the messages conveyed by the arrangement of a room where a small group of people are meeting. Chairs in rows facing one separate chair (perhaps with a table in front of it) imply that one person will dominate and control the meeting, whereas chairs placed in a circle without a table to act as a barrier imply that everyone is encouraged to join in and that no one individual is expected to dominate.

Level

This refers to differences in height between people. Generally, communication is more comfortable if people are on the same level; so it feels better to bend down or sit down to talk to a child or a person in a wheelchair,

for example. Talking to someone on a different level can leave one or both parties feeling disadvantaged. Sometimes this is done deliberately; for instance, not offering a chair to someone entering an office conveys a message that the visitor is not welcome to stay.

Posture

Posture is how people stand, sit or lie. For example, are they upright or slouched, arms crossed or not? Posture can convey a message of tension and anxiety, for example, by being hunched up with arms crossed or one of welcome by being upright with arms outstretched.

Physical Appearance

All kinds of messages may be conveyed by physical appearance, such as a person's social standing, personality, tidy habits or concern with fashion. Physical appearance can be very important to health promoters because of the messages it conveys. A uniform may convey an impression of professional competence but may also convey an unwelcome image of authority. Casual dress in a formal committee may convey the impression (perhaps a false one) that the committee's work is not being taken seriously.

Facial Expression

Facial expression can obviously indicate feelings, such as sadness, happiness, anger, surprise or puzzlement.

Hand Movements and Head Movements

Movements of the hands and head can be very revealing. Nods and shakes of the head obviously convey agreement and disagreement without the need for words. It is important to note that movements of the head and hands do not convey the same meaning in all cultures. Clenched fists, fidgeting hands (and sometimes tapping feet) reveal stress and tension, whereas still, open hands usually denote a relaxed frame of mind. Mental discomfort, such as confusion or worry, is often shown by putting the hands to the head and playing with the hair, stroking a beard or rubbing the forehead.

Direction of Gaze and Eye Contact

Direct eye contact is significant. As a general rule, a speaker looks away from the listener for most of the time when talking (because they are concentrating on what they are saying) and looks directly at the listener when they wants a response. The general rule is that the listener will look the speaker straight in the eye while they are paying attention to what they say but will look elsewhere if their attention has wandered. This is particularly important if you work with people on a one-to-one basis; a person who is talking to you will infer that you are not listening if you are looking anywhere other than at them. It is critical when counselling someone in distress; the counsellor needs to be giving the client full attention, and if the client looks up and sees the counsellor gazing elsewhere, the implication is that they are not listening (see Hough 2014 for more details on the counselling process).

Nonverbal Aspects of Speech

Consider how many ways a word like 'no' can be said. The way in which it is said can convey meanings such as anger, doubt or surprise. Tone and timing are two nonverbal aspects of speech which convey messages to the listener.

Raised awareness of NVC can help you to improve communication between you and the people you work with. For example, a person who says 'Yes, I understand' in a doubtful tone of voice with a puzzled frown clearly requires further explanation. Words alone are only part of a message and can be misleading. See Williams (2016) for more information and insights into NVC and undertake Exercise 10.6 to explore NVC in your work.

EXERCISE 10.6

Nonverbal Communication in Your Health Promotion and Public Health Practice Work

Work through the following questions and exercises with a partner.

1. When do you touch people in your health promotion and public health role, if at all?
   What rules govern when it is acceptable/unacceptable to touch them?
   Would people you work with be helped if you touched them more?

2. Carry on a conversation with your partner, first standing too close for comfort, then standing too far away.
   What does it feel like? What is the most comfortable distance?
   What implications does this have for your work?

3. When you talk to an individual in the course of your work, where do you sit or stand in relation to that person? For example, is furniture a barrier between you?
   If you talk to people in groups, how do you seat them?
   Do you think communication could be improved by making changes? If so, what changes?

4. Have a conversation with your partner with one of you sitting and the other standing. Both describe your feelings.
   Do you ever communicate with people who are on a physically different level from you?
   What are the implications for your health promotion effectiveness?

5. Practise tense and relaxed postures, then welcoming and rejecting postures.
   Which do you normally adopt with people?

6. Identify a few people you have studied or worked with whom you know fairly well. Think back to your first impressions of these people.
   Do you think that your first impressions were right?
   What were the important features of their appearance which led to your first impressions?
   What is the importance of physical appearance in your health promotion work?
   If you wear a uniform or a white coat, how do you think it affects your relationships with the individuals and groups you work with?

7. Look around at other people in the room.
   What can you infer from their facial expressions or hand and head movements?
   What is the importance of noticing facial expression or hand and head movement in your job?

8. Hold a conversation with your partner while first staring into each other's eyes all the time and then without looking at each other at all. Describe your feelings.
   Watch two people talking.
   Do they look directly at each other or do they frequently look away?
   Do they look more at each other when speaking or listening?
   How important is eye contact in your job?

9. Say 'I don't know' in as many ways as possible, trying to convey a different feeling each time, such as despair, confusion and irritation.
   How important is it for you to pick up on nonverbal aspects of speech in your health promotion work?

To consolidate your understanding of NVC, read Williams 2016 and watch the TED talk under the YouTube references at the end of this chapter.

OTHER FORMS OF COMMUNICATION

Writing is a craft, as well as an art, which all health promoters and public health practitioners need to develop. The 12-point guidelines in Box 10.2 may help with written communication, and Box 10.3 offers guidelines for all forms of public health communication including multimedia.

Public health communication and campaigns apply integrated strategies to deliver messages designed, directly or indirectly, to influence health behaviours of target audiences. The communication of messages

---

BOX 10.2
GUIDELINES ON PROFESSIONAL WRITING

1. The point of writing is clear communication. On the whole, the more simply and briefly you write, the more effective your writing is likely to be.
2. Think about what kind of document you are writing. For example, is it a paper for a formal committee, a memo to your manager or a letter to a client? This will help you to know what style to write in: formal in a set lay out for a committee, brief and to the point for a manager, business-like but friendly to a client.
3. Think about who is reading what you write, and what sort of communication they will welcome: how long should it be, how detailed, how formal or chatty, first-person or third-person?
4. Use clear, simple language, and avoid long or obscure words if you can find shorter or more familiar ones.
5. Avoid technical terms if you can. If you must use them, explain them in the text or a footnote the first time you use them.
6. Keep sentences short.
7. Break the text up with paragraphs. A paragraph should usually deal with one point and its immediate development. A new point needs a new paragraph. In formal papers and reports, use numbering, headings and subheadings to break up the text and guide the reader through.
8. Use active rather than passive verbs where possible as this is stronger and simpler. For example, write 'the health promoter advised the client on healthy eating' rather than 'the client was advised on healthy eating by the health promoter'.
9. Make sparing use of adjectives and adverbs to make your writing more striking. For example, 'the client was really very upset, cried and sobbed a lot and said they would never, ever come back to the smoking cessation programme again' (25 words) could be better expressed as 'the client was distressed and said they would never return to the smoking cessation programme' (15 words).
10. Use language accurately.
11. Use a spell and grammar checker on a word processor or ask someone to proofread.
12. If you have the time, finish a piece of writing and then put it aside for a few days. This gives your subconscious mind a chance to think about it, and you can take a fresh look and edit it. Check for clarity, simplicity and coherent structure.

BOX 10.3
A GUIDE TO EFFECTIVE PUBLIC HEALTH COMMUNICATIONS ACROSS CONTEXTS

Attributes of effective health communication
- **Accuracy:** The content is valid and without errors of fact, interpretation or judgement.
- **Availability:** The content (whether targeted message or other information) is delivered or placed where the audience can access it. Placement varies according to audience, message complexity and purpose, ranging from interpersonal and social networks to billboards and mass transit signs to prime-time TV or radio, to public kiosks (print or electronic), to the internet.
- **Balance:** Where appropriate, the content presents the benefits and risks of potential actions or recognises different and valid perspectives on the issue.
- **Consistency:** The content remains internally consistent over time and also is consistent with information from other sources (the latter is a problem when other widely available content is not accurate or reliable).
- **Cultural competence:** The design, implementation and evaluation process that accounts for special issues for select population groups (for example, ethnic, racial and linguistic) and also educational levels and disability.
- **Evidence base:** Relevant scientific evidence that has undergone comprehensive review and rigorous analysis to formulate practice guidelines, performance measures, review criteria and technology assessments for telehealth applications.
- **Reach:** The content gets to or is available to the largest possible number of people in the target population.
- **Reliability:** The source of the content is credible, and the content itself is kept up-to-date.

BOX 10.3
A GUIDE TO EFFECTIVE PUBLIC HEALTH COMMUNICATIONS ACROSS CONTEXTS *(Continued)*

- **Repetition:** The delivery of/access to the content is continued or repeated over time, both to reinforce the impact with a given audience and to reach new generations.

- **Timeliness:** The content is provided or available when the audience is most receptive to, or in need of, the specific information.
- **Understandability:** The reading or language level and format (including multimedia) are appropriate for the specific audience.

Source: Healthy People 2010 Archive (2016)

comes through various channels that can be categorised as: mass media (such as television, radio, billboards), small media (for example, brochures and posters), social media (Facebook, Twitter, blogs) and the interpersonal communication (one-on-one or group education) previously covered. Box 10.3 offers guidelines for effective communication across all forms of public health communication including mass media, small media and social media.

Health Literacy and Health Communications

One of the aims of effective communication in health promotion and public health is to improve health literacy, both in individual clients and with target groups and whole populations. The World Health Organization has defined health literacy as the personal characteristics and social resources needed for individuals and communities to access, understand, appraise and use information and services to make decisions about their health (WHO 2016). Healthliteracy (2016) claim that levels of functional health literacy are low in the UK. Health information in current circulation is written at too complex a level for 43% of working age adults (16 to 65 years); this figure rises to 61% if the health information includes numeracy. We do not know how many people are additionally burdened by low interactive and critical health literacy skills, but numbers are likely to be even higher.

The important point to note here is that health literacy has been shown to have an effect on health and illness. For example, research from the United States shows that those with low health literacy are more likely to have a long-term health condition (Berkman et al 2011). Health literacy is a social determinant of

health and is strongly linked with other social determinants such as poverty, unemployment and membership of a minority ethnic group (Healthliteracy 2016). Where health literacy differs from these other social factors is that it is, potentially, open to positive change through health promotion and public health interventions. Improving health literacy, therefore, should be a goal for health promoters and public health practitioners. For further reading on health literacy Sorensen et al (2012) offer a systematic review which integrates definition and models of health literacy, and Crondahl and Karlsson (2016) discuss the link between health literacy and empowerment.

PRACTICE POINTS

- The quality of your relationships with your clients is at the heart of your health promotion and public health role. It is important to review and consider how your attitudes and values are reflected in your professional communication.
- Good communication and the development of health literacy are fundamental to health promotion and public health goals.
- Words, whether verbal or written, are only a small part of public health interaction, and it is important to consider all aspects of communication.
- Written and multimedia communication are core competencies in health promotion and public health practice, and need to be reviewed and developed.

REFERENCES

Berkman ND, Sheridan SL, Donahue KE, Halpern DJ, Crotty K 2011 Low health literacy and health outcomes: an updated systematic review. Annals of Internal Medicine 155(2):793–4.

Crondahl K, Karlsson LE 2016 The nexus between health literacy and empowerment: a scoping review. Sage Open http://dx.doi.org/10.1177/2158244016646410. Published 2 May 2016.

Gamble SK, Gamble MW 2013 Interpersonal communication: building connections together. London, Sage.

Gamble TK, Gamble MW 2005 Contacts: interpersonal communication in theory, practice, and context. Cambridge, Pearson.

Harvey K 2012 Exploring health communication language in action. Abingdon Oxon, Routledge.

Healthliteracy 2016 Why is health literacy important?. https://twitter.com/LiteracyHealth?ref_src=twsrc%5Etfw.

Healthy People 2010 Archive 2016 Health Communication. http://www.healthypeople.gov/2010/document/html/volume1/11healthcom.htm.

Hough M 2014 Counselling skills and theory, 4th edn. London, Hodder Education.

Kale E, Kumar BN 2012 Challenges in healthcare in multi-ethnic societies: communication as a barrier to achieving health equity, public health. In Maddock J (ed.) social and behavioral health. ISBN: 978-953-51-0620-3, InTech, Available from http://www.in-techopen.com/books/publichealth-social-and-behavioral-health/communication-and-dialog-in-a-multiethnic-population.

Mind 2016 How to increase your self-esteem. http://www.mind.org.uk/information-support/types-of-mental-health-problems/self-esteem/#.V5X0uVVTGUk.

NICE 2012 Patient experience in adult NHS services: improving the experience of care for people using adult NHS services. https://www.nice.org.uk/guidance/cg138/chapter/1-guidance.

Rowan C 2013 Listening to need. The Achievement Centre. http://www.tac-focus.com/article/listening-needs#.V5dKTVVTGUk.

Sorensen K, Van den Broucke S, Fullam J et al 2012 Health literacy and public health: a systematic review and integration of definitions and models. BMC Public Health 2012, 12:80. http://www.biomedcentral.com/1471-2458/12/80.

Wikipedia 2016 Health communication. https://en.wikipedia.org/wiki/health_communication.

Williams K 2016 Body languages: the art of non-verbal communication. Amazon, CreateSpace Independent Publishing Platform.

World Health Organization 2016 Health literacy and health behaviour. http://www.who.int/healthpromotion/conferences/7gchp/track2/en/.

WEBSITES

Centre for Disease Control and Prevention Gateway to Health Communication & Social Marketing Practice with examples of communication campaigns. http://www.cdc.gov/healthcommunication/campaigns/.

For health literacy, see http://www.healthliteracy.org.uk/.

YOUTUBE

TED talk by Body Language Expert Mark Bowden at TEDxToronto – The importance of being inauthentic published on 27 Oct 2013. https://www.youtube.com/watch?v=rk_SMBIW1mg.

TED talk Your body language shapes who you are | Amy Cuddy published on 1 Oct 2012. https://www.youtube.com/watch?v=Ks-_Mh1QhMc.

TWITTER

Healthliteracy tweets. https://twitter.com/LiteracyHealth?ref_src=twsrc%5Etfw.

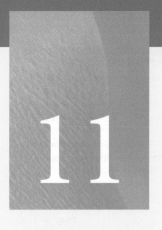

11

USING COMMUNICATION TOOLS IN HEALTH PROMOTION AND PUBLIC HEALTH PRACTICE

CHAPTER CONTENTS

SUMMARY

The first part of this chapter offers some principles governing the choice of communication tools and a summary of the uses, advantages and limitations of the main types of health promotion communication resources. There are guidelines for making the most of display materials, for producing written materials (including guidance on nonsexist writing) and for presenting statistical information. This is followed by a section on mass media including identifying the key characteristics of mass media, the variety of ways in which the mass media and the social media are channels for health promotion and public health, what they can be expected to achieve and how they can be used effectively. Guidelines are given for working with radio, television and the local press. There is a case study on the use of mass media advertising and exercises on writing plain English, preparing and presenting material on television and radio, writing a press release and writing a letter to the editor. The chapter ends with a section on using social media to promote health.

The range of communication tools outlined in Table 11.1 are used extensively by health promoters and public health practitioners in their health promoting activities but may not always be employed with maximum effectiveness. How communication tools are selected and used is as crucial as the quality of the resources themselves.

SELECTING PUBLIC HEALTH RESOURCES

There are a range of different types of communication tools available with a constant turnover as items become out of date or out of print and new ones come on the market. You could find yourself with the task of selecting a leaflet, poster, display or DVD from a range of possibilities. Or you may find that there is very little available, and you have to decide whether the one item you have found is suitable.

The following guidelines are designed to help you select any kind of material, such as leaflets, audiovisual

157

TABLE 11.1
Health Promotion Resources

Type of Resource	Uses and Advantages	Limitations
Leaflets and handouts	Clients can use at their own pace and discuss with other people. Educator and client can work through together. Can be easy and cheap to produce basic written information. Can reinforce points in a talk and add further detailed information. Can be produced in different languages	Commercially produced leaflets can be expensive and may contain advertising. Mass-produced leaflets are not tailored to everyone's needs. Not durable, easily lost. Mass distribution can be wasteful
Posters and display charts	Can raise awareness of issues. Can convey information and direct people to other sources (addresses, tel. numbers, 'pick up a leaflet'). Simple posters and information displays can be cheap to produce	High quality posters and display materials are expensive to make or buy. They are difficult to maintain. Need to ensure any writing is big enough to be read at the distance most people will see it. Displays need changing frequently to attract attention
Flip-charts, whiteboards.	Good for brainstorming and involving groups in producing ideas which can be stuck up round the room for discussion. Useful for recording notes to be written up later. Can be prepared in advance. Useful where no whiteboard available. Cheap	Educator needs to turn back to audience to write on board. Flip-chart paper easily torn and dog eared
PowerPoint presentation	Useful in large rooms or lecture theatres with a big screen. Complex information (such as graphs) can be seen clearly	Needs equipment and screen, and blackout
DVDs	Can be used to convey real situations otherwise inaccessible (e.g. childbirth), convey information, pose problems, demonstrate skills, trigger discussion on attitudes and behaviour. Can be used for self-teaching. Can be stopped, started or replayed to allow discussion	Normal TV-size screen too small for large audiences. Educator relies on equipment working properly. Equipment expensive and not easily transported. May need partially darkened room
CDs	Good for certain skills development, e.g. relaxation, exercise routines. Equipment cheap, easy to use and transport	Lack of visual material requires extra concentration to hold attention
Health websites	Websites have the potential of reaching a worldwide audience and are useful for raising awareness of health issues, conveying information and delivering self-help materials	There is an enormous amount of health information that can be accessed on the internet and no control over the quality
Facebook	Reaches a mass audience, can be accessed easily from websites, leaflets can carry the URL, health information posts can be updated daily and shared amongst large audiences for very little financial costs	The quality has to be evaluated and judgements have to be made about its suitability as a resource
YouTube	Reaches a mass audience. Can contain visual public health campaign material and a wide variety of health information that spreads the dissemination of a campaign	If you direct your clients to YouTube, they will also have access to other YouTube videos which may not be health enhancing
Micro Blogs and twitter	Dynamic and concise flow of information. Web logs (blogs) and numerous micro blogging platforms such as Twitter, allow users to publish messages (such as tweets). Tweets can be supplemented with hyperlinks to other online media, such as videos (for example those on YouTube) or websites. Tweets can also include 'hashtags', a form of information indexing that allows people to search for tweets that are related to a particular discussion or topic	It is difficult to control the quality if a range of people are accessing the microblogging platforms. It might increase inequality of access for those people who are not proficient in the social media

or social media, and you can also use them as a checklist when producing your own.

Is It Appropriate for Achieving Your Aims?

Think about the item in the context in which you intend to use it. For example, if you are working with a group of young smokers who are not motivated to stop, a leaflet on how to stop smoking may be ineffective. Materials which trigger discussion (perhaps a YouTube video) or setting up a stop smoking community blog (see the quit smoking community blog in the references at the end of this chapter) with the aim of challenging attitudes might be better.

Is It the Most Appropriate Kind of Resource?

Will something else be cheaper and just as effective, such as photographs instead of a DVD? Could you use the real thing, such as a young person who has successfully stopped smoking talking about their experiences instead of a DVD in a smoking cessation group, actual food instead of pictures or models in a nutrition talk with a weight management group?

Is It Consistent With Your Values and Approach?

If your approach is to work in a nonjudgemental partnership with your clients, the materials you use should reflect your values. You need to avoid material that is patronising, authoritarian, scaremongering or victim-blaming. Resources should not attribute or imply blame to individuals experiencing ill health when that ill health is rooted in their socioeconomic circumstances, for example, low income or poor housing.

See section on exploring relationships with clients in Chapter 10.

Is It Relevant for Your Clients?

Does it take account of the values, culture, health concerns, age, ethnic group, sex and socioeconomic circumstances of your clients? Does it reflect local practice and health services available?

Obvious examples of irrelevance are DVDs portraying lifestyles of affluent families, which are unhelpful if you are working with people who have limited financial resources. Materials designed for one ethnic group may not be appropriate for another, not just because

of language but because some aspects (such as sexual behaviour or attitudes to bereavement) are seen differently in different cultures.

Is It Racist, Sexist, Ageist?

All resources should be nonracist, nonsexist and non-ageist. Racist materials stereotype people, attributing certain roles or character attributes based on ethnic group alone. Implicit in this are the assumptions that one ethnic group is superior to another and represents the desired norm (see Liu et al 2012 for research on communicating with ethnic groups). Sexist materials stereotype gender roles, behaviours or character attributes. Resources should also not make assumptions about sexual orientation. Guidance on nonsexist writing is provided later in this chapter. Resources should reflect the fact that we live in a multiracial society where the roles of men and women have changed and continue to do so. Strong, positive messages and images should be provided of people of all ages, ethnic groups and both sexes.

Will It Be Understood?

Is it written in plain English, which people will readily understand? Are there any incorrect assumptions about the level of literacy or existing knowledge? Does it need to be produced in other languages to make it accessible to people from minority ethnic groups? Do leaflets and other visual material need to be produced in other formats so that they are accessible to people with disabilities, such as in large type or Braille, or for audiovisual media, for example, with sign language or subtitles inserted on the screen?

Is the Information Reliable?

Is information in the materials accurate, up-to-date, unbiased and complete? Or does it contain one-sided information on controversial issues and out-of-date or incomplete messages?

Does It Contain Advertising?

Commercial companies, such as drug companies, baby food manufacturers or makers of safety equipment, who produce material will produce leaflets and posters that will carry the name of the company or its products, or include advertisements. Using these resources can imply that you (or your employer) are endorsing the product. It may also damage your image as a credible source of unbiased health information, and lead people to doubt the value of the information.

For these reasons, resources containing company names, products and advertising should be avoided whenever possible. However, the item may be just what you want, and there may be no alternative. In which case:

- the product or service advertised must be ethically acceptable as healthy and environmentally friendly. This excludes tobacco, alcohol and confectionery advertising, for example.
- the advertising content must be low key. The company name on the front or back cover is acceptable, but constant references to name-brand products are not.

THE RANGE OF PUBLIC HEALTH RESOURCES: USES, ADVANTAGES AND LIMITATIONS

Table 11.1 summarises the wide range of communication resources available for promoting health and the key points about their uses, advantages and limitations. It is also important to note:

- resources are aids and should generally not be seen as substitutes for the health promoter or public health practitioner. Leaflets should be used in conjunction with face-to-face discussion. Audiovisual aids, including YouTube and social media, are best presented with an introduction and, when appropriate, a follow-up discussion and evaluation.
- it takes time and competencies to become familiar with developing and using all the health promotion and public health communication resources available.

See the section on public health teaching and learning in Chapter 12.

PRODUCING HEALTH PROMOTION AND PUBLIC HEALTH RESOURCES

Some resources, particularly posters, leaflets, audiovisual and web based materials, come ready made, but you might want to work with a community group to help them to produce materials that target their particular need or produce some yourself.

See also Chapter 10, section on written communication, and Chapter 12, section on improving patient communication.

This chapter does not offer a comprehensive guide on how to produce materials, but approaching the task in a systematic way using the planning and evaluation flowchart in Chapter 5 may be helpful. If you are producing a resource such as a public health leaflet, you will need to consider who will write the draft, who will edit it, whether and how to pilot the draft, what it will cost and whether you need the services of a desktop publisher, designer, illustrator, translator or printer.

Making the Most of Display Materials: Posters, Charts, Display Boards and Stands

Be brief and to the point. Keep the public health goal firmly in mind. Do not include material that is irrelevant; it will only distract from the main message.

Emphasis the key point(s). Use size of lettering, style or colour to achieve this. Place the important messages just above the centre of a display, which is the point of maximum visual impact.

Use language the audience understands. Explain any unfamiliar technical terms. If possible, express the message in both pictures and words. Test it out on a few people to ensure that you have no unexpected ambiguities in your message.

Be bold. Words and pictures should be as large as possible.

Make the most of colour. Colour can create continuity; for example, a repetition of background colour can link a series of posters. Colour can be used to identify parts of a diagram or highlight important information. Choose colours with care, because responses to colour are emotional (for example, green is soothing) and because colours may be associated with certain messages, images and places (such as red for danger, purple for funerals, white for clinical cleanliness).

Improve the display site. If all you have is a blank wall or a wall covered with distracting wallpaper, fix a rectangle of coloured card to the wall as a background display board. If a display board has a rough or marked surface, give it a coat of paint or a covering of coloured paper, hessian or felt.

Use the display site to best advantage. Busy corridors can only be useful sites for posters with immediate appeal and few words. More information can be conveyed in a waiting area, and it may be possible to supplement displays with leaflets to take away. Ensure that writing on displays is at eye level and large enough to read without people having to move from the queue or their chair.

Be aware of lighting. Daylight is unreliable; spotlights directed onto a display are ideal.

Making the Most of Written Materials: Instruction Sheets and Cards, Leaflets and Booklets

Pilot materials on a sample of consumers. Do not assume that you know what they like, want or need. *Ask them.*

Use colour, layout and print size to improve clarity. Larger print may be helpful for those people with a visual impairment.

Use plain English. Use everyday words; avoid jargon and explain any technical or medical words. Aim for short sentences of 15 to 20 words. Use active rather than passive verbs, for example, say 'Increase your fruit and vegetable consumption …' rather than 'Your fruit and vegetable consumption should be increased …'. Undertake Exercise 11.1 to practise plain English.

EXERCISE 11.1
Writing Plain English

Write plain English versions of the following. The first two are very similar to the instructions found on the packages of medication bought over the counter in chemist shops. The last two are very similar to passages in health promotion and public health leaflets.

1. *Wheezoff* paediatric syrup is specially formulated for children. It is indicated for the relief of cough and its congestive symptoms and for the treatment of hay fever and other allergic conditions affecting the upper respiratory tract. Contraindications, warnings, etc. Hypersensitivity to any of the active constituents. If symptoms persist, consult your doctor.

2. *Notwinge* cream – Directions for use. Apply a sufficient quantity of balm to the part affected. Massage lightly until penetration is complete.

3. The baby lies curled up in what is called the fetal position. It lies in a bag of water, and the membranes which make up this fluid-filled balloon are enclosed in the womb.

4. Vitamin B1, also called thiamin, is required for the functioning of the nervous system, digestion and metabolism. Insufficient vitamin B1 can cause anorexia and fatigue.

Do a readability test on your written materials. Many word-processing packages are able to give readability statistics, as well as the average sentence length and the percentage of passive sentences used. They give a rough measure of readability for adult readers based on the principle that the combination of long sentences and long words is harder to comprehend. But note that many other factors that affect readability are not taken into account, such as how the text is laid out, the use of illustrations and the size of print.

Nonsexist Writing

The importance of material being nonracist and nonsexist has already been discussed, but using language in a nonsexist way presents particular challenges. One is the use of 'man' as a generic term for a person. For example, people talk about manning an exhibition stand when it is just as likely to be staffed by a woman. Many job titles end with 'man' and date from the time when only men performed these duties, for example, postman.

Another problem is the generic use of the male pronoun. For example, 'Each doctor presented a case from his own practice', assumes that all the doctors are men. Although it may seem clumsy to say 'he' or 'she', it can sometimes usefully emphasis that both sexes are involved. An alternative which has been used in this book is to turn the singular into a plural and use the words 'they' or 'their', changing 'A health promoter and public health practitioner must be a fluent communicator. He must also be a good listener.' To 'Health promoters and public health practitioners must be fluent communicators. They must also be good listeners.'

It may be possible to rephrase a passage to eliminate the pronouns altogether. So, instead of 'Information given to a social work agency is confidential in the same way as communications between a doctor and his patients', say '… in the same way as communications between doctors and patients'.

Another way is to use 'you' instead of 'he', 'she' or a noun that implies male or female. For example, in a leaflet on parenting, you could change 'A mother often finds difficulty in persuading her 2-year-old to eat' to 'You may find difficulty in persuading your 2-year-old to eat' or 'Parents may find difficulty …' This avoids the implication that only mothers (not fathers) have a parenting role.

Or avoid 'he' by finding another noun. Thus, in 'You may find it difficult to persuade your 2-year-old to eat. He may prefer throwing his food around' instead you could say '… A child at this age may prefer throwing food around instead.'

It is also important to avoid sexism when speaking and writing. So, for instance, a health promoter or public health practitioner who refers to the women who attend a smoking cessation programme as 'the ladies' could affront the women in the group. It is far better to refer to the women who attend as 'patients' or 'clients'.

For further discussion of language barriers, see the section on overcoming language barriers in Chapter 10.

PRESENTING STATISTICAL INFORMATION

Numbers may be meaningless to lay people unless they are carefully presented in a visual way, such as in Fig. 11.1. A wide range of computer software programmes facilitates the production of information in

ways that are visually arresting and easy to understand. National Health System (NHS) organisations and local authorities are likely to have the equipment and expertise to support this production, and there are internet sites which also contain statistics reproduced visually. See, for example, Public Health England data in the web references at the end of the chapter.

Consider Figs 11.1 and 11.2 and analyse how effective these figures would be as a resource for use by health promoters and public health practitioners in their work with clients who smoke or who are overweight and obese. Discuss:

1. how they might be used.
2. how you might modify them for use.
3. how you might combine them with other resources.
4. whether there are any ethical issues with using figures such as these.
5. overall, how effective you think they are as public health resources.

For additional reading to support this exercise, see Walls et al (2011).

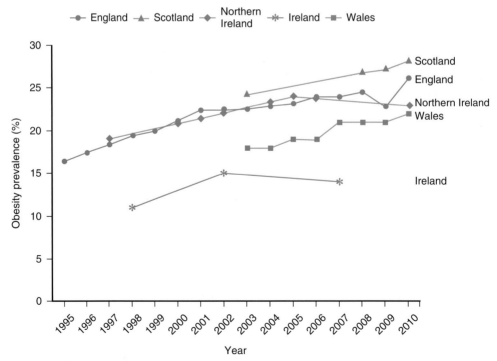

FIG. 11.1 ■ Trends in adult prevalence of obesity in the UK and Ireland. Adult (aged 16+) obesity: BMI ≥ 30 kg/m2 *(Source: Public Health England 2016a, taken from Scottish Health Survey, 2010; Health Survey for England, 2010; Health and social wellbeing survey & Health Survey for Northern Ireland; 2010 Welsh Health Survey, 2010; Survey of Lifestyles, Attitudes and Nutrition (SLAN), 2007.)*

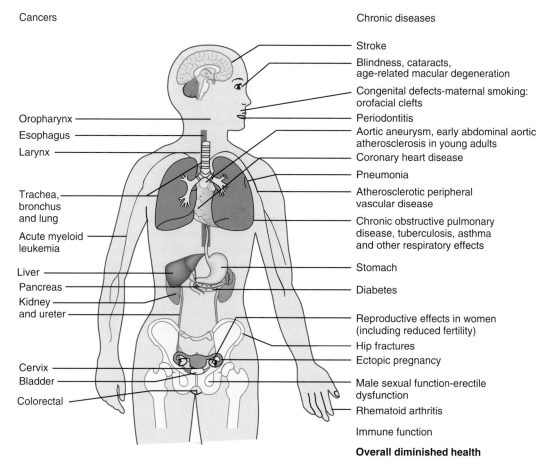

Cancers

Chronic diseases

- Stroke
- Blindness, cataracts, age-related macular degeneration
- Congenital defects-maternal smoking: orofacial clefts

Oropharynx
Esophagus
Larynx

- Periodontitis
- Aortic aneurysm, early abdominal aortic atherosclerosis in young adults
- Coronary heart disease
- Pneumonia

Trachea, bronchus and lung

- Atherosclerotic peripheral vascular disease

Acute myeloid leukemia

- Chronic obstructive pulmonary disease, tuberculosis, asthma and other respiratory effects

Liver
Pancreas
Kidney and ureter

- Stomach
- Diabetes

- Reproductive effects in women (including reduced fertility)
- Hip fractures

Cervix
Bladder

- Ectopic pregnancy
- Male sexual function-erectile dysfunction
- Rhematoid arthritis

Colorectal

- Immune function

Overall diminished health

FIG. 11.2 ■ The health consequences of active smoking.

USING THE MASS MEDIA TO PROMOTE HEALTH

The mass media are channels of communication to large numbers of people and include television, radio, the internet (see the section on social media in the following section), magazines and newspapers, books, displays and exhibitions. Leaflets and posters are also mass media when they are used on a stand-alone basis, as opposed to use as a learning aid in face-to-face communication with an individual or a group. However, usually when people talk about the media they are referring to television, radio, newspapers and magazines.

Health promoters and public health practitioners are most likely to become involved with mass media when undertaking public health programmes or campaigns with the public, or when a public health

issue becomes a news item. Probably most involvement will be with local newspapers and local radio or television. However, it is useful to put this into a wider context and to appreciate the range of ways in which health issues and messages are portrayed via mass media.

Mass Media as Tools for Health Promotion and Public Health

Health messages and information are sent through the mass media in a number of different ways:

- Planned, deliberate health promotion from posters, leaflets, displays and exhibitions on health themes, such as all of the mass media resources available for *Change4life* campaign, a campaign that aims to prevent people from becoming overweight by encouraging them to eat a healthy diet and take more exercise (NHS 2016), to advertisements and campaigns on television and the social media, such as the One You campaign focusing on encouraging lifestyle changes (Public Health England 2016b and Triggle 2016), and in newspapers (see, for example, Robinson et al 2013).

■ Health promotion by advertisers and manufacturers of healthy products and services, for example, Boots the chemist conveys a number of health and wellbeing messages through an advertising campaign (Swift 2016).

■ Books, television, newspapers and magazine articles about health issues which follow new research disseminated in academic conferences or journals or government publications. The problem here is that the media may distort the evidence with attention-grabbing headlines which can give out unhealthy messages, such as the example in Box 11.1.

Further ways health is addressed in the media are:

■ discussions of health issues as a byproduct of news items ('Rock star dies from drug overdose') or entertainment programmes, notably soap operas/serial dramas where a character has a health problem, such as being abused as a child or suffering from cancer.

■ health (or anti-health) messages conveyed covertly or incidentally, such as well-known personalities or fictional characters refusing cigarettes or, conversely, smoking. The portrayal of alcohol on television, for example, can convey a norm of heavy drinking and associates consumption of alcohol with benefits rather than costs.

■ planned promotions of anti-health messages such as advertisements for alcohol (see Alcohol Concern 2013 for alcohol advertising regulations).

■ sponsorships of health-promoting events and services by organisations or commercial companies,

BOX 11.1
NEW HEALTH RESEARCH REPORTED IN THE MEDIA CAN MISLEAD WITH ATTENTION-GRABBING HEADLINES

Low or Moderate Dietary Energy Restriction for Long-Term Weight Loss: What Works Best?

Theoretical calculations suggest that small daily reductions in energy intake can cumulatively lead to substantial weight loss, but experimental data to support these calculations are lacking. A 1-year randomized controlled pilot study was conducted of low (10%) or moderate (30%) energy restriction (ER) with diets differing in glycemic load in 38 overweight adults. Food was provided for 6 months and self-selected for 6 additional months. Measurements included body weight, resting metabolic rate and adherence to the ER prescription. The 10% ER group consumed significantly less energy than prescribed over 12 months, while the 30% ER group consumed significantly more. Changes in body weight, satiety and other variables were not significantly different between groups. However, during self-selected eating (6 to 12 months), variability in % weight change was significantly greater in the 10% ER group and poorer weight outcome on 10% ER was predicted by higher baseline BMI and greater disinhibition. Weight loss at 12 months was not significantly different between groups prescribed 10 or 30% ER, supporting the efficacy of low ER recommendations. However, long-term weight change was more variable on 10% ER, and weight

change in this group was predicted by body size and eating behaviour. These preliminary results indicate beneficial effects of low-level ER for some but not all individuals in a weight control programme and suggest testable approaches for optimising dieting success based on individualizing prescribed level of ER.

(Adjusted from the abstract of an article by Das et al (2009). Please refer to the article for full details.)

When the research previously described was published, the *Sunday Times* ran an article with the following misleading title:

Can crash diets be good for you? New research shows that crash diets can be a safe and effective way of keeping the pounds off

(Goodman 2009)

The *Daily Mail* also covered the research with an even more misleading headline:

Why crash dieting DOES work: Surprise evidence suggests it's the best way to slim

(Roberts 2009)

See Blumenthal and Pruthi (2016) for a discussion of a range of problems associated with health in the media and the misleading consequences of exaggerated headlines, and Robinson et al (2013) for an analysis of health stories in daily newspapers in the UK.

such as sponsorship of sporting events by alcohol companies (see, for example, Campbell 2014) or public health events by commercial companies (see NHS Commissioning Board 2012 for standards of business conduct including commercial sponsorship). By associating with a health-promoting event or service, the sponsor's product or service is brought to the public eye with an implied stamp of approval and a sense that it is somehow associated with health.

Using Mass Media to Promote Health

The fact that the message is sent via a medium, such as television, makes it difficult to obtain immediate feedback and modify the message to respond to the needs and characteristics of the audience. There can be some two-way communication through audience phone-ins, but mostly it is one-way, which has implications. For example, it is not possible for the sender to repeat, clarify or amplify the message, so in general it is best to use mass media to convey simple, rather than complex, messages.

There is research focusing on the efficacy of mass media for public health interventions and communications. Whilst reviews have found that mass media campaigns in public health can be effective, there are exceptions which note inconsistent findings (Newbold & Campos 2011). It is important for you to know what success you can realistically expect when you use mass media in your health promotion and public health work. The research evidence tells us how mass media can be used effectively, and what it cannot be expected to achieve, as follows.

Mass media *can* be an effective health promotion and public health tool if it fulfils the following criteria:

1. The information portrayed is:
   - perceived as relevant
   - supported by other approaches such as one-to-one advice
   - new and presented in an appropriate context.
2. The aim should be to:
   - raise awareness of health and health issues (for example, to trigger action to raise awareness about the impact of smoking on family members)

- deliver a simple message (for example, to make quitting easier by providing details of a national helpline for people who want to stop smoking)
- change behaviour (for example, to reinforce motivation and make quitting easier by phoning for a leaflet or other support).
3. The use of mass media is part of an overall strategy that includes face-to-face discussion, personal help and attention to social and environmental factors that help or hinder change. For example, mass media campaigns are just one strand in a long-term programme to combat smoking (Department of Health 2011).

What mass media *cannot* be expected to do is:

1. convey complex information
2. teach skills
3. shift people's attitudes or beliefs
4. change behaviour unless it is a simple action, easy to do, and people are already motivated to change.

For examples of mass media use in health campaigns, see O'Hara et al (2012) for an analysis of the use of the mass media to increase population usage of the Australian Get Healthy Information and Coaching Service, and Durkin et al (2012) for research into the effectiveness of a mass media campaign to promote smoking cessation.

Creating Opportunities

You may be motivated to use the mass media, but you may have misgivings and feel the need for further training. For example, you may feel apprehensive of interviews with reporters from the local news media because of concerns about being misquoted or that the media might sensationalise the issue or that you will not perform effectively.

What can be done to overcome these concerns? Many NHS organisations, local authorities and Non-Government Organisations (NGOs) have guidelines for dealing with the media (for example, Mind 2016, Solent NHS Trust 2016), and some professional bodies offer advice to their members in terms of media involvement. Contact local journalists to establish a mutually beneficial relationship. You can give exposure to health topics, and they want items for their reading, listening or viewing public. Get to know how they work and their special areas of interest. Also, remember that it is in both your interests to have good skills in communicating via the mass media, so ask for help with training needs. Short courses on using the media may also be available.

Keep a record of what you find out about local media and update it regularly. Include information on names and special interests of journalists and the copy dates (deadline for submitting written information) for each of the media in your area. The daily newspapers should be able to respond immediately to a press release; radio often needs a few days to prepare coverage; television may need longer advance notice to allow time for booking a film crew.

Working with Radio and Television

Using radio or television effectively requires research, preparation and skill. The following checklists are prepared to help you get your health promotion story to the right person and have the best chance of getting coverage. You need to monitor your local radio and television to see which programmes might be interested in your kind of news.

Basic Information

- What hours do they broadcast?
- What region do they cover?
- Who are the listeners/viewers? Does the profile alter according to the time of day?

The Programmes

- What is covered on the news items?
- How many minutes of current affairs and local interest items are broadcast?
- Are interviews used or is it straight reporting?
- What are the different kinds of programmes, and what is the proportion of time they occupy (news, current affairs, weekly events, phone-ins, music)?
- Which programmes use guests or experts?
- Is there any local programme that regularly covers health issues?
- Is there a round-up of events in the week ahead? What is the deadline for information?
- How much detail do they give? What sorts of events are covered?

Interviews

- Which programmes use interviews?
- How many minutes?
- What is the tone (bland, chatty, aggressive)?
- How long is the average answer before the next question? Time it!
- Are they on location or in the studio?
- Are they recorded or live?
- Who are the presenters or interviewers on the programmes who might be interested in health? What is their style?

Finding Out About a Specific Programme

- What programme is it? What sort of approach does the programme have? How long is it? When is it transmitted? What kind of audience does it have?
- Why is your topic of interest *now*? Is there some local or national controversy or news item that sparked off interest? If so, do you know all about it?
- How are you going to be presented: an information spot, an interview or a discussion panel?
- If you are going to be interviewed, who will do it? Will it be in the studio, on location or a telephone interview?
- If you are going to take part in a discussion, who else will be taking part?
- Will it be broadcast live or recorded first?
- How much time are you likely to have on the programme?
- When and where is the broadcast or recording to take place?

Preparing the Message

- Do your homework. You may know a lot or a little about the subject, but in either case you need to identify exactly what it is you want to get across and to have this very clearly in your mind *before* you go on air.
- Be positive. Emphasis the good news, *not* a series of don'ts. Tell people what they *can* do and emphasis the benefits.
- You should have two or three key points to put across, and *no more*. You can expand on these and describe them in different ways but do not overload your audience with too much detail or

too many points. They will not remember the additional information and may even forget the key points.

- Use anecdotes and analogies to illustrate what you mean; simple messages do not have to be bald and boring. Tell stories (short ones) and use real-life experiences. Put complex points over with everyday analogies.
- Avoid technical terms (unless these are essential in which case use them and explain them) and jargon, but do not be patronising. It helps pitch the level right if you imagine that you are talking to an intelligent 14- to 15-year-old whom you have never met.

Presenting Your Message

- If you are nervous, regard it as positive; it means that you will be keyed up to do your best. Remember that the interviewer is there to help you tell your story and to put you at ease.
- Perform with liveliness and conviction. Be alert and (if you are on television) look alert at all times. Always assume that the camera is on you even when you are not talking. Make sure you look convincing and involved.
- Speak with your normal voice; if you have a regional accent, this will make you more interesting to listen to. Speak clearly and distinctly, and (especially on radio) vary the pitch and speed.
- Make sure you say what *you* want to say. You do not have to follow the line of the interviewer's questions if, for good reason, you do not wish to. Provided you stick to the broad framework of agreed subjects, you have every right to steer the interview or discussion in such a way that you get over what you want to say. Regard the questions as springboards from which to make your points. For example, if you do not like a question you can say:
'I can't really answer that question without explaining first that ...'
'The real problem behind all this is ...'
'We don't know the answer to that at the moment, but what we do know is ...'
- When the interview is over, remain still, quiet and alert until you are *told* it is over.
- On television, wear what makes you feel comfortable and confident. Avoid wearing blue or bright red, predominant stripes, small patterns or flashing jewellery. As the camera will be on your face for most of the time, pay special attention to what you wear in the neckline area.

Practise your media skills by undertaking Exercise 11.2.

EXERCISE 11.2
Being Effective On Television And Radio

1. Prepare your message.

Select a health promotion topic that you are familiar with, such as healthy eating, sensible drinking, breastfeeding, keeping fit or avoiding home accidents.

Identify *three* key points you would want to put across in a 5-minute radio or television interview. Be clear in your mind:

- What the three key points are.
- How you will explain them in an interesting way and what illustrations, analogies or anecdotes you could use.
- How you will develop your point further if you have time.

2. Practise your presentation.

Get a colleague to act as your interviewer, and record your interview on an audio or a videotape. Ask a third person to be an observer. Play the tape back and assess your performance:

- Did you sound/look lively, alert and convincing?
- Was your voice clearly understandable? What did it sound like for speed and pitch?
- Did you get your key points across? Did you do so in an interesting way?
- Were you able to deal with difficult questions?

Working With the Local Press

Local community newspapers are an excellent medium for promoting health, and journalists will be interested in newsworthy health issues. This is a checklist of what to look for when researching a newspaper.

Basic Information

- Is it published daily or weekly?
- What are the copy deadlines?
- What locality does it cover?
- How many readers, and who are they?

The Copy

- What is the style (bright, sober, campaigning)?
- What is the average length of articles (often different for news, business, features)?

- What percentage of articles have photos?
- How many photographs per page?
- How are photographs used generally?
- How are quotes used?

The Subjects

- What sorts of stories are used (local, controversial, educational) and how are they treated?
- What is the ratio of coverage for news, features, business, diary and advertisements?
- How long and how full is the section publicising events ahead?
- Are there special sections or supplements on health, education or women? How long and on what day?
- Are there regular columnists? What are their special interests?

The Language

- What is the average length of sentences?
- What is the average length of paragraphs?
- What kind of language is used (multisyllabic, slang, turgid, lively, short and simple)?

Your Special Interests

- Anything in the papers that may be of special use to you or to your organisation?

Gradually build up expertise with a fact sheet on each newspaper. This will be indispensable for targeting your press releases.

How to Write a Press Release

To write a press or news release, you need to consider the following:

Headline. Create a catchy headline that is short and simple using less than 10 words. It should convey the key point made in the opening paragraph in a light-hearted manner that catches imagination and attention but doesn't mislead or sensationalise.

Collate and organise your facts. A simple rule is to find answers to questions pertaining to the five Ws: Who, What, When, Where, Why and then How. Identify your story's angle. A good story angle must have the following attributes. It must be the most important fact in your story;

it must be timely; it must be unique, newsworthy or contrary to trends. The story angle must be presented in the first paragraph. Make your points in order of importance. Use short sentences, brief paragraphs and easy language with no abbreviations or jargon. Put the most important message down into a quote. Journalists use quotes from the newsmakers to add an authoritative voice to their reports. If the press release contains quotes that are important and relevant, they have more chance of being replicated in full in the published article.

Keep to one page if possible. If longer, type 'More follows …' at the bottom right hand corner. Do not carry over paragraphs or sentences to the next page. Type 'ends' after the last line of the release. End the press release with brief background information on your organisation and who to contact for further information.

Be specific. Focus on people rather than making generalised statements or quoting dry statistics. For example, say 'Last week, three Bloggsville children were admitted to the Royal Infirmary after accidentally swallowing weed killer. This brings the number of children accidentally poisoned this year to over 100. Sister Florence Nightingale, in charge of the Accident and Emergency Department, said: "It is heartbreaking to see the needless distress this causes" …'

Timing is vital. Your press release may not be used if a) it comes out on a day when there is news overload, such as on the day of election of a new prime minister or b) the news is not topical or current. Alert newspapers a few days in advance so that they can send reporters to cover an interesting event. For example, contact on a Friday or Monday is usually best for a weekly paper published on the following Friday. If you want to launch a story at a particular time, use the embargo system. This means writing, for example, 'Not for use until Wednesday September 2nd 2017' or 'Embargoed 6 p.m. September 2nd 2017' across the top of the press release. If it is for immediate release, then state FOR IMMEDIATE RELEASE.

Presentation. Use A4 paper, headed with a logo if possible. Colour catches the eye, so a coloured heading or coloured paper will make your release stand out. Journalists work at speed, so make their task easier by:

- using only one side of the page, placing the text centrally on the page
- using a lay out with double spacing
- leaving at least a 1-inch (2 to 3-cm) margin on either side
- putting a release date or embargo date at the top
- giving names and telephone numbers of people in your organisation for further information (including an after-hours telephone number)
- sending it to a named journalist if possible
- not underlining any words (because this gives printers instructions to use italics; use **bold** for emphasis instead).

Photographs. If you are sending a photo, a 7×5 or 10×8, generally black and white, is preferred with a full label on the back giving names and details. Include the names of everyone on the photo the picture shows, for example, 'left to right June Bloggs, Director of Public Health, Sam Smith, Health Promotion Specialist …' and explain what they are doing 'presenting Healthy Eating awards at 3 p.m. on Tuesday March 10th at Bloggsville Town Hall'. Never write directly on the back of a photo as this will destroy its quality. Photos should be eye-catching and clear.

Communication. Send a copy of the press release to everyone who will be affected including your organisation's communication or press officer, and to everyone mentioned or otherwise involved in the story.

This section is based on ideas from *Pressbox: press release writing* (http://www.pressbox.co.uk). There are many websites with excellent ideas for writing press releases for the media. These can be found by simply using Google and the search term *press release*. See also the example of a press release in Box 11.2.

Writing Letters to the Editor

Another way of using the local paper as a medium for health promotion is by writing letters to the editor. This can keep an issue in the public eye for some time

---

BOX 11.2
PRESS RELEASE

Kofftown Local Authority Public Health Team

PRESS RELEASE 1ST JANUARY 2017 SMOKERS HOTLINE LAUNCHED

Kofftown's Smokers Hotline got off to a flying start this week when Jo Goodheart, a public health practitioner at Kofftown LA, launched the service.

The hotline has been set up as part of Kofftown's Heart Week (1st–7th January) to help people who want to stop smoking. Anyone ringing 1234 567 890 will be sent a free pack of useful ideas to help them quit including tips from ex-smokers and information about local stop-smoking groups.

'I smoked myself when I was younger, and I remember what a struggle I had to stop. Many of my clients also find it incredibly difficult', said Jo Goodheart. 'That's why I'm delighted to launch this scheme. The pack has lots of useful information to help people over the difficulties.'

Smokers have a two-to-three-times greater risk of having a heart attack than nonsmokers. At least 80% of heart attacks in men under 45 are thought to be due to cigarette smoking. Stopping smoking could lead to 150 fewer deaths each year of men and women under 65 in Kofftown.

For further information, please contact:

Jo Goodheart, Public Health Practitioner, Local Authority Public Health Team, People's Lane, Kofftown KT1 2YZ

Telephone 1234 246 802 (day) or 1234 135 790 (evenings)

---

and provides good opportunities for public debate of controversial issues. Letters to the editor should be to the point, short (some newspapers restrict length) and be on one topic only.

Practise writing a press release and a letter to the editor by undertaking Exercise 11.3.

EXERCISE 11.3
Writing for the Local Press

1. Write a press release about a public health issue you are currently concerned about or working on, such as healthy school meals, binge drinking, drug taking by young people in local clubs, lack of play facilities for young children or poor public transport.

2. Write a letter to the editor supporting a current public health campaign or drawing attention to a specific need for health promotion.

For quality criteria for consumer health information, see the Discern webpage in the reference section at the end of this chapter. These criteria can be used for judging online materials in addition to printed materials but will not judge the scientific accuracy. It is designed for healthcare contexts but can also be applied to public health information.

USING THE INTERNET AND SOCIAL MEDIA TO PROMOTE HEALTH

The internet has revolutionised the way health promoters, public health practitioners and the general public gain access to health information. Because of the massive growth of web-based health information, the global nature of the internet and the absence of real protection from harm for citizens who use the internet for health purposes, quality is regarded as a problem (Fahy et al 2014).

The internet can be used by public health practitioners and health promoters to:

■ support evidence-informed practice
■ disseminate resources and information to other professionals
■ provide information and support to the public.

See the section on evidence-based health promotion in Chapter 7.

The Social Media

Ventola (2014) offers a useful overview of social media, describing the term as generally referring to internet-based tools that allow individuals and communities to gather and communicate; to share information, ideas, personal messages, images, and other content; and, in some cases, to collaborate with other users in real time. Social media

are also referred to as social networking. Social media sites provide a variety of features that serve different purposes for the individual user. They may include blogs, social networks, video- and photo-sharing sites, wikis or a myriad of other media, which can be grouped by purpose, serving functions such as:

■ social networking (Facebook, MySpace, Google Plus, Twitter)
■ professional networking (LinkedIn)
■ media sharing (YouTube, Flickr)
■ content production (blogs (Tumblr, Blogger) and microblogs (Twitter))
■ knowledge/information aggregation (Wikipedia).

Participation in social media by the general public has increased sharply. In the United States, for example, the proportion of adults using social media has increased from 8% to 72% since 2005. The use of social media is prevalent across all ages and professions and is pervasive around the world (Ventola 2014). Because of this global increase in people accessing social media, there are many public health benefits, but also risks. Health promoters and public health practitioners can use social media to engage people in an interactive way on public health issues and facilitate individual's and group's access to information about health and wellbeing including news about services. An example of its potential is shown by Public Health England, who use social media to share news and information about their work and engage with other social media users. As well as their national social media accounts, they maintain a number of Twitter accounts which deal with specialised public health subjects. See Public Health England Facebook, Blog, Twitter and YouTube activity in the reference list at the end of this chapter.

CASE STUDY 11.1

The Mums2Be Smokefree Facebook Support Group

Case study produced by Tracey Hellyar, N.N.E.B, Smoking in Pregnancy Coordinator, Solutions 4 Health LTD

BACKGROUND

Women who smoke during pregnancy often experience feelings of embarrassment, guilt and fear. Attending a group is often deemed uncomfortable

because of a feeling of being judged. In Somerset, as a result of the rural nature of the landscape, a group was not viable. Web-based support groups offer a number of advantages including convenience, increased access to care for individuals who would not attend groups residing in remote areas or for those suffering from social anxiety. Additionally, fewer resources are required thus reducing costs.

The Mums2Be Smokefree Facebook Support Group *(Continued)*

AIM

Each client who engages with the Mums2Be Smokefree programme has the opportunity to receive peer support. By using an online platform, support is available continually for 24 hours a day, 7 days a week. An advantage to remaining in the group post-delivery is that each woman has continued support potentially reducing the chance of relapse.

SET UP AND ADMINISTRATION

To protect the clients' anonymity, the group was set up as a secret Facebook group. This meant that the group could not be searched for, that nothing in the group is shown on the clients' timeline and no one could see that the client was in the group except for other group members.

To join the group, the client is sent a friend request by the administrator and, once accepted, they are added to the group. The friend acceptance is then removed.

There are two administrators in the group and three practitioner moderators. The group also has four users who are nominated Champions who post regularly.

Clients may stay in the group for as long as they wish as there is no time frame as it is important for the support to continue post delivery.

HOW IS THE SUCCESS EVALUATED?

An online survey was carried out 11 months after the initial group was set up. The survey was anonymous, and a link was posted within the group for members to complete. The group at the time had 73 client members. There was a 31.5% response rate.

- 95.85% strongly agreed or agreed that participation in the group provided support and encouragement.
- 100% strongly agreed or agreed that participation in the group helped them to realise that any problems they encountered were not unique.
- 87.5% strongly agreed or agreed that participation in the group enabled them to confront difficult problems.
- 96% strongly agreed or agreed that participation in the group supported them to quit.
- 75% strongly agreed or agreed that participation within the group helped to avoid relapse.
- 96% would recommend the group to friends.
- 96% felt safe within the group.

Mums2Be Smokefree is an intensive Smoking in Pregnancy programme, offering one-on-one support and free Nicotine Replacement Therapy (NRT) with a named Practitioner throughout the clients' pregnancy and up to 6 months post-delivery within the clients' home. The online support group is an extension of this service enabling the client to gain further support around the clock from their peers and maintain support post-delivery to prevent relapse.

See Chapter 13 for guidelines on setting up a Facebook page.

Assessing the Quality of Health Information on the Internet

The potential health risks of social media are well documented (for example, Fahy et al 2014 and Ventola 2014). Guidelines issued by public health organisations and professional bodies provide sound and useful principles that health promoters and public health practitioners should follow to avoid pitfalls. It is important that health promoters and public health practitioners evaluate the quality of any website or social media such as blogs or Facebook pages they use and/or advise their clients to use before trusting the information it provides. The following guidelines offer some insights into what you should be evaluating (adjusted from Georgetown University Library 2016):

Author

- Is the name of the author/creator on the page?
- Are his/her credentials listed (occupation, years of experience, position or education)?
- Is the author qualified to write on the given topic? Why?
- Is there contact information, such as an email address, somewhere on the page?
- Is there a link to a homepage and, if so, is it for an individual or for an organisation?

- If the author is with an organisation, does it appear to support or sponsor the page?
- What does the domain name/URL reveal about the source of the information, if anything?

Purpose

Knowing the motive behind the page's creation can help you judge its content:

- Who is the intended audience?
  - Specialist audience or experts?
  - General public?
- If not stated, what do you think is the purpose of the site? Is the purpose to:
  - inform or teach?
  - explain or enlighten?
  - persuade?
  - sell a product?

Objectivity

- Is the information covered fact, opinion or propaganda?
- Is the author's point-of-view objective and impartial?
- Is the language free of emotion-rousing words and bias?
- Is the author affiliated with an organisation?
- Does the author's affiliation with an institution or organisation appear to bias the information?
- Does the content of the page have the official approval of the institution, organisation or company?

Accuracy

- Are the sources for factual information clearly listed so that the information can be verified?

- Is it clear who has the ultimate responsibility for the accuracy of the content of the material?
- Can you verify any of the information in independent sources or from your own knowledge?
- Has the information been reviewed or refereed?
- Is the information free of grammatical, spelling or typographical errors?

Reliability and Credibility

- Why should anyone believe information from this site?
- Does the information appear to be valid and well-researched, or is it unsupported by evidence?
- Are quotes and other strong assertions backed by sources that you could check through other means?
- What institution (public health agency, government, charity such as Mind) supports this information?

Currency

- If timeliness of the information is important, is it kept up-to-date?
- Is there an indication of when the site was last updated?

Links

- Are links related to the topic and useful to the purpose of the site?
- Are links still current?

Undertake Exercise 11.4 and read Case Study 11.1 to consider the benefits and risks of using social media to promote health.

EXERCISE 11.4

Does Social Media Pose a Threat to Public Health?

Read the following interview with a retiring Director of Public Health. Do you agree that social media is a threat to public health? List the ways social media could be both a threat and offer opportunities to promote public health. Do the benefits outweigh the threats?

Social media could pose one of the biggest threats to public health in the future, a leading doctor has warned.

Tom Scanlon, the outgoing director of public health for Brighton and Hove, issued the warning as he prepares to leave the position after 15 years. He said emerging evidence shows that, in some areas of mental health, the use of Facebook, websites and Twitter can have a detrimental effect. Although social media can be used as a force for good, Dr Scanlon said the existence of websites that promote anorexia and other eating disorders are harmful. He said cyberbullying and the increased access to images of super-skinny celebrities could all also have a negative impact. He said, 'The public health science on social media is in its infancy. We have managed to mine some social media use locally for our annual report and my view is that in certain areas of mental wellbeing: eating disorders, self-harm, anxiety and depression, there is emerging evidence that the use of social media can have a detrimental effect. This has previously been suggested in some cases of suicides, although I haven't seen any local instances of this, and we know there can be a copy-cat effect. My feeling is that some of the imagery/texts/memes posted on social media becomes aspirational, particularly to certain vulnerable young people and that this select group behaviour, probably hidden from external influences like parents/teachers, feeds the problem rather than provide any positive support or solutions. This is something we are just on the cusp of, and we don't really know how it will develop. It is a real challenge.'

Dan Raisbeck, co-founder of the internet bullying charity the Cybersmile Foundation, said the organisation recognised the risks associated with social media and the promotion of some websites. He said: 'Safeguarding is something that each user needs to learn about, how security and profile settings can be applied and the use of filtering tools or monitoring home internet use, especially if young people are involved. Learning about the risks and finding out how you can keep yourself and your family safer online is a very important part of dealing with the problem.'

Source: The Argus 2016.

Chapter 13 has more information on establishing social media groups.

PRACTICE POINTS

- Communication tools for health promoters and public health practitioners are wide ranging and need to be selected carefully and used effectively with an assessment made of the advantages, uses and limitations of each kind of resource.
- Consider factors such as location, colour, language and style when creating displays.
- Written materials should be nonsexist, nonracist, in plain English and accessible to everyone, for example, ethnic minority languages, large type or alternative formats such as audiotape instead of written materials.
- Present statistical information with appropriate use of graphics to ensure clarity.
- The mass media can be used to raise awareness of health issues and deliver simple messages.
- Work effectively with local media by researching potential opportunities and carefully preparing TV presentations and press releases.
- The social media offers a potentially effective way of promoting health but needs to be used with caution.

REFERENCES

Alcohol Concern 2013 Stick to the facts: alcohol advertising regulation that balances commercial and public interest. http://www.alcoholconcern.org.uk/wp-content/uploads/woocommerce_uploads/2014/12/stick_to_the_facts_report.pdf.

Blumenthal S, Pruthi N 2016 Health and the headlines, The Huffington Post. http://www.huffingtonpost.com/susan-blumenthal/health-and-the-headlines_b_9749588.html.

Campbell D 2014 Ban alcohol firms from sponsoring sports clubs and events, doctors urge. The Guardian. https://www.theguardian.com/society/2014/dec/25/ban-alcohol-firms-sponsoring-sports-clubs-doctors.

Das SK, Saltzman E, Gilhooly CH et al 2009 Low or moderate dietary energy restriction for long-term weight loss: what works best? Obesity 17(11):2019–2024.

Department of Health. 2011. Healthy Lives, *Healthy People: A Tobacco Control Plan for England*. Stationary Office, London.

Durkin S, Brennan E, Wakefield 2012 Mass media campaigns to promote smoking cessation among adults: an integrative review. Tobacco Control 21:127–138. http://dx.doi.org/10.1136/tobaccocontrol-2011-050345.

Fahy E, Hardikar R, Fox A, Mackay S 2014 Quality of patient health information on the internet: reviewing a complex and evolving landscape. Australasian Medical Journal 7(1):24–28.

Georgetown University Library 2016 Evaluating internet resources. http://www.library.georgetown.edu/tutorials/research-guides/evaluating-internet-content.

Goodman J 2009 Can crash diets be good for you? New research shows that crash diets can be a safe and effective way of keeping the pounds off. Sunday Times. http://www.timesonline.co.uk/tol/life_and_style/health/article6415198.ece.

Liu JJ, Davidson E, Bhopal RS, White M, Johnson MRD, Netto G, Deverill M, Sheikh A 2012 Adapting health promotion interventions to meet the needs of ethnic minority groups: mixed-methods evidence synthesis. Health Technology Assessment 16(44).

Mind 2016 How to report on mental health. http://www.mind.org.uk/news-campaigns/minds-media-office/how-to-report-on-mental-health/.

Newbold KB, Campos S 2011 Media and social media in public health messages: a systematic review. Ontario, McMasters Institute of Environment and Health.

NHS 2016 Change4life campaign pages and resources. http://www.nhs.uk/change4life/Pages/change-for-life.aspx.

NHS Commissioning Board 2012 Standards of Business Conduct. https://www.england.nhs.uk/wp-content/uploads/2012/11/stand-bus-cond.pdf.

O'Hara B, Bauman AE, Phongsavan P 2012 Using mass-media communications to increase population usage of Australia's Get Healthy Information and Coaching Service®. BioMed Central Public Health 12, 762. http://dx.doi.org/10.1186/1471-2458-12-762.

Public Health England 2016a Trends in adult prevalence of obesity in the UK and Ireland. https://www.noo.org.uk/NOO_about_obesity/adult_obesity/UK_prevalence_and_trends.

Public Health England 2016b One You Home page. https://www.nhs.uk/oneyou#P0mSdG3yOs5qIQs8.97.

Roberts S 2009 Why crash dieting DOES work: Surprise evidence suggests it's the best way to slim. Daily Mail http://www.dailymail.co.uk/femail/article-1189956/Why-crash-dieting-DOES-work-Surprise-evidence-suggests-best-way-slim.html.

Robinson A, Coutinho A, Bryden A, McKee M 2013 Analysis of health stories in daily newspapers in the UK. Public Health 127(1):39–45.

Solent NHS Trust. 2016 Media Policy. http://www.solent.nhs.uk/_store/documents/pr01-mediapolicy.pdf.

Swift J 2016 Boots channels 'chemist of the nation' heritage for new brand campaign. http://www.campaignlive.co.uk/article/boots-channels-chemist-nation-heritage-new-brand-campaign/1394844#HLyeOS27aqKuBdvS.99.

The Argus 2016. 2016 Social media could pose one of the biggest threats to public health in the future, a leading doctor has warned. Published on 29th March 2016. http://www.theargus.co.uk/news/14388589.Social_media_poses_one_of_the_biggest_threats_to_public_health/?ref=twtrec.

Triggle N 2016 Middle age risk unhealthy retirement, BBC News. http://www.bbc.co.uk/news/health-35728990.

Ventola CL 2014 Social media and health care professionals: benefits, risks, and best practices. Pharmacy and Therapeutics 39(7):491–499 520.

Walls HL, Peeters A, Proietto J, McNeil JJ 2011 Public health campaigns and obesity – a critique. BioMed Central BMC Public Health http://dx.doi.org/10.1186/1471-2458-11-136. http://bmcpublichealth.biomedcentral.com/articles/10.1186/1471-2458-11-136.

WEBSITES

Change for life resources. http://www.nhs.uk/change4life/Pages/change-for-life.aspx.

Public Health England for statistics on health trends such as obesity smoking. https://www.noo.org.uk/search.php?f = 14&q = smoking + trends&x = 22&y = 13.

Public Health England homepage. https://www.gov.uk/government/organisations/public-health-england.

The Discern site for quality criteria for health information. http://www.discern.org.uk/.

BLOGS

Public Health England blog. https://publichealthmatters.blog.gov.uk/.

Quit Smoking Community blog. https://quitsmokingcommunity.org/blog/.

FACEBOOK

Public Health England Facebook Page. https://www.facebook.com/publichealthengland.

TWITTER

Public Health England on Twitter. https://twitter.com/PHE_uk.

YOUTUBE

Public Health England on YouTube. https://www.youtube.com/user/PublicHealthEngland.

12

EDUCATING FOR HEALTH

CHAPTER CONTENTS

SUMMARY

The first section of this chapter involves a discussion on the principles of learning. An exercise is used to analyse the qualities and abilities of an effective public health educator, and some principles of facilitating health learning are outlined. Subsequent sections contain guidelines on giving public health talks, strategies for patient education and teaching practical skills for health. A role-play exercise is used to focus on skills of effective patient health education.

This chapter is about the skills and methods used in planned public health learning experiences. These events are underpinned by theories that aim to empower by providing individuals, groups or communities with the opportunity to acquire health information and the skills needed to make quality health decisions. Health education is an important area of health promotion, and public health and many health professionals have a remit for public health education. Examples are: a health promotion specialist giving a talk on a locally identified health topic to a large community group; an environmental health officer teaching an adult education class in food safety; school nurses facilitating a sexual health programmes in schools; cardiac rehabili-

tation teams running cardiac rehabilitation sessions for patients recovering after heart attacks; a diabetes nurse giving information to a diabetic patient on a one-to-one basis about diagnosis, treatment and self-care; or a public health practitioner teaching a small group of colleagues about the techniques and procedures used in a smoking cessation programme.

PRINCIPLES OF LEARNING FOR HEALTH

Some aspects of education, teaching and learning are relevant for health promoters and public health practitioners. Health promoters, public health practitioners and other health, local authority and voluntary organisation professionals generally have credibility because of their training and expert knowledge which is likely to be valued and respected by clients, but expertise alone does not make a good public health educator. To get results in the form of measurable learning achievements, such as greater retention and application of health information and skills, public health educators need to understand some principles of learning, such as the importance of participation. The basic principles of learning as applied to health are

BOX 12.1

PRINCIPLES OF LEARNING AS APPLIED TO PUBLIC HEALTH EDUCATION

- Learning for health is most effective when the learner identifies their own learning needs and sets their own goals.
- The public health educator's role is to enable or facilitate learning rather than to direct it. Public health educators who adopt this approach often refer to themselves as facilitators.
- Learners are generally most ready to learn things that they can apply immediately to existing health problems or to their own situation.
- Learners bring with them life experience, which should be seen as a resource and to which new health learning should be related.
- Learners can help each other, because of their experiences, and should be encouraged to do so.
- Health learning is best when active (not passive), by doing and experiencing, for which learners need a safe environment where they feel accepted.
- Learners should be encouraged to carry out continuous evaluation of their own learning. Public health educators should use this evaluation to fit the learning process to the learners' needs.

summarised in Box 12.1. There are more than 80 learning theories, models and frameworks that address how people learn. If you want to read more on these and how they can be applied in practice, see Bates (2015) and for health education concepts, principles and models, see WHO (2012).

FACILITATING HEALTH LEARNING

Exercise 12.1 will help you to identify factors that have helped and hindered your learning and to assess your own qualities and abilities.

Plan Your Session

However skilled and knowledgeable you are about the public health topic, it is vital to put thought and time into preparation. You need to think through what you aim to achieve, how you are going to introduce and develop your session and how you will involve your audience. Preparation is especially important when facilitating health learning is new to you, but even the most experienced and self-confident public health educator needs to spend some time in preparation. Active participation is a more complex process and will require greater attention to planning.

EXERCISE 12.1
What Helps and Hinders Health Learning?

Think of two occasions when you have been a learner, such as when you were a health promotion or public health student, in the audience listening to a public health talk or when you were being taught on a one-to-one basis. These learning occasions need not have been connected with work, for example, listening to an art lecture or taking a driving lesson. One should be when you felt, overall, that the session was *good* and the other when it was *bad*. The aim of the exercise is to identify the factors that made them good or bad for you.

In each of your two situations in turn, identify factors that helped you to learn and factors that hindered your learning. Think of these factors in three categories:

1. Those to do with the learning *environment* (e.g. too hot? noisy? uncomfortable chairs? a spacious, comfortable room?).
2. Those to do with the *qualities of the health educator/facilitator* (e.g. sense of humour? contagious enthusiasm? seemed unfriendly?).
3. Those to do with the *presentation* (e.g. talked too long? used relevant illustrations? involved audience? muddled? used words you didn't understand? used audiovisual and media aids effectively?).

Enter these factors on this chart:

	Environment	Health educator	Presentation
Factors that helped			
Factors that hindered			

If you are working in a group, compare your chart with those of other people:

- What have you learnt about the importance of the environment?
- What qualities of a good public health educator do you think you already possess?
- What helpful points about presentation do you think you already use, or will use, in your own work?
- What points about your own qualities or presentation skills would you like to improve?

Work from the Known to the Unknown

Time is wasted in teaching people something they already know, so the starting point is finding out what your clients know. If you cannot do this in advance, spend some time at the beginning of the session asking a few questions. If you have a mixed audience with varying degrees of knowledge, it may be best to acknowledge that some people know more than others, and you will have to make a decision about the level at which to pitch your information: 'Some of you will probably know this, but I'll talk about it briefly because it will be new to others …'.

Your aim is to add new health information and awareness, or new skills, to what is already known.

Aim for Maximum Involvement

People learn best if they are actively participating in the learning process and are, not just passive listeners. For an example of participatory health learning in practice, see WHO (2014) and Proust et al (2013) for an analysis of the effectiveness of participatory approaches.

First, where appropriate, involve your clients in deciding the aim and content of the session. If you are running a course, such as a series of antenatal classes or one on food hygiene, you might begin by explaining your aims, asking for comments and suggestions, and then going on to discuss the content. This will help to increase motivation by stimulating clients to think about their own needs and to take some responsibility for their own learning. The goals and content of a one-to-one session can be established by mutual agreement at the outset. As a general rule, it is worth considering how much room for negotiation there is in your public health education role and spending time to find out what people really want. Ask yourself 'Is what I cover what *I want to teach* or what *my clients want to learn*?'

Second, keep your clients involved as much as possible during sessions. This is a challenge if you are giving a talk or a lecture to a large audience, but there are possibilities, such as asking people to respond to a question, such as 'I'd like you to put your hand up if you made a new year resolution to take more exercise this year'. Or ask them to respond to a series of statements, for example, as an introduction to a talk on nutrition, ask the audience to stand up, then ask them to sit down if they:

usually eat white bread …
add sugar to tea and coffee …
regularly eat fried food …
add salt at the table …
and so on.

Most of them will be sitting down by now but will feel alert and involved. Another way of keeping an audience involved is to give them time to talk. This can be done by having question-and-answer sessions or by allowing short breaks when they can talk about something in groups of two or three for a few minutes. In a talk on passive smoking, for example, you could give your audience a couple of minutes to tell their neighbours how they are affected by other people's smoke.

You can also keep people involved with eye contact, making sure that you look around at everybody, not just the people immediately in front of you.

Vary Your Learning Methods

It is natural to consider health educating from the public health educator's point of view, but it may be more helpful to look at it from the learner's point of view. For example, talking for half an hour demands concentrated effort and total involvement on your part; but all your audience is doing is listening, which involves only one of their senses and is highly unlikely to hold their full attention.

Variety can be brought into health teaching in many ways including strategies that can be used with individuals, groups, large audiences, children or adults; see Table 12.1 for ideas.

Devise Public Health Education Activities

Listening is passive; activities are the means by which you help learners to think through what is being said and act on it in their own way. It is not sufficient to ask a group 'What do you think?' at the end of a health talk or after viewing a DVD; planned activities are necessary to help people to explore and apply ideas, feelings, attitudes and behaviour. It is more effective to have a mix of activities that are specifically tailored for a particular group of learners, so where possible develop the skill of devising your own activities rather than relying on learning aids made for general audiences. There is an almost infinite range of possibilities. Some of the more common types of activity are set out in Table 12.2. There are also ideas in some of the exercises used throughout this book.

TABLE 12.1	
Learning Methods Involving Clients	
Client Involvement	**Materials and Methods**
Listen	Lectures, audiotapes, one-to-one or small group information giving
Read	Books, booklets, leaflets, handouts, posters, whiteboard, flip-chart, PowerPoint slides, websites, blogs
Look	Photographs, drawings, paintings, posters, charts, material from media (such as advertisements)
Look and listen	DVDs, PowerPoint, demonstrations, YouTube
Listen and talk	Question-and-answer sessions, discussions, informal conversations, debates, brainstorming
Read, listen and talk	Case studies, discussions based on study questions or handouts
Read, listen, talk and actively participate	Drama, role-play, games, simulations, quizzes, practising skills
Read and actively participate	Programmed learning, computer-assisted learning
Make and use	Models, charts, drawings
Use	Equipment
Action research	Gathering information, opinions, interviews and surveys
Projects	Making public health education materials – DVDs, leaflets, etc.
Visits	To health service premises, fire station, sewage works, playgroups, voluntary organisations
Write	Articles, letters to the press or politicians, stories, poems

For discussion of some of these methods, see Chapters 13 and 14; for discussion on the use of audiovisual and media aids, see Chapter 11.

TABLE 12.2	
Common Types of Public Health Learning Activities	
Type of Activity	**Example**
Guidelines for discussions with particular people about particular topics	Guidelines on 'what to do if you think your child is offered drugs' for discussion at a parent–teacher meeting
Analysing and discussing diary records	Ask people to keep a diary or write down what they ate or the alcohol units they consumed in the last 24 hours. Ask them to talk about what they are pleased about and not pleased about
Sentence completion	Ask people to complete a sentence such as 'I feel really stressed when ...'
Using checklists	Have a list of 'ways to make small changes to my lifestyle', such as taking the stairs and not the lift, walking (or cycling to work) or joining an exercise class, and discuss how many you use
Identifying your own thoughts/feelings/behaviour in particular situations	Ask people to think about and discuss what they feel when visitors to their home ask if they can smoke and how they respond
Generate lists	Ask a group to make a list of all the ways they could deal with an obese family member who will not comply with advice on healthy eating
Answer sheets	A quiz with yes/no or multiple answers on 'How much do you know about sensible drinking?'
Drawing charts or bubble diagrams	Draw a stick-person picture of yourself in a supermarket in the middle of a page. Draw bubble thoughts about all the things that influence what foods you buy
Writing instructions	Ask a group learning about food hygiene to write down instructions for someone else on how to store food safely in a fridge
Practical skills development	Practise bathing a baby using a doll or a real baby

Ensure Relevance

You should ensure that, as far as possible, what you say is relevant to the needs, interests and circumstances of the clients. For example, recommendations about health-promoting activities that cost money may not be useful to an audience which has no money for extras. A discussion on childhood vaccination may be irrelevant to a pregnant woman whose overwhelming concern is the birth itself; she may not relate to an issue that will not meet her immediate needs.

You will help your clients to see the relevance of your subject if you use concrete examples, practical problems and case studies to explain and illustrate your points. It may be more difficult for your clients to relate to abstract generalisations, quotations of statistics or epidemiological evidence. For example say '1 person in 10' instead of 'X million people in this country'; tell the story of a home accident rather than describe a list of risk factors; and describe 'increasing the risk' by saying 'It's like driving a car with faulty brakes, there's no guarantee that you will have an accident, but your chances of having one are greater'.

Identify Realistic Health Goals and Objectives

In Chapter 5, there was a discussion on the importance of clearly identifying health promotion aims and objectives, but it is worth emphasising again that it is essential to be clear about what you are trying to do (raise awareness of a health issue? give people more health knowledge?) and what you want your clients to know, feel and/or do at the end of your session. As previously mentioned, your clients should be involved in these decisions (see Chapter 5, section on setting aims and objectives).

Three or four key points are all that clients can be expected to assimilate from a session. Including more than that does not mean that they learn more; it usually means that they forget more. For example, if you are asked to give a talk on a huge theme, such as food for health, you will need to select what you feel to be the few points most relevant for your audience and avoid the temptation to include everything.

Use Learning Contracts

In some public health educational settings, the learner is told what objectives or targets to work towards. This can conflict with some people's psychological need to be self-directing and may induce resistance, apathy or withdrawal. Learning contracts are an agreement, decided together, about what is to be learnt. By participating in the process of diagnosing needs, formulating goals, choosing methods and evaluating progress, learners can develop a sense of ownership of the plan and feel more committed and empowered.

The stages of developing a learning contract are described in the following text.

Step 1: Diagnose Health Learning Needs With the Learners

First, decide the competencies required to carry out actions, behaviour or roles. A competency can be thought of as the ability to do something, and it is a combination of knowledge, understanding, skills, attitudes and values.

For instance, the ability to ride a bicycle from home to school involves knowledge of how a bicycle works and of the route from home to the school; understanding of the risks inherent in riding a bicycle; and skills in mounting, pedalling, steering and stopping. It is useful to analyse competencies in this way, even if it is crude and subjective, because it gives the learners a clearer sense of direction.

Next, assess the gap between where learners are now and where they should be with regard to each health-related competency. Learners may wish to draw on the observations of friends, family or experts to make this assessment. Each learner will then have an idea of the competencies needed and a map of their health learning needs.

Step 2: Specify the Learning Objectives of Each Learner

Translate the health learning needs identified in Step 1 into objectives that describe what each learner wants to *learn*. All learners should state their health learning objectives in terms most meaningful to them. For example, to ride a bicycle from home to school, learners may decide that they need knowledge of how to work the bicycle gears and improved skills of steering and stopping safely.

Step 3: Specify Learning Methods

Review the learning objectives of the learner or (if you are working with a group of learners) all the members of the learning group, perhaps through listing them on a flip-chart and identifying shared objectives and areas of difference. Now think about how you could go about accomplishing these objectives. Specify the methods you would use. In the bicycle example, you could specify that practical demonstration followed by supervised practice in a traffic-free area would be the way to learn. Ask learners to suggest the methods they prefer.

Step 4: Evaluate Learning

Now describe what evidence you will need to show that these objectives have been achieved. For example, health knowledge can be tested through quizzes; understanding can be tested through problem solving; skills can be tested through demonstrations of performance; attitudes can be tested through role-play and simulation exercises; values can be tested through line debates and value-clarification exercises (see also Chapter 5, section on planning evaluation methods).

An example of a learning contract for a group is provided in Box 12.2. Individuals in a group can have their own personal version of the learning contract (see Chapter 14, section on strategies for increasing self-awareness, clarifying values and changing attitudes).

Organise Your Public Health Education Material

Whether you are talking to a group or an individual, it helps if you organise your material into a logical framework and tell your client(s) what this is, both at the beginning and during your health education session. For example, with an individual client in a smoking cessation group, say:

'We are going to:

- look at your smoking behaviour and the reasons why you smoke
- identify the barriers to you giving up smoking
- measure where you are in terms of your motivation to stop smoking.

First, let us discuss your smoking behaviour and what prompts this behaviour.
Second, what do you think will prevent you from stopping ...
Finally, let us see where you stand in terms of you wanting to stop smoking ...'

The same principle applies if you are talking to a group. You tell them what you are going to tell them, tell them and then tell them what you have told them! This helps both you and the audience to know where

---

BOX 12.2
LEARNING CONTRACT FOR A YOUNG PARENTS' GROUP ON HEALTHY EATING

Group members said they wanted to know more about how to cook cheap, interesting, healthy meals for their families as a change from the usual ready prepared foods such as frozen fish fingers, cans of beans or frozen chips. Facilitator and group members worked out the following learning contract.

Learning objectives	Learning methods	Evaluation of achievement of objectives
Know what to eat to be healthy	Keep food diaries for 2 days. Facilitator to produce guidelines and members discuss how far their food matches up to guidelines	Be able to say what sort of food each member should aim to eat more or less of
Know where to buy healthy cheap food	Group members share experience of where they buy food, its price and quality	Two weeks later, members identify changes in where they buy food and whether it is better quality and value for money
Be able to cook healthy meals that their families enjoy eating	Facilitator and group members bring recipes, choose some to try out and cook together	Have cooked new healthy meals at home

you are and where you are going. Recapping where you are at intervals is helpful: 'That's all I've got to say on the benefits of yoga; now, to move on to how you can get started ...' or 'Now I'd like to move on to my third and final point, which you may remember I said was about ...'

Evaluation, Feedback and Assessment

It is important to get feedback, so that you can assess how much your client is learning and improve your own performance in the future (see Chapter 5, section on planning evaluation methods, and Chapter 10, section on asking questions and getting feedback).

Assessing Your Own Performance

You need to ask yourself what went well, what didn't and why and how things could be improved next time. You may find it helpful to use a simple form to record your thoughts. This is especially useful if your session is part of a course with a team of people involved. An example is given in Box 12.3, a form used by a group facilitator to record issues after a group session on healthy eating and cooking.

Getting Feedback

You could include oral feedback as part of your session. For example, at the end, ask people to do a round of sentence completion:

BOX 12.3
NUTRITION AND COOKING PROJECT MONITORING FORM

Session no:
    Date:
    Time:
    Facilitator:
    Number of attendees:
    Number in crèche:
    Activity:
    Positive outcomes:
    Negative outcomes:
    Feedback/comments from participants:
    Crèche issues:
    Issues needing further action:
    Action plan:
    Completed by:

(From Hartcliffe health and environment action group and health visitors from Hartcliffe and Withywood, Bristol. Reproduced with permission.)

BOX 12.4
EVALUATION FORM A

Title of session:
    Date:
    Please help me to get the session right for you by completing the following sentences about how you feel. Thank you.
It helps me when ....
It is difficult for me when ....
I would like more of ....
I would like less of ....

'The thing I liked best about today's session was ...'
'The most important thing I am taking from this session is ...'
'The thing I liked least about today's session was ...'

However, some people may find this intimidating and might not feel comfortable with expressing what they feel. You may wish to use a written evaluation form; see the two examples in Boxes 12.4 and 12.5.

Assessing the Health Learning Outcomes

Assessing learning outcomes is an important aspect of evaluation in health education. It is the process of measuring the extent and quality of your clients' learning: judging how successful they have been in progressing towards goals which they set themselves. It may be carried out very informally through getting apparently casual feedback from clients about how they have applied the learning to real-life situations or it may involve setting tests in formal situations. Here are two examples of ways in which health promoters assess how well they are doing:

1. Sandra is a smoking cessation advisor. She evaluates the effectiveness of her support group activities by using the self-reported number of cigarettes smoked per month, taken at the outset of the 3-month programme, at the conclusion of the programme and 6 months after the termination of the programme.
2. Marleen teaches cookery and healthy eating to adults with learning difficulties. She keeps records of their progress in relation to their previous level of competence in choosing healthy menus and cooking healthy meals.

Monitoring clients' progress by keeping records of achievements can be valuable for helping them to see what they have achieved. If your public health

---

BOX 12.5
EVALUATION FORM B

Title of session:
Date:
   We would like your views to help us assess this session and make plans for similar sessions in the future. All your comments will be valued and used, and treated confidentially.

	Yes	No	Partly
1. Overall, have you found this session beneficial? (please tick)			

	Yes	No	Partly
2. Did the session match up to your expectations?			

3. What did you expect to gain from the session?
Please comment:

4. Which parts of the session have you found most beneficial?

5. Which parts of the session have you found least beneficial?

6. How do you think the session could be improved?

7. Do you have any other comments you would like to make?

   Please write your name here (or leave blank if you prefer to remain anonymous).
   Thank you very much for filling this in.

---

education is geared towards people learning to change behaviour, it can help to keep diary-type records of what they ate or drank, or their physical activity levels. If they are learning practical creative skills, photographic records can help. For example, on a course designed to help people cook and eat healthier food for their families, you could give them a single-use camera to make a pictorial record of the dishes they cooked and their family enjoying the meals.

GUIDELINES FOR GIVING PUBLIC HEALTH TALKS

Giving a formal public health talk is often part of a health promoter's work. There are considerable

disadvantages in this method. A talk is largely a one-way communication process with little opportunity to assess how much people are learning or understanding and with only a small proportion of it likely to be remembered at the end (and still less a few days later).

Despite these limitations, talks and lectures can be valuable for several reasons. A talk can be used to introduce a public health topic by giving a broad overview of it, and this may lead people to take further action. For example, an introductory talk on first aid may lead people to enrol for a first aid course. A talk may also be an important source of health information and awaken a critical attitude in the audience, for example, by drawing their attention to issues such as traffic pollution or misleading information on food labels. Giving talks is also a relatively economical way to use a health promoter's time, because large numbers of people can be addressed at one time. To ensure success, the following points need to be addressed:

Check the Facilities

If possible, visit the place where you are going to give your talk and check the seating, lighting and audiovisual equipment including electric power points and extension leads. On the day of the talk, arrive early so that you can arrange chairs, open windows and check that the equipment is working. Get your audiovisual and media equipment ready for use. If you need blackout, check that you can turn the lights on and off quickly so that you do not lose rapport with the audience while they are left in the dark.

Make a Plan for the Session

It can be useful to make an outline plan of your whole session, indicating the sections, times and any audiovisual or media aids you are using. This is particularly useful if you are sharing a session with a colleague so that you are both clear what you are doing. See the example in Box 12.6 and either use this as a skeleton overall plan to guide you when you make detailed notes to speak from (see following section) or it might be enough to enable you to speak from the plan itself.

Making and Using Notes

It is generally best to give a public health talk from notes. The more experienced you are, the fewer notes you are likely to need, unless your talk is full of technical detail or likely to be taken down and quoted

BOX 12.6
PLAN FOR GIVING A TALK

Talk on 'Sense in the Sun – Preventing Skin Cancer'
Bloggshire Secondary School Parent–Teachers Meeting
21 February 2017: An hour at the end of a curriculum meeting, 8:00–8:45 p.m.

SN (school nurse) and DH (deputy head)
AIM: To give parents basic information on risks and prevention of skin cancer

Time	Section	Content	Audiovisual aids PowerPoint (PP)	Who
8:00	Intros	Intro JAS & SNS. Why we are now concerned about skin cancer – rising incidence?	TED YouTube lesson – Why do we have to wear sunscreen? PP graph showing rise in skin cancer in UK	DH
8:05	What is skin cancer?	Different types of skin cancer. How you spot it? Who is most at risk (fair skin, sunburn, etc.)?	PP key points	SN
8:15	Prevention	Key message: Respect the sun – avoid exposure at hottest times, use good sunscreen, cover up with sun hats and light clothing. Be a mole-watcher	Examples of sun hats, light clothing (big, long-sleeved, cotton shirts, etc.). Examples of sunscreen creams	SN
8:25	What the school can do?	Encourage the use of cover-up and sunscreen creams in outdoor PE. Include topic in PHSE and science teaching	Main points on PP	DH
8.30	Summary	Aim for school and parents to work together. Main points to remember: Care in the sun, Cover up, use sunscreen Creams	PP: 3 Cs to remember: Care in the sun, Cover up, Creams. Leaflets to take away	SN
8:35	Any questions?			SN
8:45	Concluding remarks and further information	Further reading: Facebook page – sun safety* BBC webpage – sun safety* Blog – Sunsense*	PP	SN

* See references at the end of the chapter.

verbatim (for example, by the press). However, very few people can give a successful talk with no notes at all, and beginners may find it helpful to write out a talk in full before they transfer the main points to notes.

If you are writing out your talk in full to begin with, it is useful to know that a 50-minute lecture consists of about 5000 words, allowing for pauses and an estimated speed of delivery of about 110 words per minute. You can then try transferring the key points as notes to cards or paper.

Never give a talk by writing it out in full and then reading it. Unless you are an exceptional orator, it will sound flat and stilted. Furthermore, you will find it difficult to look at your audience, because you will need to keep your eyes on the notes, and if you look up, you are likely to lose your place.

Prepare Your Introduction

Secure the attention of your audience with your opening words. Some ways of doing this are to:

- state a surprising fact or an unusual quote
- ask a question that has no easy answer
- use a visual image to trigger interest
- get the audience to do something active (some suggestions are discussed in the earlier section on aiming for maximum involvement)
- tell a joke if you have the confidence to do it successfully.

Establish eye contact with your audience and, if necessary, ask them whether they can see and hear you.

State your aim and theme at the beginning of your talk. It should be a brief statement, not a complex summary of the whole talk. For example, say 'I'm going to talk about the benefits of incorporating more physical activity into your life and ways of making small changes to ensure you are getting sufficient exercise', but do not go into detail at this point; save that for the main part of the talk.

By the time you have finished the introduction, you should have:

- established your aim and theme with the audience
- obtained their interest and commitment
- ensured that they can hear and see you clearly.

Prepare the Key Points

Identify the three or four main points you wish to make, and prepare your talk around each point in turn. Illustrate and support your points with evidence from your experience or from research with examples, audiovisual materials, and other materials (see Chapter 11, on using and producing audiovisual materials including leaflets, handouts and DVDs).

Plan a Conclusion

Some ways of concluding your talk are:

- a very brief recapitulation of what you've said, such as 'We've now covered the basics of exercising and lifestyle change'
- a statement of what you hope the audience will do with the information you have given

them, such as 'I hope that you can confidently make changes to your lifestyle to include more exercise'
- a suggestion for further action: 'If you'd like to find out more about exercise and health, please come to see me afterwards or contact me at … (giving email, telephone and/or office address)'
- a question, such as 'What small lifestyle changes can you make to include more physical activity into your life?'
- thanking the audience for their attention and/or participation.

Ask for Questions

If possible, include a question-and-answer session in your talk. It gives you feedback and gives the audience a chance to participate.

When you ask for questions, allow people time to think; do not assume that there are to be no questions just because one is not instantly forthcoming. When a question is asked, it is often helpful to repeat it or summarise. This gives you a little time to consider the question and ensures that everyone else in the audience has heard it. Never ignore or refuse to answer a question. If you don't know the answer, admit this and ask whether anyone else in the audience does. In any case, this helps involve the audience; you could also ask for comments on answers: 'Does anyone else have suggestions for the person who asked that question?'

Work on Your Presentation

Important points about presentation include pace and timing, which can mean consciously having to slow down your rate of speaking; the nervous beginner can speak too quickly. Other factors are looking at the audience and using notes appropriately.

Thorough preparation will help you to feel confident, but however nervous or inexperienced you may feel, do not apologise for being there. For example, if you have been asked to give a talk about your work, *do not say* 'I'm going to talk about the work of health visitors, but I'm afraid I've only been qualified for a year so there's a lot I don't know yet'. Instead, present yourself positively: 'I'm going to talk about the work of health visitors. I've been qualified for a year now, and I'd like to share my experience of the work with you'.

The way to improve presentation is practise. Practise giving your talk out loud or to friends or colleagues. Ask a trusted colleague to sit in when you give a talk and to give you feedback afterwards. It is also helpful to have your talk recorded so that you can assess your own strengths and weaknesses.

Plan for Contingencies

A major fear when giving a talk is that you might lose your place or your train of thought. If this is a possibility, it is better to think beforehand about what you will do if it should happen. It is best to acknowledge that you have a problem rather than leave an embarrassing silence. For example, say 'Sorry, I've lost my place'. Remember that an audience is likely to be friendly rather than hostile. So let them help by asking for time: 'Excuse me for a moment while I look through my notes' (see also section on dealing with difficulties in Chapter 13).

Another fear is that audiovisual equipment may not work. You cannot insure against this, so it is best to have a contingency plan ready. For example, 'As we can't see the sequence on PowerPoint as I'd hoped, I'll write the stages up on the flip-chart and talk through them instead', or you may wish to ensure you have a back-up, such as overhead projector slides of the PowerPoint presentation.

IMPROVING PATIENT EDUCATION

Evidence suggests that patients want health information, but some have difficulty in understanding and remembering what they have been told by their doctor, nurse or other health worker. Obstacles that prevent understanding of and action on health information include literacy, culture, language, age and physiological barriers (Beagley 2011). Patients who feel dissatisfied with the communications aspect of their encounters with health professionals may be reluctant to ask for more information and/or may not comply with the advice and treatment prescribed for them (see, for example, McNaughton and Shucksmith 2015).

There may be complex reasons for these apparent failures, but some of the cause will be the way in which information, advice and instructions are given to patients. Often, the circumstances are less than ideal,

because patients are distressed or feeling unwell, and there may be little time in a busy surgery, health centre, outpatient clinic or hospital ward. This is all the more reason to ensure that the best possible use is made of the time and opportunities for patient education.

All the basic communication skills discussed in Chapter 10, and the principles of helping people to learn outlined in this chapter, are important. There is also now a growing body of evidence in the field of patient education and imparting health information. The Cochrane website provides various systematic reviews on patient education (http://www.cochrane.org). For examples of some of these reviews, see Attridge et al (2014) for a review of culturally appropriate health education for people in ethnic minority groups with type 2 diabetes mellitus and Brown et al (2011) examining patient education in the management of coronary heart disease.

Some particular principles that have been found helpful in patient education are set out in Box 12.7.

Exercise 12.2 is designed to help you practise the skills of patient education and supplements the basic communication skills outlined in Chapter 10. Another useful way of learning to improve communication skills is to record and then analyse an interview with a patient.

TEACHING PRACTICAL SKILLS FOR HEALTH

Health promoters in a number of health-related settings are often called upon to teach practical skills, such as relaxation or physiotherapy exercises, how to bathe a baby or change a nappy, and how to give an injection or test urine.

Teaching a skill is not just about giving the client information and teaching new practical skills. It is also necessary to pay attention to what clients *feel*. If people are afraid to do something because they are worried about looking foolish or doing it incorrectly, they are unlikely to succeed; encouragement and step-by-step progress are needed. Confidence-building is as important a part of the health educator's role as developing practical skills.

To develop clients' abilities to perform a skilled task, a three-stage approach is most effective:

Stage 1. Demonstrate
Stage 2. Rehearse
Stage 3. Practise.

BOX 12.7
SOME PRINCIPLES OF PATIENT EDUCATION

- Say important things first: Patients are more likely to remember what was said at the beginning of a session, so give the most important advice and instruction first whenever possible.
- Stress and repeat the key points: Patients are more likely to remember what they consider to be important, so make sure they realise what the important points are. For example, say:
  - 'The most important thing for you to remember today is …'
  - 'The one thing it's really essential to do is …'

Repetition of key points also helps people to remember them.

- Give specific, precise advice: Sometimes it is appropriate to give general guidance, but specific, precise advice is more likely to be remembered than vague guidance. For example, say:
  - 'I advise you to lose 5 pounds in the next month' rather than 'I advise you to lose weight'.
  - 'Try to take 30 minutes exercise every day' rather than 'Take more exercise'.
- Structure information into categories: This means telling the patient headings and then categorising your material under these headings as you present it. See 'Organise Your Public Heath Education Material' discussed previously in this chapter.

- Use plain language. Avoid jargon and long words and sentences: If you need to use medical terms or jargon, make sure the patient understands what they mean. Never use a long word when a short one will do. Use short sentences. See Attridge et al (2014) for the plain language report on their study as an example of the difference between professional language and plain language.
- Use visual aids, leaflets, handouts and written instructions (see Chapter 11 on using communication tools).
- Avoid saying too much at once: Three or four key points are all that you can expect someone to remember from one session. See 'Ensure Relevance' discussed previously in this chapter.
- Ensure advice is relevant and realistic to the patient's circumstances.
- Get feedback from patients to ensure that they understand (see the section on asking questions and getting feedback in Chapter 10).

EXERCISE 12.2

Skills of Patient Education

Work in groups of three, taking each role in turn.

The **first person** takes the role of the public health educator. She selects the topic to be taught, drawing on her own experience, and tells the patient their medical history before role-play starts.

The **second person** plays the patient. This patient should have one of the following sets of characteristics:

- Intelligent but with very limited understanding of spoken English, no ability to read or write English and no one available to translate
- Extremely worried, tense and anxious about their medical condition and prognosis
- Has some learning difficulty, finds great difficulty in understanding and remembering instructions although they try hard to be cooperative.

The **third person** takes the role of the observer, using the observer's checklist in the following text.

Role-play the scene in which the health promoter is teaching the patient for 10 minutes. The observer keeps time. Then give constructive feedback as follows:

- First, the health promoter assesses their own performance, saying what they felt they did well, and identifying points they feel they need to work on in the future.

- Second, the patient describes how it felt to be the patient, identifying what the health promoter did or said which made them feel at ease, put down, anxious, reassured, more confused, and so on.
- Finally, the observer gives feedback using the checklist as a guide.

Communication checklist

1. Nonverbal aspects of communication (e.g. tone of voice, posture, gestures, facial expression and use of touch)
2. Sequence and structure of key points (e.g. important things first, logical sequence, information in categories)
3. Choice of language (e.g. appropriately simple and short, use of jargon or idioms, medical terms)
4. Two-way communication (e.g. encourage patient to talk and express feelings, get feedback about how much is understood, open/closed/biased/multiple questions)
5. Amount of information (e.g. too much or too little)
6. Clarity of objective(s)
7. Use of repetition
8. Use of emphasis to stress important points
9. Any assumptions made but not checked (e.g. about previous knowledge, facilities for carrying out instructions, willingness to comply)
10. Anything else?

Clients will be watching and listening in Stage 1, but they become actively involved in doing in Stages 2 and 3.

It may be useful to begin by using a dummy, for example, when teaching safe lifting techniques, or to use an orange instead of a person when teaching injection techniques. As skills develop, the techniques can be tried in real-life situations (lifting people, for example) and perhaps under more difficult circumstances.

Individual learners need to progress at their own pace and build up confidence at each stage. For this reason, teaching practical skills needs time and patience, but it is worth the investment to get the right skills programme from the beginning. People who have lost confidence in their ability to do something are sometimes more difficult to help than a new learner.

PRACTICE POINTS

- To be successful in public health education with clients you need to understand principles of learning and factors that help and hinder the learning process. You may find it helpful to use informal learning contracts.
- Giving talks on public health topics requires detailed planning, preparation and practise.
- You can help patients to understand and remember more if you take account of some key principles of patient education.
- Use a three-stage approach of demonstration, rehearsal and practice when you are teaching practical health-related skills.

REFERENCES

Attridge M, Creamer Ramsden JM, Cannings R, Hawthorne JK 2014 Culturally appropriate health education for people in ethnic minority groups with type 2 diabetes mellitus. http://onlinelibrary.wiley.com/doi/10.1002/14651858.CD006424.pub3/full.

Bates B 2015 Learning theories simplified: …and how to apply them to teaching. London, Sage.

Beagley L 2011 Educating patients: understanding barriers, learning styles, and teaching techniques. Journal of Perianesthesia Nursing 26(5):331–337.

Brown JPR, Clark AM, Dalal H, Welch K, Taylor RS 2011 Patient education in the management of coronary heart disease. http://onlinelibrary.wiley.com/doi/10.1002/14651858.CD008895.pub2/full.

McNaughton RJ, Shucksmith J 2015 Reasons for (non)compliance with intervention following identification of 'high-risk' status in the NHS Health Check programme. Journal of Public Health 37(2):218–225.

Proust A, Colbourn T, Seward N et al 2013 Women's groups practising participatory learning and action to improve maternal and newborn health in low-resource settings: a systematic review and meta-analysis. The Lancet 381(9879):1736–1746.

WHO 2012 Health education: theoretical concepts, effective strategies and core competencies. Geneva, WHO.

WHO 2014 WHO recommendation on community mobilization through facilitated participatory learning and action cycles with women's groups for maternal and newborn health. Geneva, WHO.

WEBSITE

BBC webpage on health advice, such as sun safety, referenced in Box 12.6. http://www.bbc.co.uk/programmes/articles/YDD2fTqHVfWJbV5qkHPL7D/sun-safety.

For systematic reviews on patient education on the Cochrane Library. http://onlinelibrary.wiley.com/cochranelibrary/search.

YOUTUBE

The Ted Lesson on sun safety referenced in Box 12.6. https://www.youtube.com/watch?v=ZSJITdsTze0.

FACEBOOK

Facebook page on sun safety referenced in Box 12.6. https://www.facebook.com/search/top/?q=sun%20safety%20.

BLOG

Sun Sense Blog with up to date tips and recommendation referenced in Box 12.6. http://www.sunsense.co.uk/blog/2014/stay-sun-safe-on-the-slopes.aspx.

13

WORKING WITH GROUPS TO PROMOTE HEALTH

CHAPTER CONTENTS

SUMMARY

This chapter is about working with clients in groups (including social media groups) and begins by discussing the range of groups in health promotion and public health, potential benefits of group work and when it is appropriate to use it as an approach. Group leadership styles and responsibilities and individual group behaviour are considered. The last part of the chapter focuses on the competencies needed for working successfully with people in groups including the practicalities and skills of setting up a group, getting groups established, discussion skills and dealing with difficulties. Exercises focus on identifying the benefits of joining a group, looking at your leadership style and planning a group meeting.

Health promoters and public health practitioners work with many different kinds of groups in a variety of settings. Working with groups of colleagues is considered in Chapter 9; in this chapter, the focus is on the public health promoter's work with groups of clients, but many of the skills discussed in Chapter 9 (such as coordination, teamwork and working effectively in meetings and committees) may also apply when working with client groups (see Chapter 9).

Group work encourages clients to be active participants in their own health issues and with their communities. Many of the groups with which health promoters and public health practitioners are involved will already exist, where members have come together for a common purpose and health issues form part, or the whole, of the agenda. The role of the health promoter or public health practitioner may vary widely, from leading a one-off session to facilitating the development of a new group, or leading a group with a defined lifespan. Whatever the role, competencies in group work are needed. Leading therapeutic groups are excluded from the discussions in this chapter. Therapy requires in-depth professional training in a range of possible approaches, which is outside the scope of this book (see Group Therapy 2016 for further details on therapeutic group activities including what group therapy can do in terms of promoting health).

TYPES OF GROUPS

Groups are formed for a variety of purposes and are not simply a random collection of individuals. Members generally have a sense of shared identity, common objectives, defined membership criteria and their own particular ways of working. The term *group work* can be applied to a range of activities such as group therapy, social action or self-help. Groups in the context of health promotion and public health are usually formed for one or more of the following purposes:

For raising awareness. To increase members' interest in, and awareness of, health issues through group discussion. This may be a group already in existence, such as a women's group, which may agree to discuss a health issue.

For mutual support. To support members in difficult decision making, to help each other to cope with shared health problems/disabilities or to change a health-damaging behaviour. Examples are self-help groups, such as patients' associations and Alcoholics Anonymous.

For social action. To use collective power to campaign for social change, for example, tackling a local problem of drug misuse, housing standards or community facilities.

For education. To impart skills, offer information and sometimes to prepare members for specific life events like, for example, becoming a parent.

For group counselling. To help members to find solutions through exploring a shared problem with a counsellor, for example, a group of menopausal women.

Being clear about the purpose of a group is important. Confusion can result if the tasks of a group are changed, especially if this means that individual members have to adopt different roles. For example, an individual will have difficulty if she attends a group to obtain support and finds the task has changed to campaigning. A new group is required for the new task.

The type of task will determine the most effective size for the group; for example, educational groups may be larger than support groups.

Different kinds of groups may also require the health promoter or public health practitioner to take on different roles and use different skills. Leading and facilitating groups or administrating or moderating social media

groups requires special skills and methods; later in this chapter, group leadership and the skills you need to be effective as a group leader are discussed.

WHEN TO USE GROUP WORK

Whilst health promoters and public health practitioners may be unsure about when it is appropriate to use a group work approach to promote health, there is a growing evidence base that these types of intervention work (see, for example, Tang et al 2012, research into self-management groups for diabetes). Group work is appropriate when your plans fulfil the following criteria (see also Chapter 5, section on deciding the best way of achieving your aims):

■ You have looked critically at what other health promotion opportunities exist, and you have concluded that group work is needed to meet the particular needs of specific groups of people.

■ You have strong evidence that group work is effective for this particular client group.

■ You are going to be working with a defined group of people over a period of time, which will allow the group to build up trust and be able to help each other, for example, a group of teenage mothers, a self-help group of patients who are recovering after heart attacks or people who have been diagnosed as HIV-positive.

■ You have access to a comfortable, private and relaxed environment in which to run the group; for example, a community centre.

■ You have access to support and supervision to provide you with assistance when you need it and help you to develop your group work.

In some circumstances, group work may be particularly helpful. For examples:

■ you are planning to work with people who are already in a close small group and possibly already used to group work; for example, a group of young people who are in a residential drug rehabilitation setting.

■ you are establishing a connection with a number of people who have a common interest and wish to develop an equal and respectful partnership with them; for example, a group of people with mental health problems who have recently moved into a group home.

you want to work with a particular ethnic minority community, but you do not come from that group yourself and are faced with issues of differences in culture and language. In this case, it could be helpful to run a group to look at health issues in partnership with a link worker or health advocate who can offer culturally sensitive help and skills in translation and interpretation.

There are times when it may not be advisable to embark on group work or to continue to run an existing group. These may include situations when:

- you have not consulted with prospective clients to establish their needs
- group members are from such a diverse range of backgrounds that they have little in common and feel uncomfortable with one another
- the cultural or psychosocial background of the group will make it difficult for them to adapt to group work
- the group will meet only once or twice, which means that people will not have long enough to get to know and trust one another
- the membership of a group is not stable, and people are constantly leaving or joining
- your aim is solely to transmit information, so a talk with questions and answers would be better
- the aim of the group is to encourage a change towards a healthier lifestyle but the people concerned do not have the opportunity to make changes because of lack of money, skills, support or facilities
- you do not have suitable accommodation for meetings; for example, you only have available a large, tiered lecture theatre
- you do not yet have the competencies to facilitate group work or access to the necessary training and support.

GROUP LEADERSHIP

Two aspects of group leadership are useful to consider. One is your leadership style and the other is your responsibility as a group leader.

Leadership Style

It is important that all the members of the group are agreed upon who is the leader and support the leader in this role. The leadership style needs to be compatible with the group members, especially if the group has to work together to complete complex tasks. For example, a group of highly motivated and trained professionals will work best with a leader who encourages participation and shared decision making. It is essential for leaders to be aware of which style members prefer and to develop the ability to adjust their style if the situation demands it.

A key dimension of leadership style is where the leader stands on a continuum from authoritarian to participative.

An authoritarian style is directive with the group leader acting as a source of expertise. If you adopt this approach, you rely on your status, credibility and expertise to ensure acceptance of your views and leadership role.

The strength of this style is that children and vulnerable people (such as those who are sick or distressed) may feel secure, reassured and protected from harm.

The weaknesses of this style are that clients may become fearful, anxious and reluctant to take independent action; it does not develop their ability to take responsibility for their own decisions and actions. Furthermore, clients may respond by rebelling and rejecting your guidance.

A participative style involves shifting power from the group leader so that it is shared between the leader and the group members. This means using all the skills and knowledge of the group members, as well as the leader who is more likely to choose the title of facilitator. As a facilitator, you will need to show warmth and empathy, encourage group members to express their feelings and provide counsel and encouragement. You will need to be tolerant of different viewpoints, showing fairness and impartiality. You will need skills and the ability to confront difficult issues and resolve conflict using a problem-solving approach (see Chapter 9, section on understanding conflict).

The strength of this style is that clients learn to trust their own judgements and at the same time to appreciate other people's rights and opinions.

The weaknesses of this style may be that strong feelings are uncovered and distress experienced by the client and yourself, which might be difficult to manage. Also, clients who are used to being told what to do may feel confused and dissatisfied because they are not receiving advice and direction. They will need to have the approach explained to them and be given suitable learning experiences to show them that it works.

Group leaders can operate somewhere between the two extremes, providing some authoritative leadership while also encouraging a degree of participation. Successful group leadership depends on a variety of factors such as:

- the leader's preferred style of operating and personality. For example, if you have been used to being perceived as the expert with the authority of professional knowledge that you want to pass on, you will probably feel (and look) uncomfortable if you try to switch to a facilitator style without sufficient training, and this may produce tension in the group.
- the group members' preferred style of leadership in the specific circumstances of the group. For example, if group members are low in confidence, they may need you to be more authoritarian to start with so that they feel secure. You can then gradually encourage participation and adopt a more facilitative style as members learn to trust you and each other, and feel confident enough to join in.
- the group's objectives and tasks. For example, a group that has the objective of learning new skills (such as an exercise class) will need a more authoritarian leader who will tell them how to do the exercises properly, whereas a group of parents in a support group that aims to help them recover from the death of a child will need a facilitator to help members to express and work through their grief.
- the wider environment, such as the culture of the group members and of the organisations they belong to. For example, the cultural norm of some ethnic minorities may be passive, and they may not only lack confidence about active participation in groups but may also perceive it as inappropriate.

You need to consider these factors and how they might be modified so that the group achieves its purpose. The easiest thing to modify in the short term should be your own style, but in the long term it may also be possible to make other changes; for example, develop the group members' confidence so that they are willing to take on more responsibility and in-

crease participation (see Chapter 4, section on analysing your aims and values: five approaches).

The participative style fits best with the self-empowering client-centred approach to promoting health. However, some health promoters and public health practitioners will have been trained in an authoritarian style and will have modelled themselves on this experience. If this is true in your case, you will need to learn how to work in a participative style to become more effective in empowering your clients.

Finally, a participative style must be distinguished from a permissive style. A permissive style lets clients come to their own conclusions and aims to avoid conflict and keep everyone happy. Helping the clients to enjoy the experience is more important to the leader than achieving the goals of the group. Difficulties and conflict are not confronted, and the clients may feel neither nurtured nor secure.

Leadership Responsibilities

The responsibilities of group leaders will depend on the role they take; for example, whether they are responsible for the practical organisation such as booking a venue. But whatever the role, a leader's responsibilities may include:

- helping members to identify and clarify their interests and needs, and what they would like to gain from the group in the short and long term
- helping to develop a relaxed atmosphere in which group members feel able to be open and trusting with each other, and able to participate freely
- offering expertise to the group on the understanding that members are free to accept or reject the offer
- accepting and valuing all contributions from group members.

But it is not only the group leader who has responsibilities: group members have them too. They may include:

- participating in clarifying the aims of the group
- choosing whether and how much to participate
- identifying personal health goals and concerns
- deciding which challenges and risks they are prepared to take. For example, how much are they prepared to expose their own weaknesses and vulnerability to other people in the group?

GROUP BEHAVIOUR

Health promoters and public health practitioners will be able to work with a group more effectively if they are aware of the group dynamics and the ways in which people are likely to behave when they come together in groups. There are three aspects of group behaviour that you may find particularly useful: the pattern of behaviour that usually develops in a group's life, the different roles group members may perform and the concept of hidden agendas.

Group Development

Groups tend to show a particular pattern of behaviour as they mature and develop. An early and much quoted study characterised small group developmental process into four stages (see Bonebright 2010 for an historical review of Tuckman's model of small group development):

1. *Forming.* The group is forming. People meet each other and get to know one another with individuals establishing their own identity and role within the group. The group's purpose and way of working are established.

2. *Storming.* Most groups go through a conflict stage when the leadership and ways in which the group is working are challenged. For example, people may question how things are being done and what the leader's role is, and may get into heated discussions with each other. This can be a difficult period for both leader and members, but it is a vital stage in the group's maturing process rather like the period of rebelling and questioning during adolescence. Successful handling of this period leads to the development of open communication, trust and shared responsibility for achieving the purposes of the group (see Chapter 9, section on understanding conflict).

3. *Norming.* At this stage, the group settles down with the norms and accepted practices of the group established.

4. *Performing.* The group is fully effective at this stage and is able to concentrate on its tasks.

When the developmental process fails in some way, attempts to sabotage the group may occur. It is thus worth investing time and effort to help new groups to develop successfully.

Many groups have a limited life, meeting for a set number of sessions or until a particular task or aim has been achieved. At the end of a group's life, it may be helpful to have a final session, which could give group members an opportunity to express their appreciation and perhaps arrange a follow-up or reunion.

Group Members' Roles

An early study established the characteristics of team members, identifying that a mix of nine roles is needed for full effectiveness (Belbin 1981). These roles are also relevant to a group's effectiveness and are outlined in Box 13.1.

BOX 13.1
ROLES NEEDED FOR EFFECTIVE GROUPS AND TEAMS

The Coordinator – clarifies goals, promotes decision making, delegates well to enable the group to work effectively.

The Shaper – is action oriented and encourages the group to get on with its tasks.

The Plant – is the creative source of ideas and proposals.

The Monitor/Evaluator – is good at analysing and criticising.

The Resource Investigator – has a good network of contacts and liaises with other people and agencies.

The Company Worker – is good at organising and administration.

The Team Worker – supports the members of the group and is a good listener.

The Specialist – provides specialist knowledge and skills.

The Finisher – contributes foresight and perseverance to ensure that the group completes its tasks.

At different times, each group member may play a variety of these roles, and most people have personal characteristics which might result in more affinity with a particular role. If one or more of these roles is lacking, the facilitator can help to make a group more successful by consciously adopting a new role or encouraging other group members to adjust their roles.

Hidden Agendas

People will have their own individual reasons for joining a group, which may be in addition to, or instead of, the reason expected. For example, a woman may attend a women's health group because she is lonely and sees the group as a way of meeting people; she has not joined because she is particularly interested in health issues. Or a group member may seek a prominent position in a group, such as being the Chair or Secretary, to fulfil their need to feel valued and useful; they may or may not also be committed to the work itself and the aims of the group. In these examples, fulfilling these personal objectives are hidden agendas.

Most people bring their own hidden agendas to groups in addition to the agreed group objectives; these commonly include meeting the need for social contact or making a particular alliance. Members will work together best when there is communication about individual objectives or agendas and agreement about shared objectives. Otherwise members may promote their own interests at the expense of the group. You will be more effective as a group leader if you are aware of the hidden agendas in the group and can find ways of dealing with them.

SETTING UP A GROUP

Planning and preparation are essential for successful group work. The following sections take you step-by-step through the thinking and planning you need to do when setting up a group.

Why Are You Proposing to Run the Group?

- Are you reacting to a demand from clients, other professionals, a community or your own observations?
- Are you trying to develop your health promotion role and see this group as a way of progressing?
- Are you aiming to provide advice and support, to supply information or to help people to change health-related behaviour?
- Are you aiming to satisfy your own needs or your clients' needs? (Your reasons can include both, but it is helpful to distinguish between them.)

Who Will the Members Be?

- Will the members be referred (from their GP, for example), will they be coerced into joining or will membership be entirely voluntary?
- Have you given everyone an equal opportunity to join (such as ensuring facilities for wheelchairs, disabled toilets, signing for those hard of hearing, hearing loops, translation into appropriate minority languages)? Have you made provision for people to let you know of any special needs?
- How will you identify the potential members of your group – from individuals requesting a group, from local or national registers, from people with shared characteristics (such as age, sex, lifestyle, culture, job, health concern) or by other means?
- How will you recruit your members? Do you need to advertise?
- How many members do you aim to have? What is the ideal number, bearing in mind the purpose of the group and any constraints imposed by your location?

What Are the Group's Aims and Objectives?

- Are these within the realistic abilities of yourself and the members?
- Can all the potential membership understand them?
- Are you clear about your own objectives in setting up the group and whether these are different from the members' objectives?
- Are all members clear about their individual objectives (i.e. the specific outcomes they hope to achieve through attending the group)?

Where Will the Group Meet?

- Is the location appropriate? For example, a health centre or hospital could appear clinical and cold and remind people of illness. Neutral territory, such as a room in a community centre or someone's house, may be more relaxing and inviting.
- What is the seating like? If you are aiming for participative group work, seating people in a circle is best (see Fig. 13.1) with physical barriers to communication such as tables or desks removed. Can you put chairs in a circle where all group members can see each other?
- What are the facilities like? Is there enough space for the activities you plan? Is the floor covering suitable for the purpose? Is the temperature suitable and adjustable if necessary? Are the facilities adequate for the purpose (for example, access for pushchairs, toilets, catering facilities,

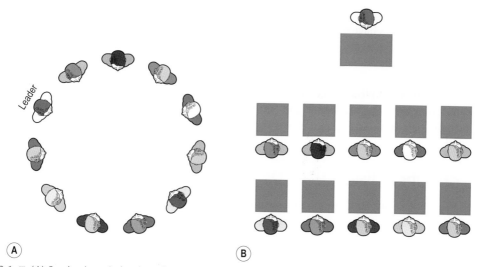

FIG. 13.1 ■ (A) Seating in a circle – best for group work; (B) traditional seating in rows – not suitable for group work.

washing/shower rooms, crèche)? Are there facilities for people with special needs (for example, wide access for wheelchairs, disabled toilets, hearing loops, signs in minority languages)?

■ Is access good? Is the venue accessible by local transport? Do you have transport for members who cannot manage on public transport? Are parking arrangements satisfactory?

■ What are the security arrangements? Where the fire extinguishers and what is the fire drill? In case of an emergency, who do you contact? Do you need insurance coverage?

What Resources Do You Need?

■ Do you need any special equipment, for example, audiovisual media equipment? Are you familiar with the equipment and confident you can operate it? Does the equipment have to be booked in advance? If so, are you familiar with the booking system?

■ Do you need any additional resources or facilities such as WiFi, DVDs, leaflets, posters, books or outside speakers? If so, have you made all the necessary arrangements in advance?

■ Do you need to pay for anything? If so, have you identified a source of funding (for example, a charge to the group members or a sponsor)?

When Will the Group Meet?

■ Is the time you have chosen the best one for the clients or have you chosen it to suit yourself?

■ Does the length of meetings suit members and take into account their other commitments?

■ Have you consulted potential members about timing and tried to satisfy the majority?

How Will the Group Be Run?

■ Will it be a self-help group and directed by the members or led by a public health-related professional?

■ To what extent will the structure be flexible and the content negotiable?

■ Will the group be open (anyone can join at any time) or will there be restrictions on admitting new members once the group has started?

How Will the Group Be Evaluated?

■ At the end of each meeting? At the end of the group? Or both? (See also Chapter 12, section on evaluation, feedback and assessment.)

■ Verbally, or in writing, or both? How will you ask questions to obtain accurate feedback from members (for example, by providing opportunities for anonymous feedback)?

- How will you know that the group, individual and your own objectives have been achieved?
- Were there any unplanned outcomes of the group? Were these desirable or undesirable? What caused them?
- What have you learned? What would you do differently next time? (See DeLucia-Waak and Nitza 2013 for more details in setting up a group and group work in general.)

GETTING GROUPS GOING

Some people may feel nervous about going to a group meeting for the first time, especially if they are unlikely to know other members. The initial task for the group leader is to help people to feel at ease.

Before the First Meeting

If you know in advance who is coming to a group meeting, it may be helpful and welcoming to confirm by email (a group's email list would be the most time efficient), Facebook post or messenger alert, letter or telephone text that you are expecting them, and the time and place. If anyone has let you know they have special needs, contact them in advance to discuss their needs and let them know what facilities will be available.

On Arrival

It helps if clients can be greeted personally, introduced to other people or given something to do: 'There are some books and leaflets on the table if you'd like to look at them until everyone has arrived'. Ensure that anyone with special needs has appropriate facilities and assistance.

Getting to Know Each Other

Knowing each person's name and something about them is the first step towards constructive group work because it helps them to feel valued as a member of the group and is the beginning of openness and trust between members.

There are many ways of going about this, some of which are as follows.

Introduction in Pairs

Ask each person to sit next to someone they have not met before. One person in each pair then interviews their partner. After a few minutes (the leader keeps the time), the partners swap roles. Then, in turn, each member of the group introduces their partner by name and says something about them. You may like to remind people that no one has to answer any questions if they do not wish to.

The leader could also suggest appropriate questions. For example, in groups for prospective parents, the leader could suggest that partners find out if this is the first baby, where the mother goes for antenatal check-ups or where she is booked to have her baby.

Name Games

Group members sit in a circle and you, the leader, take an object, such as a pen, and hand it to the person on your left, saying 'My name is A and this is a pen'. You ask the person who now holds the pen to say 'My name is B and A says that this is a pen'. B then passes the pen to the person on his left, who says 'My name is C and B says that A says that this is a pen'. This continues until the pen gets back to the beginning. If group members forget someone's name, the rest of the group can prompt them. This helps establish a cooperative and supportive atmosphere, as well as helping people to learn each other's names. Any tension and embarrassment is relieved by laughing and tension is effectively broken.

At subsequent group meetings, it is often helpful to do a quick round of names at the beginning, for example 'Who would like to have a shot at naming every member of the group?' or 'I'm going to try to see if I can remember everyone's name'.

You might like to set the tone by suggesting how people are addressed, by first names or more formally. The important thing is to encourage people to use whatever feels comfortable: 'My name is Ann Jones, and I'm happy for you to call me Ann'.

Sharing Initial Feelings and Expectations

People may be helped to relax if they know that others also feel nervous or shy. So ask 'What did you feel about coming here today? Did anyone feel nervous? Did anyone almost *not* come?' This can open the way for people to express their anxieties. You can also encourage them to say why they have come to the meeting and what they expect to gain from it. It might help to ask members to complete a checklist, ticking statements that are true for them. Such statements could include the following:

- I'm worried I won't have anything to say.
- I'm afraid I'll talk too much.
- I'm worried I'll make a fool of myself.
- I'll be too embarrassed to join in.
- I'm afraid I might get upset.
- I'm concerned I may be bored.
- I want to meet other people in the same situation.
- I enjoy talking to others.
- I enjoy a good debate.
- I want to get out of the house.
- I want to go somewhere different.
- I enjoy listening to other people.

People can then compare their list with that of one or two other people, and then it may be helpful to share what has been discovered with the whole group.

Setting Ground Rules

People joining a group will have different expectations and assumptions about how the group will run. Problems can arise if these are not brought out in the open and clarified at the beginning. For example, people may assume that what they say in a group will be treated confidentially and then be upset if they find that another member did not realise this and had discussed the issue elsewhere. Or some members might expect the group leader to take all the responsibility for organising the group and may feel let down if they later discover that the leader expects them to do some of the work.

To prevent these difficulties, it is often helpful to establish a set of ground rules. Early on in the group's life, members need the opportunity to explore their expectations and reach agreement about issues, such as the following:

- How members are expected to behave in the group.
- Are any rules and sanctions to be set, for example, about nonattendance at group meetings or whether members can join in if they arrive late?
- What is confidential to the group?
- Can new members join at any time, or is the group closed to new membership?

- How will the leader and the members exercise control in the group?
- Who has responsibility for the practical aspects of running the group, such as bringing refreshments along or booking the room?

For example, in a self-help group, mutual rights and responsibilities will be agreed on the basis of equality of leader and clients, but in reality the power balance will not be completely equal and a contract will help with power sharing. In a counselling group, the power of the counsellor is much greater than that of the clients, and the leader has a duty to respect the members and to promote their autonomy.

DISCUSSION SKILLS

A discussion may not happen just by putting a group of people together and saying 'Let's discuss …'. Discussion needs planning and preparation, and there are many ways of triggering it off and providing structures that will help everyone to participate.

Trigger Materials

Discussion can be triggered by providing a focus, preferably a controversial one. This can simply be a question 'What do you think about the ban on child-in-car smoking?', but it might also be a leaflet, a poster, a health promotion campaign film or an item in a newspaper or magazine ('What do you think the makers of this alcoholic drink are trying to convey in this advertisement?'). Choose something that people are likely to have strong views about.

Some health promotion campaign films are specially made as trigger materials, presenting situations for people to talk about. Helpful notes for group leaders often accompany such campaign films.

Brainstorms/Think Sessions

Brainstorming is a useful way to open up a subject and collect everyone's ideas. Ask an open question to which there is no single right answer, such as 'Why do some young people binge drink?' or 'What do you feel you need to know before your baby is born?' Accept every suggestion, without comment or criticism, and write them down in a list on a flip-chart or blackboard. Ask the group not to start discussing the ideas until everybody has finished. You can make your own suggestions and write them down along with others.

In this way, all members' contributions are equally valued and everyone has a chance to participate. Encourage shy members by asking 'Anything else?' and allowing silent pauses while people think.

Then you can set the group to work by asking them to put the ideas into categories and to identify the key features of each category. For example, people might categorise reasons for binge drinking into a *constructive* category: 'It helps me to socialise' or 'It helps me to relax, to feel good', and an *escape* category: 'I can forget my problems' or 'It stops me from feeling upset'.

Rounds

A round is a way of giving everyone an equal chance to participate. You invite each group member in turn around the circle to make a brief statement. You might like to start the round yourself or join in when your turn comes in the circle. For example, ask everyone to make a brief statement about one of the following:

'My first feelings when I knew I was pregnant were …'

'What I think about jogging is …'

'The main reason why I can't lose weight is …'

'The thing that has helped me most in my efforts to give up smoking is …'

There are four essential rules for successful rounds, which must be explained and gently enforced if necessary. These are:

- no interruptions until each person has finished his statement
- no comments on anybody's contribution until the full round is completed (no discussions, interpretation, not even 'I think that too' remarks)
- anyone can choose not to participate. Give permission, clearly and emphatically, that anyone who does not want to make a statement can just say 'pass'. This is very important for reinforcing the principle of voluntary participation
- it does not matter if two or more people in the round say the same thing. People should stick to saying what they had intended even if someone else has said it already; they do not have to think of something different.

Rounds are also useful ways of beginning and ending sessions. For example:

'One thing I've put into practice since last week is …'

'The main thing I've got from today's session is …'

'One thing I'm going to find out by next time we meet is …'

It is also a useful way of getting feedback. For example:

'One thing I really liked about today's session was …'

'One thing I didn't like about today's session was …'

'One thing I wish we'd done is …'

Buzz Groups

Buzz groups are small groups of two to six people who discuss questions or topics for short periods, usually about 10 minutes. It is especially useful for large groups to be divided up in this way as it gives everyone more chance to talk. Form the groups first of all, then say what you would like each one to do, such as 'Make a list of the times when you want a cigarette' or 'Talk about the things you find helpful when you feel stressed', and how long they have in which to do it. If you want people to share ideas with the rest of the group as a whole afterwards, it may be helpful to provide large sheets of paper and felt-tip pens, so that feedback posters can be put up for everyone to see and discuss.

Safe Revelations

Sometimes people may hesitate or refuse to say what they really feel for fear of looking silly, being embarrassed or getting upset. One way of overcoming this is to give everyone a piece of paper and ask them to write down, for example, what their biggest worries are or what they really want to know. All the papers are then folded and put in a receptacle, such as a waste-paper basket or a shopping bag. Each person in turn picks out one piece of paper and reads aloud what is written on it. Tell people not to say if they happen to pick out their own piece of paper, and that, of course, nobody needs to identify themselves as the author of any of the statements.

The aim is to find out the concerns of the group members in the security of anonymity. Make sure that everyone listens and does not comment until all the papers have been read out. Then you can discuss what was discovered.

DEALING WITH DIFFICULTIES

Acknowledge the potential difficulties of running a group and work out strategies for coping should the problem actually arise. Some common problems and possible strategies for coping are as follows.

Silence

Silence can be useful; it can be time that group members need to think. Silence often does not feel as threatening to group members as it may do to the facilitator; however, you may find it helpful to:

- run a group with a partner so that you can help each other out if either of you gets stuck
- ensure thorough preparation so that you have planned activities and questions. Write down a plan and a list of questions to ask (such as at the end of showing a DVD)
- have an additional activity ready to use if the reason for the discussion closing down is that what you have planned does not seem to be working.

Disasters

Unexpected disasters include such things as arriving late or finding that too few or too many people have turned up. There is no blueprint strategy to cope with the unexpected, but it will help if you acknowledge what has happened and share it with your group: 'I'm delighted that so many of you have come along, but I wasn't expecting such numbers, so we may be a bit crowded this week'. Also share your plans for dealing with the disaster ('I'm going to try to get a bigger room next time' ... 'I'm going to start 10 minutes late'). Sharing the problem and enlisting cooperation can have the positive benefit of encouraging mutual support; *not* sharing it can leave your group feeling angry.

Distractions

Distractions can take many forms: noises outside the room (such as road works), noises inside the room (such as crying babies, coughing), people coming in late or leaving early or interruptions. Distractions can also be caused by group members themselves, for example, by someone becoming very angry or upset.

As a rule, there are three choices for you as group leader:

- **Ignore them.** This is seldom a good idea as it leaves people wondering whether you are going to do anything, and this in itself is a distraction.
- **Acknowledge and accept them.** This is generally best with things you cannot change: 'I know the traffic is really noisy, but there's nothing we can do about it, so I think we'll just have to put up with it this time and I will find a different room/ venue for future meetings'.
- **Do something about them.** It is preferable to involve the group in the decision: 'As so many of you found it difficult to get here by 2 o'clock, shall we start at 2:15 next week?' or 'Do you think it would be helpful if you took it in turns to look after the babies in the next room?'

If someone is showing emotion, such as crying, acknowledge it: 'I can see that you're upset' and offer reassurance that it is OK to show emotion: 'There's no need to be embarrassed ... we don't mind if you cry ...'. Offer the opportunity to talk about it: 'Would you like to tell us what is upsetting you?' or to take some time away from the group, accompanied by you or someone else: 'Shall we go outside for a few minutes?' Do not put any pressure on people in distress. Help them to do what they want to do, whether it is cry, talk, keep silent, stay, leave or be by themselves. But *do not* ignore a show of emotion; ignoring it will only cause tension and embarrassment.

Difficult Behaviour

How group members behave can pose difficulties for the public health leader. There are two broad categories of difficult behaviour: nonparticipation and talking too much. The latter category takes many forms: The person who dominates and always responds with the answers and prevents other people contributing, people who launch into long stories, people who interrupt, people who talk off the point, people who always disagree and people who always crack jokes. Note that people often change their behaviour as they get to know others and feel more comfortable in a group, but here are some points about dealing with people who talk too much and about encouraging quiet members to engage:

- Think about why dominant people are behaving like this. Are they nervous, threatened or worried? Are they desperately in need of attention? If you can deal with the underlying cause, the situation is likely to improve.
- Get people to work in pairs or small groups, which can help quiet members to join in and give others a break from the constant talker.
- Use structures in your discussion such as rounds or make a point of asking for other people's opinions: 'Would someone else like to say what he thinks?' or 'Would you like to give us your opinion, Ann?'
- Finally, it may be necessary to confront a person who talks too much but not in front of the rest of the group. For example, you could say: 'I've noticed that you contribute a great deal to the group discussions. That makes me concerned about whether other people are getting enough chance to talk. I'd like to suggest that you keep your comments to just a couple of sentences. Would you feel OK about doing that?'

Exercise 13.1 offers you the opportunity to apply all the previous points when planning a group meeting. Case Study 13.1 is an example of good practice in the use of group work.

VIRTUAL GROUPS

Social media, including Facebook, have become a pervasive part of people's lives and offer a way that virtual groups can be formed to exchange public health-related information and support. Research has shown that some public health Facebook groups that are used for support exchanges between group members contained a) highly specialised health-related information including information about health services use, symptom recognition, compliance, medication use, treatment protocols and medical procedures and b) tailored emotional support through comparison, empathy, encouragement and hope. These findings have implications for group health communication practice and offer evidence to tailor interventions that leverage existing social media platforms to enhance group work support for public health target groups, patients and caregivers (Gage-Bouchard et al 2016a, 2016b). See also Park et al 2016 for research on the use of Twitter for health promotion and public engagement.

Setting Up a Social Media Group

When setting up and using a Facebook (or other social media) group, you will be the group Administrator or Moderator. It is important to abide by the communications protocol of your organisation. See, for an example of this, Merton Council Social Media Protocol on their website referenced at the end of this chapter. It is also important to establish a set of guidelines for group conduct. See Box 13.2 for an illustration of social media guidelines.

BOX 13.2
EXAMPLE OF GUIDELINES FOR FACEBOOK AND TWITTER GROUPS

DO:

- Stay on-topic. Don't post messages that are not related.
- Be reasonably concise and not constitute spamming of the site.
- Post in English – unfortunately, we do not currently have the resource to moderate comments in other languages.
- Respect other people. Comments should not be malicious or offensive in nature.

DON'T:

- Incite hatred on the basis of race, religion, gender, nationality or sexuality or any other personal characteristic.
- Reveal personal details, such as private addresses, phone numbers, email addresses or other online contact details.
- Impersonate or falsely claim to represent a person or organisation.
- Be party political.
- Include swearing, hate-speech or obscenity
- Break the law – this includes libel, condoning illegal activity and breaking copyright.
- Advertise commercial products and services – you can mention relevant products and services as long as they support your comment.

Adjusted from NHS England Social media and comment moderation policy (see website at the end of the chapter). Please note these guidelines are for Twitter use but are equally applicable to Facebook.
See Case Study 11.1 in the chapter on using communication tools for an example of setting up and running a Facebook support group.

EXERCISE 13.1
Planning a Group Meeting

1. Identify a public health issue that you have encountered or are likely to encounter where informal group work would be appropriate For example, this could be a group of food handlers, a preretirement group, an antenatal group, a group of hospital patients recovering from a heart attack, a stop-smoking group or a group for healthy eating and weight control. Assume that your group consists of about 12 people who do not know each other, and that this is the first of several meetings.

What do you think would be the best place and time to meet and the best physical features of the meeting room?

What are your aims for the first meeting?

What are your objectives for your group members for the first meeting?

Complete the following:

At the end of the first meeting, each group member will:

1. ....

2. ....

3. ....

etc. ....

2. Make a plan for what you will do:

■ as people start to arrive

■ to get people to become acquainted with each other

■ in the main part of the group meeting

■ to round off the meeting at the end

■ to evaluate whether you have achieved the objectives you set.

CASE STUDY 13.1
Group Practice And Support For Adult Weight Management – Counterweight

Case study produced by Sarah Button, Health Improvement Service Manager, Sirona Care & Health, Bath, UK.

In Bath and North East Somerset (UK), Sirona Care & Health's Healthy Lifestyle Service is currently commissioned to provide weight management interventions that are evidence-based for adults who are overweight and obese. Criteria for joining these programmes (which are delivered via a group or one-on-one) are based on a 30-plus body mass index (BMI) with the aim to engage people to lose at least 5% of their initial body weight.

One of the weight management programmes is called Counterweight. Counterweight is a national evidence-based programme which was initiated 15 years ago involving a team of dietitians and doctors and collaboration between seven UK Universities (http://www.counterweight.org/Programmes).

GROUP SUPPORT

There is a strong evidence base for the effectiveness of group interventions which offer the opportunity to learn behavioural techniques for losing and maintaining weight loss (for example, Counterweight Project Team 2012). Groups are also effective in allowing people to share their experiences and to provide each other with mutual support. Being part of a group also adds competition to weight loss and can help to keep people motivated.

Counterweight involves six interactive, motivational and social/peer support group sessions, followed by long-term support at 3, 6, 9 and 12 months. At the start of the programme, group participants are assessed on motivation, readiness and self-efficacy for weight management change. A different topic is covered at each of the six sessions. The content

Continued on following page

CASE STUDY 13.1

Group Practice And Support For Adult Weight Management – Counterweight (Continued)

combines advice on beliefs and attitudes around food preferences, healthier eating, energy intake, food labelling, portion size and physical activity. Ten to fifteen participants are recruited for each group, and the sessions are based around the principles of adult learning, which are very much designed to encourage group interaction and active learning.

The focus is on developing people's personal knowledge and skills in behaviour change to enable and empower them to make small lifestyle changes to lose weight which can be embedded into their everyday life. Building people's self-confidence and motivation to change is key. A range of evidence-based approaches are incorporated into sessions including patient-centred goal setting, problem solving, self-monitoring and other behavioural approaches.

Goal setting is used in promoting changes in health behaviours and has been shown to be effective in adopting dietary and lifestyle change. Helping clients set personal goals is crucial to success. Goal setting involves the public health practitioner and client working together to mutually agree upon goals for dietary and lifestyle change. For many clients, being part of a group gives them the social support and increased motivation to remain focused. Group members are encouraged to discuss previous or ongoing strategies that they use to manage their weight, to plan for situations that might get in the way of change and to share their behaviour change goals with others.

The weight management groups are designed to support and equip people with the skills they need to maintain their weight loss. This is enabled by providing support to our clients beyond 12 weeks. Counterweight is effective because longer-term follow-up of at least 12 months is included. This ensures that clients who achieve initial weight loss are encouraged to continue to lose weight or maintain a healthy weight. We also discuss relapse prevention techniques and support clients to become more self-dependent by promoting self-help opportunities and incorporating peer support activity when appropriate.

There are a number of outcomes that are expected from the group-based weight management programmes. The overall aim of is for clients to achieve a modest weight loss of 5% to 10% of initial body weight with improved dietary intake, improved physical activity levels, improved mental health and wellbeing, and weight maintenance.

Group weight losses are reported using a range of outcome measures so that the effectiveness of the different services can be compared. The measurements that are recorded are height, weight, waist circumference and BMI.

Source: Counterweight Project Team 2012 The implementation of the Counterweight Programme in Scotland, UK Family Practice 29: i139–i144.

There are two important issues to bear in mind when setting up a Facebook page. First, the mission statement should create a sense of belonging, and second, you will need to protect the group's privacy. The privacy setting of the Facebook page is crucial. There are three privacy settings: Public, Closed and Secret. A closed or secret group might work best, but this would depend on the aim and mission of the group. See Facebook Help pages under the web references at the end of this chapter for more information on setting up a group. A set of guidelines as in Box 13.2 will enable the efficient administration of the virtual group.

You can also practice setting up a Facebook group page for the same issue if you feel a virtual group would be more appropriate or would be a useful supplement to a group meeting.

See Case Study 13.1 for an example of working with groups to promote health.

PRACTICE POINTS

- In health promotion and public health, groups in a number of forms, including social media, are useful for raising awareness of health issues, mutual support, social action, education and group counselling.

- Group work covers a wide range of activities and has a number of potential benefits for individual group members.
- Group work is not always the most appropriate health promotion or public health practice method to use; you need to be sure that it is right for your particular clients and public health issue.
- You need to develop skills of group leadership and facilitation, appreciate the range of leadership styles and understand the roles and responsibilities of both leaders and members and the way in which groups develop over time.
- Thorough planning and preparation are essential for successful group work, which includes having a clear rationale and aims, and paying attention to recruitment, venue, facilities, resources, timing and evaluation.
- If you facilitate groups, you will find it helpful to develop a range of competencies and strategies for getting groups established, encouraging discussion and dealing with difficulties.

REFERENCES

Belbin RM 1981 Management teams. London, Heinemann.

Bonebright DA 2010 40 years of storming: a historical review of Tuckman's model of small group development. Human Resource Development International 13(1):111–120.

DeLucia-Waak JL, Nitza AJ 2013 Effective planning for groups (group work practice kit). London, Sage.

Gage-Bouchard EA, LaValley S, Mollica M, Beaupin LK 2016a Cancer communication on social media: examining how cancer caregivers use Facebook for cancer-related communication. Cancer Nursing 2016 Jul 20. [Epub ahead of print]. http://www.ncbi.nlm.nih.gov/pubmed/27442210.

Gage-Bouchard EA, LaValley S, Mollica M, Beaupin LK 2016b Communication and exchange of specialized health-related support among people with experiential similarity on Facebook. Health Communication 2016 Aug 2:1–8. [Epub ahead of print]. http://www.ncbi.nlm.nih.gov/pubmed/27485860.

Group Therapy 2016. http://www.counselling-directory.org.uk/group-therapy.html.

Park H, Reber BH, Chon M 2016 Tweeting as health communication: health organizations' use of Twitter for health promotion and public engagement. Journal of Health Communication: International Perspectives 21(2):188–198.

Tang TS, Funnell MM, Noorulla S, Oh M, Morton BB 2012 Sustaining short-term improvements over the long-term: Results from a 2-year diabetes self-management support (DSMS) intervention. Diabetes Research and Clinical Practice 95(1):85–92.

YOUTUBE

How to Create A Facebook Group – Facebook tutorial. https://www.youtube.com/watch?v=8KO3tK8YBJc.

WEBSITES

Facebook Help Centre https://www.facebook.com/help/220336891328465.

Merton Council Social Media Protocol. http://www.merton.gov.uk/community-living/online-communities/social-media-protocol.htm.

NHS England Social media and comment moderation policy. https://www.england.nhs.uk/comment-policy/.

14 ENABLING HEALTHIER LIVING THROUGH BEHAVIOUR CHANGE

CHAPTER CONTENTS

SUMMARY

This chapter considers the approaches used to support people in making changes to their health-related behaviour. In the first section, there is a synopsis of two behaviour change models. This is followed by an overview of working with a client's motivation, working towards client self-empowerment, increasing self-awareness, clarifying values and changing attitudes. Public health strategies for decision making and changing behaviour are outlined. The chapter ends with principles for using behaviour change approaches effectively and summarises the barriers to change. Exercises, examples and a case study are interspersed throughout the chapter.

Human behaviour linked to alcohol, smoking and other substance misuse, poor dietary habits, unprotected sexual practices and physical inactivity is an important influence on overall health and wellbeing and plays a key role in the global growth of noncommunicable diseases and related mortality (Davis et al 2015). Because of this, enabling healthier living

through behaviour change approaches has been a consistent focus in promoting public health, and there is a growing body of recommendations and guidance on interventions related to changing behaviours around alcohol use, eating patterns, physical activity, sexual behaviour and smoking. For example, NICE guidelines and recommendations cover what public health teams should do in terms of their overall strategy for behavioural change approaches (see NICE 2014). This chapter focuses on the competencies you need when you are enabling people to make changes to their health-related lifestyles. Health behaviour may have developed without conscious decision making and in response to individual and group circumstances and external events. Active control of behaviour is different because it involves committing time and effort (yours and your client's) to understanding the factors that influence health choices and behaviour, and to taking considered decisions and actions.

However, it has to be accepted that people may carry on with behaviours that seems unhealthy as the benefits may outweigh the risks, or the socioeconomic circumstances in which a person lives might have resulted in them being trapped and having limited choices. The Marmot review into health inequalities in England demonstrates that the social determinants of health – the conditions in which people are born, grow, live, work and age – may lead to certain behaviours, such as dietary choices and substance use, and ultimately to health inequalities. It is important to recognise when engaging in behavioural change approaches that the socioeconomic environments in which some people live, learn, work and play also need to be changed alongside individual behaviours (Marmot 2010).

Respect for people's values, opinions and their right to choose are fundamental to establishing relationships between health promoters and public health practitioners and their clients. You also have to consider that a person's right to individual freedom of choice has to be balanced against the effect of that choice on other people; for example, a parent choosing to smoke could affect their children's health by subjecting them to passive, secondary smoking. Furthermore, choosing a healthy behaviour does not automatically lead to practising it. Changes such as taking more exercise, eating healthier foods and stopping smoking can require self-discipline and overcoming barriers which make these changes difficult (see the section on barriers to change at the end of this chapter).

Bearing in mind these limitations, it is still important to enable people to look at their motivations, beliefs, values and attitudes relating to health and, where possible, to make and implement decisions that will lead to improved health and wellbeing.

MODELS OF BEHAVIOUR CHANGE

Health-related behaviour change is a very complex process involving a web of psychological, social and environmental factors. Health behaviour change refers to a replacement of health-compromising behaviours (such as sedentary behaviour) by health-enhancing behaviours (such as physical exercise). To describe, predict and explain the behaviour change process, a number of theories or models have been developed. Health behavioural change theories are designed to examine a set of psychological constructs that aim at

explaining what motivates people to change and how they take preventive action (see Davis et al 2015 and Kelly and Barker, 2016 for an overview and full discussion of the issues). Using behaviour change theories and models will help you to clarify your thinking and make your practice more effective. Models are simplified ways of describing reality and to provide frameworks and routes to help you know where to start and what to do. The Health Action Process Approach (HAPA) and the Stages of Change Model are examples of models that can be used by health promoters and public health practitioners.

The Health Action Process Approach

HAPA is a psychological theory and an open framework of various motivational and volitional constructs that explain and predict individual changes in health behaviours such as quitting smoking or improving physical activity levels. HAPA suggests that the adoption, initiation and maintenance of health behaviours should be conceived of as a structured process including a motivation phase and a volition phase. The former describes the intention formation while the latter refers to planning and action (initiative, maintenance, recovery). The model emphasises the particular role of perceived self-efficacy at different stages of health behaviour change (see Fig. 14.1 and the user page for HAPA in the webpages in the references at the end of this chapter). The following explanation of the model is adapted from the HAPA user page:

The Motivation Phase

In the motivation phase, the individual forms an intention to change risk behaviours in favour of other behaviours. Self-efficacy and outcome expectancies are seen as the major predictors of intentions. Outcome expectancies can be seen as precursors of self-efficacy because people usually make assumptions about the possible consequences of behaviours before inquiring whether they can really take the action themselves. The influential role of risk perception (or threat) in the motivation and volition process may have been overestimated in past research and interventions. Fear appeals are of limited value; rather, the message has to be framed in a way that allows individuals to draw on their coping resources and to exercise skills to control health threats. In persuasive communications, a focus

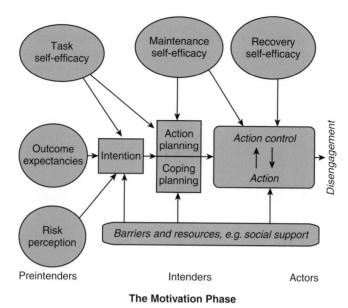

The Motivation Phase

FIG. 14.1 ■ The Health Action Process Approach (HAPA). (*Source: Schwarzer 2016*)

should be made on self-percepts of personal coping capabilities to manage effective precaution strategies. This suggests a causal order where threat is specified as a distal antecedent that helps stimulate outcome expectancies which further stimulate self-efficacy. A minimum level of threat or concern must exist before people start contemplating the benefits of possible actions. The direct path from threat to intention may become negligible if expectancies are already well established.

In establishing a rank order among the three direct paths that lead to intention, it is assumed that self-efficacy and outcome expectancies dominate, whereas threat (or risk perceptions) may fail to contribute any additional direct influence. As indirect factors, however, threat may be of considerable significance within the motivation phase (Schwarzer 2016).

The Volition Phase

Correlations between intentions and behaviours vary tremendously. The right-hand part of Fig. 14.1 consists of three levels: cognitive, behavioural and situational. The focus is on cognitions that instigate and control the action, a volitional process which is subdivided into action plans and action control. When a preference for particular health behaviour has been shaped,

the intention has to be transformed into detailed instructions of how to perform the desired action. If, for example, someone intends to lose weight, it has to be planned how to do it: what foods to buy, when and how often to eat which amounts, when and where to exercise. Thus, a global intention can be specified by a set of subordinate intentions and action plans that contain proximal goals and action sequences. Self-efficacy beliefs influence the cognitive construction of specific action plans, for example, by visualizing scenarios that may guide goal attainment. Once an action has been initiated, it has to be controlled by cognitions to be maintained. The action has to be protected from being interrupted and abandoned prematurely due to incompatible competing intentions which may become dominant while behaviour is being performed. Daily physical exercise, for example, requires self-regulatory processes to secure effort and persistence and to keep other motivational tendencies at a distance (such as the desire to eat or socialise).

When an action is being performed, self-efficacy determines the amount of effort invested and the perseverance. People with self-doubts are more inclined to anticipate failure scenarios, worry about possible performance deficiencies and abort their attempts prematurely. People with an optimistic sense of self-efficacy, however, visualise success scenarios that guide the action and let them persevere in face of obstacles. When running into unforeseen difficulties, they quickly recover.

Performing intended health behaviour is an action. The suppression of health-detrimental actions requires effort and persistence as well and therefore is also guided by a volitional process that includes action plans and action control. If one intends to quit smoking, one has to plan how to do it. For example, it is important to avoid high-risk situations where there are pressures to relapse. If someone is craving a cigarette, action control helps him or her to survive the critical situation. For example, individuals can make favourable social comparisons, refer to their self-concept or simply pull themselves together. The more these meta-cognitive skills and internal coping dialogues are developed and the better they are matched to specific risk situations, the easier the urges can be controlled. Finally, situational barriers and opportunities have to be considered. If situational cues are overwhelming, the temptation cannot be resisted. Actions are not only a function of intentions and cognitive control, they are also influenced by the perceived and the actual environment. A social network, for example, that ignores the coping process of a quitter by smoking in his presence creates a difficult stress situation which taxes the quitter's volitional strength. If, on the other hand, a friend or partner decides to quit too, then a social support situation is created that enables the quitter to remain abstinent in spite of lower levels of volitional strength.

In sum, the action phase can be described along three levels: cognitive, behavioural and situational. The cognitive level refers to self-regulatory processes that mediate between the intentions and the actions. This volitional process contains action planning and action control, and is strongly influenced by self-efficacy and also by situational barriers and support (Schwarzer 2016).

Transtheoretical Model and Stages of Change

One way of supporting people in making health-related decisions and changing their behaviour is to consider all the stages in the process and how people move from one stage to another. The Transtheoretical Model

(TTM) developed by Prochaska and DiClemente (1982) is rooted in extensive research and integrates a range of psychological theories. The TTM has evolved over time and now contains five core constructs: stages of change, processes of change, decisional balance, self-efficacy and temptation (Prochaska 2008), which provides a valuable conceptual framework for how people naturally change their behaviour. However, there is controversy and debate about whether this can consistently be translated into an intervention programme (see, for example, Aveyard et al 2009 and Prochaska 2009). Studies based on this model, such as Aveyard et al (2006), found no evidence that the smoking cessation intervention based on the model was more effective than a control intervention that was not tailored for stages of change. Armatage (2009) offers a useful critique of the model and an assessment of three studies that deemed to have successfully utilised the processes of change to reduce alcohol consumption, encourage smoking cessation and increase physical activity. It is important before using the approach to be abreast of the controversy and the systematic reviews on its effectiveness. A useful summary with a full set of up-to-date references is presented on Wikipedia (http://en.wikipedia.org).

The stages of change component of the TTM identifies a number of stages that a person can go through during the process of behaviour change. It takes a holistic approach, integrating factors such as the role of personal responsibility and choices, and the impact of social and environmental forces that set very real limits on the individual potential for change. It provides a framework for a wide range of potential interventions by health promoters, as well as describing the process individuals go through when acting as their own agents of change, for example, when someone stops smoking without any professional support. The main stages identified in the model are set out in Fig. 14.2.

The key to the model is to regard the cycle in the centre as a series of stages that people go through in the process of changing health behaviour, such as stopping smoking, taking more exercise regularly or adopting healthier eating. A crucial point is that the cycle can be thought of as a revolving door, because people usually go around more than once before emerging to a permanently changed state. It is also important to

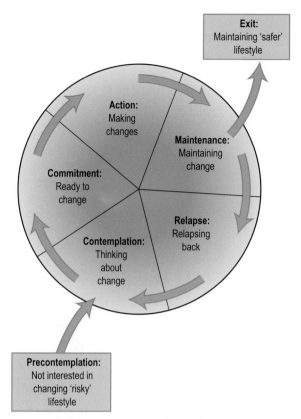

FIG. 14.2 ■ Stages of changing health behaviour. *(Adapted from Prochaska & DiClemente 1984 and Neesham 1993)*

recognise that some people may never get as far as entering the revolving door.

Precontemplation stage. The stage that precedes entry into the change cycle is referred to as precontemplation. At this stage, a person has no awareness of a need for change, or does not accept it, and has no motivation to change habits or lifestyle.

Contemplation stage. This stage is the way into the revolving door cycle of stages of change. People enter this stage when they have enough motivation to contemplate seriously changing their habits; the entry stage is therefore called contemplation.

Commitment stage. If people continue to progress around the cycle, they enter the commitment stage in which they make a serious decision to change the particular habit concerned, such as stopping smoking or taking more exercise.

Action stage. They next enter the action stage as they actively begin to change the habit.

Maintenance stage. At this stage, people struggle to maintain the change and may experiment with a variety of coping strategies.

Relapse stage. Although individuals experience the satisfaction of a changed lifestyle for varying amounts of time, most of them cannot exit from the revolving door the first time around. Typically, they relapse; for example, they start smoking again. Of great importance, however, is that they do not stop there, but move back into the contemplation stage, engaging in the cycle all over again. Prochaska et al (1992) found that, on average, successful former smokers take three revolutions of change before they find the way to become fully free of the habit and exit from the revolving door.

Exit stage. This is the stage in which people are settled into a changed behaviour, such as stopping smoking permanently.

By identifying where clients are in the stages of change, health promoters can tailor their interventions to the particular stage. For example, behaviour change strategies are appropriate for someone in the action or maintenance stages; education and awareness raising are appropriate for someone in the precontemplation stage; working for client self-empowerment is appropriate for someone in the contemplation stage; strategies to help people to make decisions are useful for those in the commitment stage.

The model can be useful in primary healthcare settings, because clients' needs can be assessed and appropriate advice or information given within the constraints of a short consultation.

WORKING WITH A CLIENT'S MOTIVATION

Motivation is a state that changes frequently depending on many different factors. If people are struggling to maintain their new behaviour, what gets them through this difficult time without relapsing? It is thought that both the *importance* of the new behaviour (in terms of the expectation of costs and benefits) and the *confidence* of the person being able to maintain the new behaviour are essential to prevent relapse. The following suggestions can help you explore the importance of the new behaviour with clients and to build their confidence.

Ideas For Exploring Importance

- What are the positive aspects of the current behaviour?
- What are the negative aspects of the current behaviour?
- Summarise and ask 'And is there anything else?'
- Where does that leave you now?

Ideas For Building Confidence

- Get the client to identify as many solutions as possible which will help to prevent relapse.
- Ask 'What have you learned from previous attempts to change about what works (or doesn't work) for you?'
- Ask 'Are there methods that you know have worked for other people?'
- Aim to help the client develop a clear plan but explain that it can be reviewed at any time.

It is essential to listen actively to the client when exploring readiness to change. Confidence can be divided into self-efficacy and self-esteem. Self-efficacy is concerned with a person's confidence in being able to make a specific change in behaviour; self-esteem is a more general sense of wellbeing that a person has about themselves. Self-efficacy can vary in different situations, and you can help your clients look at different approaches for improving self-efficacy in situations where they feel less confident.

This section is partly based on the work of Rollnick et al and research on motivational interviews. See the Stephen Rollnick page under websites at the end of this chapter for the up-to-date research in this area and publications.

Dangerous Assumptions About Motivation

Health promoters and public health practitioners can become very focused on health issues and may forget that there are other motives for change and that health might not be one of them. The following list illustrates some of the other assumptions that are easy to make when counselling clients:

- This person ought to change
- This person wants to change
- It is the right time for this person to change
- If this person decides not to change, this intervention has failed.
- A tough approach is always best
- For this person, health is a prime motivator
- I'm the expert. This person must follow my advice.

WORKING FOR CLIENT SELF-EMPOWERMENT

Making health choices, setting health goals and carrying them out can bring benefits. These are not only the benefits that go with a healthier lifestyle, such as improved health and wellbeing, but also increased self-esteem from the feeling of taking active control over a part of life, such as being in control of the smoking habit rather than cigarettes being in control. In other words, making a positive choice about health can be a self-empowering process.

There are a number of different ways of working towards self-empowerment. Using the Stages of Change is empowering, because people can follow their own progress. It may encourage them to try to get to the next stage of the cycle, and not to see change as all-or-nothing. Also, the recognition that relapse can be part of the process of changing behaviour is important (see Prochaska et al 2013 for a discussion of the stages of changes and the position of relapse). Behaviour change messages can be tailored to individual need, for example, through using technology to provide clients with specially designed messages (EUFIC 2014). Other methods include group work and experiential learning, individual counselling and therapy, and advocacy, all of which are considered in the following sections, except therapy, which is beyond the scope of this book. Unless you are a mental health specialist, most people you work with probably do not need in-depth therapy.

The process of empowerment involves helping clients to become more self-aware and have greater insight into, and understanding of, themselves, their attitudes, values, motivations and feelings

STRATEGIES FOR INCREASING SELF-AWARENESS, CLARIFYING VALUES AND CHANGING ATTITUDES

Many of the strategies that are useful for increasing self-awareness, clarifying values, developing belief systems and changing attitudes for the contemplation stage of change are designed for group work. However, some of them can be adapted for health promoters and public health practitioners to use in one-to-one situations (see Chapter 12, helping people learn and Chapter 13 working with groups).

Deciding What to Change

Some clients could benefit from making several life-style changes to improve their health, and it can be tempting to try to address all of them at the same time. But people are often at different stages of readiness to change on different issues. For example, a person considering making improvements to his or her diet might be ready to make one change (such as eating more fruit and vegetables) but not ready to make others, such as changing to lower fat milk; an overweight person may be ready to take more exercise but not change his or her eating habits.

Ranking or Categorising

Ranking is a way of analysing an issue to distinguish the relative importance of different aspects. It is therefore useful for clarifying values. For example, in Exercise 1.1 in Chapter 1, readers are asked to rank aspects of being healthy. Health is a value, and that exercise is designed to help readers to clarify which aspects of health they value most (see Chapter 1, section on what does being healthy mean to you?).

Another approach to increasing self-awareness and values clarification is to generate a list of items and then code them into different categories. Exercise 14.1 illustrates this approach; it is designed to raise awareness of the link between enjoyment and health.

EXERCISE 14.1
Enjoyment and Health

Quickly list as many things as you can think of that you enjoy doing. Write them down the left-hand side of a piece of paper. On the right-hand side, code each item according to the following categories:

£ – any items that involve spending money
A – any items that you do alone
P – any items you do with other people
R – any items that involve some kind of risk
F – any items that help to keep you fit
C – any items that involve creativity
D – any items that involve consumption of drugs (including alcohol and tobacco)
H+ – any items that positively affect your health
H− – any items that negatively affect your health.

Items may be coded in more than one category. For example, if one of the things you enjoy is going out to the pub for a drink, this may be coded £, P and D, as well as H+ and/or H−. What have you learned about enjoyment and health through doing this exercise?

Using Polarised Views

This is a way of getting people to clarify their views about a particular issue. Views about the issue are polarised and phrased to reflect extremely different views. For example, if the issue was 'Is jogging good for you?', polarised views could be summed up as 'Jogging kills people and only very fit athletes should do it' or 'Jogging is very beneficial to health and all people would be fitter if they took it up'. Examples of polarised views can be described by the health promoter or public health practitioner or taken from writings that express opposite views. If working with a group, the public health facilitator may ask people to work in pairs with each individual acting as if he fully adopted one of the points of view for the duration of the exercise, whatever his personal opinions. First, each person writes down all the arguments he can think of that support his position without discussing it with his partner at this stage. After a few minutes, the partners are asked to start arguing the case, usually for about 15 minutes. The leader then lists the points in favour of each view by asking each pair in turn to contribute one point, until all the points have been collected. She then asks the group to comment on what they have learnt. In this way, members of the group can consider a whole range of arguments, which helps them to understand other people's points of view, tolerate differences of opinion, clarify their own views and perhaps see the issue in a new light.

Another example of a values clarification exercise using the polarised arguments approach is Exercise 4.1 in Chapter 4.

Using a Values Continuum

This is an extension of the polarised argument technique. It helps people to understand the spread of opinion on a particular issue and to clarify where they stand.

The leader describes two extremes of opinion and asks the group to imagine that these can be represented by two points, A and B, joined by a straight line. With a small group, this line can be across a room; with a large group, it could be drawn on the blackboard. The group members are then asked to mark or place themselves at a point along the line that best reflects their own view. For instance, in the jogging example discussed previously, pro-joggers place themselves at one end with the most extreme at the farthest point, whereas people with moderate views stand around the middle and the most ardent anti-joggers stand at the other end. The leader asks each person to state his views briefly as he takes up his position. Other people are asked not to interrupt or comment until everyone has taken up a position or has passed if they choose not to participate.

This technique can encourage a more detailed discussion of the range of possible options than the polarised argument technique. On the other hand, if everyone seems moderate, a better discussion may be stimulated by the polarised argument technique.

The values continuum technique is used in the last task of Exercise 4.1 in Chapter 4.

Using Role-Play

Role-play generally means taking on the role of another person in a specified situation and acting out what that other person might do and say in that situation. This helps people to understand what it feels like to be in another person's shoes. For example, health promoters or public health practitioners role-playing non-English-speaking patients visiting a clinic may be helped to understand how those patients feel, especially if the role-play is given added authenticity by using a foreign language that the health promoters do not speak.

It is also possible to role-play oneself in a new situation. This is a useful way of practising a new skill or rehearsing for a future event. For example, patients can role-play a consultation with a doctor to practise the skills of presenting their health problems to doctors.

For an example of a role-play exercise, see Exercise 12.2 in Chapter 12.

Using Structured Activities

Structured activities, usually for a group of people but sometimes for one or two people only, can be used to meet a variety of aims. One is to help people to get to know each other – icebreakers; other activities are devised to help people trust each other, communicate more openly or to increase self-awareness (see Chapter 13, section on getting groups going, for icebreaker ideas).

For example, activities can be used to help people to identify irrational beliefs. Irrational beliefs are misconceptions that hinder people from achieving their goals. For an interesting discussion of irrational beliefs, see REBT (2016). These beliefs lead to self-defeating thinking, which in turn can affect health. It can lead to health-related behaviour with destructive consequences, such as emotional disorders, heavy drinking and physical ailments. The quiz in Exercise 14.2 aims to help you identify your own irrational beliefs.

STRATEGIES FOR DECISION MAKING

As a health promoter or public health practitioner, you may be involved in counselling with the aim of enabling people to make a choice, such as which treatment to have, whether to have a blood test for HIV or how to select healthy foods in particular circumstances (see Chapter 10 on fundamentals of communication).

Basic skills of counselling to help people make decisions at the commitment stage of change are those discussed in Chapter 10: Understanding nonverbal communication, listening, helping people to talk, asking questions and obtaining feedback. For those of you who require a level of counselling skill but are not trained counsellors or therapists, see Mcleod (2013) for an introduction to counselling techniques across all disciplines.

Beliefs Quiz

Look at the following statements and put a tick in the appropriate column:

	Agree	Disagree
1. I believe in the saying, 'A leopard cannot change his spots'.	☐	☐
2. I believe that 'wait and see' is a good philosophy for life.	☐	☐
3. I want everyone to like me.	☐	☐
4. I usually put off important decisions.	☐	☐

Now identify your rational beliefs and your irrational beliefs (misconceptions):

Q1. If you agreed with this statement, you may believe that the past has a lot to do with determining the present and that people are largely unchangeable. 'I'm made that way.' The idea that you are no good at playing sports, for example, can be used to avoid trying out new behaviour and learning the skills necessary to participate in a sport. The truth is that people who take risks, experiment and work on things generally find that they can become reasonably competent at most of the things they attempt; not necessarily perfect, but good enough.

Q2. If you agreed with this statement, you may believe that human happiness can be achieved by hoping for the best and waiting to see what happens. This belief could result in you becoming merely a spectator in life, watching television every night and somnolent on a sun-lounger for the whole of your holidays. Getting more actively involved could be more satisfying and actually provide you with more energy. If you feel too exhausted, now may be the time to take a close look at how you are managing your life and make some changes.

Q3. If you agree with this statement, you may believe you are only as good as other people think you are. Because of this, you may feel worthless if, despite your efforts, people don't seem to like you. Having the approval of others is pleasant but, to run our own lives, we shall almost certainly have to do some things some people do not like. Work on giving yourself the approval you deserve.

Q4. If you agreed with this statement, you may believe that life's problems will go away if you avoid them. Don't waste your time hoping that things will work out; make them.

There are at least five stages involved (adapted from Burnard 1985 and Inskipp 1993). These stages may seem familiar to you because counselling involves a framework of planning and evaluating similar to the one used in Chapter 5 when planning a health promoting intervention. They are also similar to the stages of change (see Chapter 5, planning and evaluating health promotion).

Stage 1: Identify the Need and Create the Climate

Rogers (1983), an early pioneer of counselling, identified the qualities necessary for a counsellor to establish a climate in which a client can open up. These are warmth, openness, genuineness, empathy and unconditional positive regard. Unconditional positive regard is the quality of totally respecting the worth and dignity of a person, irrespective of whether you like the person or agree with his views or behaviour.

The practical aspects of creating the climate include ensuring that you will not be interrupted and cannot be overheard, that you have sufficient time and that you are comfortably seated in chairs of the same height with the counsellor adopting an open posture and making direct eye contact when appropriate.

Stage 2: Explore the Needs and the Concerns

Through giving full attention and actively listening, by encouraging the client to talk and by asking questions, the counsellor begins to establish trust and to enable the client to move from superficial issues to deeper needs and concerns.

Stage 3: Help the Client to Set Goals and Identify Options

Having gained a new perspective on the issues and concerns, it becomes possible for the client to identify goals and ways these might be achieved. The counsellor could help the client to identify themes or to get a clearer vision of the future by asking key questions, such as:

'How would you feel if …?'
'If things were exactly how you wanted them to be, how would they be different from now …?'
'Have you ever felt like that on other occasions …?'

The counsellor may also provide the client with information to establish options:

'If you do X, what's likely to happen is …'
'If you do Y, the chances are that …'
'You might find it helpful to consider that …' and so on.

Stage 4: Help the Client to Decide Which Option to Choose

The important thing about this stage is that the choice must be the client's, not the counsellor's. Making decisions – that is, choosing between alternative options – is a highly complex process. It involves:

- weighing up the pros and cons of the alternative options
- considering the likely consequences of pursuing each alternative
- deciding which is the best alternative
- having the confidence to pursue the best alternative.

If the client is reluctant to commit to a decision, then both parties need to consider whether it is worth undertaking further work at Stages 2 and 3.

If the client chooses an alternative that the counsellor feels may not work, they should nevertheless back the client's choice and help them to develop an action plan, knowing that if it doesn't work, there is still the possibility for exploring other options.

Stage 5: Help the Client to Develop an Action Plan

Having made a decision, the client now needs to think about turning that decision into action. They may need to identify coping strategies and sources of support. Once an action plan has been agreed, the final details are to set a review date and to clarify how progress will be monitored. (See next section on strategies for changing behaviour.)

STRATEGIES FOR CHANGING BEHAVIOUR

Having made a choice, people may need considerable help to carry their decision through into the action stage of change. A number of techniques developed from behavioural psychology are useful, and the philosophy behind them, that people are responsible for their own behaviour and are capable of exercising control over it, is as important as the techniques themselves. For further reading on strategies for changing behavior, see Coleman and Pasternak 2012.

A variety of material has been developed to help people to change different aspects of their behaviour. For example, the Department of Health *Change for Life* campaign (http://www.dh.gov.uk) has a range of interactive tools and information that clients would find useful in supporting their change efforts.

Some useful techniques are as follows.

Self-monitoring

Self-monitoring involves keeping a detailed and precise account, often in the form of a diary, of behaviour that is to be changed. Its aim is to help people to analyse their pattern of behaviour and become fully aware of what they are doing, which is a starting point for gaining control. Second, the diary provides a baseline against which progress can be checked.

Self-monitoring involves answering questions, such as:

- How frequently does the problem occur?
- When the problem occurs, what else is happening, both externally (in the environment) and internally (in thoughts and feelings)?
- What event leads up to the problem?
- What happens afterwards: the consequences?

Box 14.1 is an example of a smoker's diary.

Identifying Costs, Benefits and Rewards

The cost of changing behaviour can be considerable, involving deprivation of what might have become

---

BOX 14.1
A SMOKER'S DIARY

Day........................ (Complete one of these charts every day.)
Each time you smoke a cigarette, note down in the columns:
1. The time.
2. How urgent your craving for a cigarette is, on a scale of 1–10 (1, very little craving; 10, extremely high craving).
3. Where you smoke the cigarette.
4. Whether you are alone or who you are with.
5. Do you smoke it with drinks (coffee, tea, alcohol)?
6. Do you smoke it after a meal?
7. What else are you doing at the time (for example, chatting, reading the paper, working, talking on the phone)?
8. Why did you decide to smoke this cigarette?
9. What do you feel about it afterwards?

Time	Craving	Where	Who with	With drinks	After meal	Doing what	Why	Afterwards

---

support mechanisms, such as cigarettes, and pleasures, such as eating and drinking, or there may be a heavy price to pay in terms of time, effort and perhaps money. So it is helpful to identify the benefits clearly and set up a system of rewards to encourage perseverance.

Benefits may be long term, such as better health or increased life expectancy. They may be abstract: 'It will prove I've got willpower', or in other people's interests: 'For the family's sake'. These benefits may be important, but it is also necessary to find immediate, short-term rewards that people genuinely enjoy, such as small treats.

Setting Targets and Evaluating Progress

Targets should be realistic rather than idealistic. Losing up to a kilo in weight a week is realistic for most people; losing 7 kilos in a month usually is not. People may have unrealistic hopes and expectations about what can be achieved, which lead to disappointment and a sense of failure when they don't meet the target.

To evaluate progress, it is necessary to keep a record of behaviour so that achievements can be seen clearly. Progress should be assessed once the new behaviour has been given a fair trial, perhaps for 2 or 3 weeks, although short-term reviews ('How have I done today?') can also be useful.

If the target is not being achieved, possible reasons must be looked for and changes made. For example:

■ is the target too difficult? Should it be lowered?
■ are the rewards too distant? Is there a more immediate reward that could be more encouraging?

■ is there an unforeseen crisis or illness? If so, encouragement to continue self-monitoring and to look on the setback as a learning experience may be needed.
■ are other people unhelpful? More strategies to cope with the negative influence of other people may be needed.
■ are there other problems which require support, such as learning to cope with anxiety or stress, or a lack of the resources required to fund changes?

Devising Coping Strategies

Changing behaviour can mean coping with numerous difficulties, for at least a short period of time, until the new behaviour becomes a normal part of life. Someone who is stopping smoking has to cope with problems, such as the craving they feel, the need to put something in their mouth, not knowing what to do with their hands, doing without their accustomed tension reliever in moments of stress and resisting the offer of a cigarette.

People adopt a wide variety of coping strategies, and it is often useful to get a group to share their ideas about what helps them to cope. The list of strategies here is certainly not exhaustive:

■ Finding a substitute, such as substituting chewing gum for cigarettes or eating low-calorie instead of high-calorie foods.
■ Changing some routines and habits that are closely associated with the unhealthy behaviour.

Examples are drinking tea or fruit juice instead of coffee, because coffee is closely associated with cigarettes.

■ Making it difficult to carry on with the unhealthy behaviour by, for example, not keeping alcohol in the home or restricting eating to meal times, not between meals.

What all these strategies have in common is that they require only a small step to achieve a large degree of help for self-control. Other strategies may be:

■ getting support from other people in the same situation, who might be from a weight control group, a smoking cessation clinic or a self-help group. Another helpful way of getting support is by linking with another person on the understanding that each may telephone or meet the other if they need help.

■ practising ways of responding to unhelpful social pressures, for example, refusing the offer of a cigarette or a drink.

■ adopting a 1-day-at-a-time approach. The prospect of the whole of the rest of life without a cigarette may be overwhelming, but the prospect of 1 day without one is far more tolerable. Even shorter time spans may be helpful, such as putting off eating, drinking or smoking for just 15 minutes at a time.

■ learning relaxation techniques and other ways, such as exercise, of relieving stress. Simple relaxation routines that can be practised at any time and place can be helpful in coping with stressful moments when the habit would have been to reach for a drink or a cigarette.

USING STRATEGIES EFFECTIVELY

A number of different strategies have been covered that you can use when you are trying to help clients to increase their self-awareness, clarify their values and beliefs, change their attitudes and behaviour and maintain behaviour change, in other words, to move them through the Stages of Change cycle. While it may be relatively easy to influence attitudes and behaviour in the short term, it can be difficult for people to sustain behaviour change over a longer period. To use these strategies with maximum effect, there are a number of principles to bear in mind.

Advocacy and Working in Partnership

Some people may need extra help to make health choices. Advocacy is generally taken to mean representing the interests of people who cannot speak up for themselves because of illness, disability or other disadvantage. In the context of health promotion and public health, it is better seen as a variety of ways of empowering those people who are disempowered in our society. It is concerned with using every possible means to assist people to become independent and self-advocating.

There can be deep conflicts of loyalty for health promoters and public health practitioners who take on an advocacy role. There may be a need to challenge employers, or those in authority, about services that fail to meet people's needs.

For example, if a patient complains to a community mental health nurse that his drugs are making him feel drowsy and generally unwell, but the doctor insists they should continue to take them, where should the nurse's loyalties lie: with the patient, with the doctor, with the health service (their employer) or with their professional body? How can the nurse most effectively act as an advocate in this situation?

Because of such conflicts of loyalties, many advocacy schemes use nonprofessional workers who come from a similar background to those they are empowering. For example, Maternity-Links schemes provide workers as advocates and interpreters for Asian mothers who do not speak English (http://www.bfwh.nhs.uk). The workers are Asian themselves but able to speak English, as well as their own mother tongue, and the organisation may be run with health service funding but managed independently.

In order to reach and influence disadvantaged groups of people successfully, many projects involve professionals working in partnership with lay volunteers. For example, a community mothers' programme involved nonprofessional mothers as volunteers working with disadvantaged first-time mothers to improve their parenting skills (Community Mothers Annual Report 2010).

Making Healthier Choices Easy Choices

People make health choices in the context of their own environment, subject to all the pressures and influences that surround them. If this environment is conducive to a healthier lifestyle, clients have greater freedom to choose the healthier alternatives and change their behaviour. For example, the provision of

Behavioural issue	Nudging	Shoving (regulating through legislative and fiscal action)
Smoking	Make nonsmoking more visible through mass media campaigns communicating that the majority do not smoke and the majority of smokers want to stop	Ban smoking in public places
	Reduce cues for smoking by keeping cigarettes and ashtrays out of sight	Increase price of cigarettes through taxation
Alcohol	Serve drinks in smaller glasses	Regulate pricing through duty or minimum pricing per unit
	Make lower alcohol consumption more visible through highlighting in mass media campaigns that the majority do not drink to excess	Raise the minimum age for purchase of alcohol
Diet	Designate sections of supermarket trolleys for fruit and vegetables	Restrict food advertising in media directed at children; introduce sugar tax.
	Make salad rather than chips the default side order in restaurants	Ban industrially produced trans fatty acids
Physical Activity	Make stairs, not lifts, more prominent and attractive in public buildings	Increase duty on petrol year on year (fuel price escalator)
	Make cycling more visible as a means of transport, e.g. through city bike hire schemes	Enforce car drop-off exclusion zones around schools

FIG 14.3 ▪ Examples of nudging and legislative/regulating actions. *(Source: Adjusted from Marteau 2011)*

cycleways makes it easier to take regular exercise by cycling to work. National and local policies can create a climate where it is easier to adopt healthier behaviour. Nudging is a policy directive that uses a combination of persuasion and environmental and legislative action to enable change, as shown in the examples in Fig. 14.3 (see Chapter 1, section on what affects health and Chapter 16, section on changing policy and practice).

Undertake Exercise 14.3 to apply some of these ideas to an example of a behaviour change scenario.

EXERCISE 14.3
Changing Behaviour in Practice

Add to the table in Fig.14.3 with further examples of nudging and regulating for smoking, alcohol, diet and physical activity.

Would nudging work for other health issues, such as sexual health? If so how?

What are the ethical issues linked to nudging? (See Schubert 2016 and Chapter 4 for discussion on the ethics of nudging.)

Relating to Clients

Clients are more likely to change if the health promoter or public health practitioner understands the client, sees things from their point of view and accepts them on their own terms. Achieving this relationship may be the most difficult part of helping people to change (see Chapter 10, section on exploring relationships with clients).

Sometimes it is difficult to start a discussion about changing behaviour, and establishing good rapport is essential for an honest discussion and openness for change. One way you can understand your client and also assess readiness to change is to ask the client to take you through a typical day with reference to a particular behaviour.

It is important to note that the attitude and behaviour of the health promoter may influence the outcome. For example, an obese health promoter may find it more difficult to encourage an obese client to adjust their dietary habits. The experiences of health promoters in trying to change their own behaviour, however, can be valuable in helping them to understand the difficulties that their clients experience. It is important to remember that everyone is different and that, although for some people making a particular change may be easy, for others a similar change may prove very difficult.

Dealing With Resistance

It is sometimes difficult for health promoters and public health practitioners to stop providing advice when they know that a particular behaviour, such as stopping smoking, can have huge benefits for the client. It is important to recognise when your clients are showing signs of resisting the suggestion to change. When you see this resistance, it is better to express empathy, emphasising that it is the client's personal choice and that they have control over their lifestyle choices. Useful strategies for these clients at a later date are to reassess readiness to change, establish how important the behaviour change is to them and how confident they feel about making the change.

Using Methods Sensitively

People invest a great deal of emotion in their values and attitudes, which means that the exercises described here, especially those that are designed to encourage people to explore feelings, need to be handled with care and sensitivity. Special training in the use of experiential methods is recommended but, at the very least, health promoters should not attempt to use them unless they have experienced them first themselves. Some points to remember are as follows:

- Explain the activities carefully and thoroughly, and check to ensure that everybody understands what the exercise is for and what they are expected to do.
- Emphasise that participation is entirely voluntary.
- Allow plenty of time for discussion at the end. If people's opinions and cherished ideas have been challenged, they are likely to feel strongly about it. Increased self-awareness may be a very uncomfortable experience too. The group leader should ensure that people have time to express

their feelings and get any support that they need before they leave the group.
- Ensure that there is an atmosphere of confidentiality and trust so that people feel free to explore their views and feelings in safety.
- Save your own views to the end after the group members have had a chance to think things through for themselves. Be open and honest about yourself and your beliefs, and nonjudgemental of values that might conflict with your own.

BRIEF INTERVENTIONS

A brief intervention is a technique used to initiate change for an unhealthy or risky behaviour such as smoking, lack of exercise or alcohol misuse. As an alcohol intervention it is typically targeted to nondependent drinkers whose drinking may still be harmful. Brief interventions involve opportunistic advice, discussion, negotiation or encouragement. They are commonly used in many areas of health promotion and public health, and are delivered by a range of primary and community care professionals including GPs (see Case Study 14.1).

For smoking cessation, brief interventions typically take between 5 and 10 minutes and may include one or more of the following:

- Simple opportunistic advice to stop
- An assessment of the patient's commitment to quit
- An offer of pharmacotherapy and/or behavioural support
- Provision of self-help material and referral to more intensive support such as the NHS Stop Smoking Services.

The particular package that is provided will depend on a number of factors, including the individual's willingness to quit, how acceptable they find the intervention on offer and the previous ways they have tried to quit (NICE 2014). NICE (2014) provides practice recommendations and a range of other strategic and policy advice on brief interventions. For further information on alcohol brief interventions, see Barrie and Scriven (2014).

Brief Interventions in Primary Care

Case study produced by Dr Laura Jarvie, General Practitioner (GP), The Nelson Medical Practice, London (UK)

Alec is a 55-year-old window cleaner. He attended about some bothersome tendonitis in his shoulder, and my computer system prompted me to complete an AUDIT questionnaire in which he scored 14. Alec was surprised to hear that his current level of drinking could be damaging to his health; like most of his friends, he had a couple of beers in the evening, a bit more at the weekend and the occasional 'binge'. He had never seen his drinking as a problem and, at that stage, had no intentions of changing.

A few weeks later, he returned with indigestion which he thought was caused by the painkillers prescribed for his shoulder. We discussed how alcohol can also cause inflammation in the stomach and his current levels of drinking may also be contributing. I encouraged Alec to think about the benefits he might find by reducing his drinking including improved sleep and weight loss, as well as pointing out some of the longer term health benefits. We stopped the painkillers and arranged some routine blood tests and to meet again.

Alec's blood results showed evidence of excessive alcohol in both his blood count and liver function. I called him on the phone, explaining that this was nothing irreversible, and that small changes could result in big improvements in his health in both the long and short term. I explored his ideas about reducing his drinking and any strategies he had tried in the past. He seemed to recognise the problems.

I didn't see Alec for a while. When he did return many months later, his opening line was 'you've told me a few times I need to look at my drinking, now I realise I do'. It wasn't his health that had prompted this change of heart; Alec had been to the pub after work with his mates, had a few too many and got into an altercation. The police had been called, and Alec had spent a night in the cells. This had given him a fright; he had remembered the brief interventions I had employed and he now returned to me as he was ready to make the necessary changes.

As a GP, it sometimes feels like I am constantly talking to patients about their unhealthy behaviours, be it drinking, smoking, drugs or obesity. Not everyone is ready to change, and it is easy to become disheartened, prescriptive or rehearsed in your advice. However, because we see patients repeatedly, our brief interventions stand a better chance of catching them at the right point in the cycle of change, and even if they aren't there yet, our interventions, if executed effectively, may sow a seed which is remembered in the future.

BARRIERS TO BEHAVIOUR CHANGE

To engage successfully in enabling people to take up healthy behaviours, it is important to understand and take account of some of the obstacles that might be encountered. There is considerable research evidence which highlights some of these barriers. In a systematic review which looked at the barriers and facilitators to the uptake and maintenance of healthy behaviours by people at mid-life (aged 40 to 64), evidence was found relating to uptake and maintenance of physical activity, diet and eating behaviours, smoking, alcohol, eye care and other health-promoting behaviours and grouped into six themes: health and quality of life, sociocultural factors, the physical environment, access,

psychological factors and evidence relating to health inequalities. Barriers that recurred across the different health behaviours included lack of time (due to family, household and occupational responsibilities), access issues (to transport, facilities and resources), financial costs, entrenched attitudes and behaviours, restrictions in the physical environment, low socioeconomic status and lack of knowledge. Facilitators included a focus on enjoyment; health benefits including healthy ageing, social support, clear messages and integration of behaviours into lifestyle (see Kelly et al 2016 for the full results). Kelly and Barker (2016) offer an excellent and important discussion of what they see as the six common errors that result in unsuccessful behaviour change interventions including the notions that behaviour change is just common sense, and when people are given the health information, they will make rational choices. The complexity of behaviour change as an approach should be noted and efforts made to overcome some of the barriers and to challenge some of the assumptions on which behaviour change approaches are based.

Finally, for detailed guidance and evidence on behavioural change approaches, see the NICE website in the reference section at the end of the chapter, and for details on social marketing as a behavioural change approach, see Chapter 2.

PRACTICE POINTS

- For individuals to be ready to change a particular behaviour, they need to feel confident in being able to adopt the new behaviour. The new behaviour also needs to be important to them and have clear benefits. You may need to help clients develop a number of competencies or life skills to do with social interaction, assertiveness and time management, and possibly specific skills (such as those needed to participate in a physical exercise programme).
- To devise the appropriate strategy for each individual, you need to start by exploring clients' health knowledge and beliefs related to the issue of concern, the stage of change they are at and what outcomes they desire. Asking the client to describe a typical day in relation to the behaviour is a useful approach.
- You need to be aware that clients may be resistant to change. In these situations, it is best to emphasise that it is the client's personal choice and that they are in control. At a later date, you could go back to explore again the individual's confidence about changing and how important the change is to them.
- You need to tailor an action plan to the specific needs of each client and provide positive consequences for the desired healthy behaviour (such as praise or rewards) to maintain behaviour change.
- You can improve success by combining a number of strategies. For example, a patient who is being rehabilitated after a heart attack could have an interview with a hospital doctor, a home visit from a nurse to encourage support from family members and small-group self-help sessions to help patients to manage their problems.
- Records are important for follow-up. They are most effective if they are kept and owned by the individual concerned, for example, in the form of a diary.
- Equally important is the provision of environmental and socioeconomic circumstances that facilitate healthy choices rather than acting as barriers. And at a broader level, national and local policy needs to address the broader socioeconomic determinants of health, such as poverty and deprivation.

REFERENCES

Armitage CJ 2009 Is there utility in the transtheoretical model? British Journal of Health Psychology 2:195–210.

Aveyard P, Lawrence T, Cheng KK et al 2006 A randomized controlled trial of smoking cessation for pregnant women to test the effect of a transtheoretical model-based intervention on movement in stage and interaction with baseline stage. British Journal of Health Psychology 2:263–278.

Aveyard P, Massey L, Parsons A et al 2009 The effect of transtheoretical model based interventions on smoking cessation. Social Science and Medicine 68(3):397–403.

Barrie K, Scriven A 2014 Alcohol misuse: public health mini guides. London, Churchill Livingstone Elsevier.

Burnard P 1985 Learning human skills: a guide for nurses. Oxford, Heinemann Nursing.

Coleman MT, Pasternak RH 2012 Effective strategies for behavior change. Primary Care 39(2):281–305. http://dx.doi.org/10.1016/j.pop.2012.03.004.

Community Mothers Annual Report 2010. http://www.lenus.ie/hse/bitstream/10147/136802/1/CommMothers2010.pdf.

Davis R, Campbell R, Hildon Z, Hobbs L, Michie S 2015 Theories of behaviour and behaviour change across the social and behavioural sciences: a scoping review. Health Psychology Review 9(3):323–344. http://dx.doi.org/10.1080/17437199.2014.941722.

EUFIC 2014 Motivating Behaviour Change. http://www.eufic.org/article/en/expid/Motivating-behaviour-change/.

Inskipp F 1993 Counselling: the trainer's handbook. Cambridge, National Extension College.

Kelly MP, Barker M 2016 Why is changing health-related behaviour so difficult? Public Health 136:109–116.

Kelly S, Martin S, Kuhn I, Cowan A, Brain C, Lafortune L 2016 barriers and facilitators to the uptake and maintenance of healthy behaviours by people at mid-life: a rapid systematic review. PLoS One 11(1):e0145074. http://www.ncbi.nlm.nih.gov/pmc/articles/PMC4731386/.

Marmot M 2010 The Marmot review final report: Fair society, healthy lives. London, University College London.

Marteau T 2011 Judging nudging: can nudging improve population health? British Medical Journal 342:263–264.

Mcleod J 2013 An introduction to counselling, 5th edn. Maidenhead, Open University Press.

NICE 2014 Behaviour change: individual approaches. Guidance and Recommendations https://www.nice.org.uk/guidance/ph49/chapter/1-recommendations.

Prochaska JO 2009 Flaws in the theory or flaws in the study: a commentary on 'The effect of transtheoretical model based interventions on smoking cessation'. Social Science and Medicine 68(3):404–406; discussion 407–409.

Prochaska JO, DiClemente C 1982 Transtheoretical therapy: towards a more integrative model of change. Psychotherapy: Theory, Research and Practice 19(3):276–288.

Prochaska JO, DiClemente CC, Norcross JC 1992 In search of how people change. Application to addictive behaviors. American Psychology 47(9):1102–1114.

Prochaska JO, Norcross JC, Diclemente CC 2013 Applying the stages of change. Psychotherapy in Australia 19(2):10–15.

Prochaska JO, Redding CA, Evers KE 2008 The transtheoretical model and stages of change. In Glanz KREBT 2016. What are irrational beliefs? REBT Centre University of Birmingham. http://www.birmingham.ac.uk/schools/psychology/centres/rebt/about/beliefs.aspx.

Rogers CR 1983 Freedom to learn for the eighties. Columbus, Ohio, Charles E Merril.

Schubert C 2016 A note on the ethics of nudges. http://voxeu.org/article/note-ethics-nudges.

Schwarzer R 2016 The Health Action Process Approach (HAPA) user page. http://userpage.fu-berlin.de/health/hapa.htm.

YOUTUBE

A 2014 Ralf Schwarzer lecture on HAPA – Theoretical framework to understand constructs and mechanisms in health behavior change. The difference between motivation and action is explained, and the roles of self-efficacy, coping planning and action control are highlighted. https://www.youtube.com/watch?v=aTJ-yUl2TdE.

WEBSITES

HAPA user page. http://userpage.fu-berlin.de/health/hapa.htm.

Marmot indicators. http://www.instituteofhealthequity.org/projects/marmot-indicators-2014.

Marmot Review Fair Society Healthy Lives. http://www.instituteofhealthequity.org/projects/fair-society-healthy-lives-the-marmot-review.

NICE lifestyle and Wellbeing guides. https://www.nice.org.uk/guidance/lifestyle-and-wellbeing.

Psychcentral website for a discussion of whether the Transtheoretical Model of Change Works for Addiction? http://pro.psychcentral.com/does-the-transtheoretical-model-of-change-work-for-addiction/007272.html#.

Stephen Rollnick page – Publications using motivational interviewing. http://www.stephenrollnick.com/publications.php.

15

WORKING WITH COMMUNITIES

SUMMARY

This chapter begins with a discussion of community-based work in health promotion and public health, and an overview of the range of activities it may include. Some key terms and principles are explained before an examination of three particular ways of working with communities: community participation, community development and community health projects. Each of these includes an exercise, and there is also a case study of a community development project. The chapter finishes with a consideration of the competencies health promoters and public health practitioners need to work effectively with communities.

The challenge of promoting public health is considerable when working with people in the community who may be disadvantaged and discriminated against, and who may feel powerless to do anything about their health. This chapter is about engaging with communities in ways that enables them to take more control over their health.

COMMUNITY ENGAGEMENT IN HEALTH PROMOTION AND PUBLIC HEALTH

Community-based work in health promotion and public health involves engaging with groups of the public in a sustained way which will enable them to increase control over their health and its determinants to improve their health.

Key Terms

Community

Traditionally, a community is seen as a group of interacting people living in a common location. The word is often used to refer to a group that is organised around common values and social cohesion within a shared geographical location, generally in social units larger than a household. Essentially, a community is a network of people. The link between them may be:

- where they live (such as a housing estate or neighbourhood)

- the work they do (such as the farming community or school community)
- the way they live (such as new-age travellers or homeless people)
- common interests, shared values or beliefs (such as a church community)
- other factors they have in common (such as sexual preferences, so the gay community)

The people in the network come together on the basis of a shared experience or concern and identify for themselves which communities they feel they belong to. Networks may be formal or informal, and since the advent of the internet, the concept of community no longer has geographical limitations as people can now virtually gather in an online community and share common interests regardless of physical location. 38 Degrees is an excellent example of a virtual community that demonstrates community empowerment and action by community-identified campaigns that put pressure on politicians and those in power. See the 38 Degrees website and Facebook pages in the references at the end of the chapter, and watch the video of the work of 38 Degrees.

Community Work

This means working with community groups and organisations to overcome the community's problems. Community work aims to enhance the sense of solidarity and competence in the community. For example, a community development worker may promote health by working with particular communities to collectively bring about social change and improve quality of life. This involves working with individuals, families or whole communities to empower them to:

- identify their needs, opportunities, rights and responsibilities
- plan what they want to achieve and take appropriate action
- develop activities and services to improve their lives.

Community Health Work

This is community work with a focus on health concerns, but generally health is defined broadly to include social and economic aspects so that community health work may encompass almost as broad a range of activities as community development work.

Community Action

This means activity carried out by members of the community under their own control to improve their collective conditions. It may involve campaigning, negotiating with or challenging authorities and those with power.

Community Participation

This is about involving the community in health work that is led by someone outside the community, for example, a worker employed by a statutory agency. The degree of participation may vary (see Fig. 15.1).

Community Development

This means working to stimulate and encourage communities to express their needs and to support them in their collective action. It is not about dealing with people's problems on a one-to-one basis; it aims to develop the potential of a community as a whole. A community development approach to health involves working with groups of people to identify their own health concerns and to take appropriate action. Community development health workers are essentially facilitators, locally based, whose role is to help people in the community to acquire the skills, knowledge and confidence to act on health issues. They are usually community workers by background rather than health professionals.

Community Health Projects

This is a loose term applied to programmes of work that are organised by agencies for the improvement of health in a community or applied to local organisations aiming to improve health by supporting some combination of community activity, self-help, community action and/or community development.

Community Health Services

There are many community health services with the word 'community' often used as an adjective to describe anything that is not based in a hospital. Most community health care takes place in people's homes. Teams of nurses and therapists coordinate care, working with professions including GPs and social care. Additionally community health provides preventative and health improvement services, often with partners from local government and the third sector. Although less visible than hospitals, they deliver an extensive and varied range of services (for more information on the extent of community health services in England, see NHS confederation 2015 and the Community Health Services Forum webpage in the references at the end of the chapter).

PRINCIPLES OF COMMUNITY-BASED ENGAGEMENT

There are four key principles, as follows:

1. The Centrality of the Community

It is the community which defines its own needs. Community-based work is essentially a bottom-up process, rather than being top-down expert-led where those with power and authority make the decisions. Health promoters and public health practitioners recognise and value the health experience and knowledge that exists in the community and seek to use it for everyone's benefit. In the UK, both legislation and policy recognise the importance of community participation in their own affairs. The White Paper Healthy Lives, Healthy People (2010), for example, specifies that the public health approach will be responsive and owned by communities and shaped by their needs.

2. The Facilitator Role of Community Health Promoters and Public Health Practitioners

Community health promoters and public health practitioners do not perceive themselves as experts in health, but as facilitators whose role it is to validate, encourage and empower people to define their own health needs and to meet them. They start where the community is, recognising and valuing people's own abilities and experiences. They involve people in community health work from the very beginning, encouraging and supporting them in working together. Knowledge and skills are shared and demystified. Community health promoters aim to make people's access to statutory agencies easier and making the agencies more accountable to the people they serve.

3. The Importance of Addressing Inequalities

A central concern in community-based health promotion and public health work is the need to challenge and change the many forms of disadvantage, oppression, discrimination and inequalities that people face and which adversely affect their health (see Chapter 1, section on inequalities in health).

Work, therefore, has focused particularly on the needs of disadvantaged groups. A central way of working is to bring people in such groups together for support and information sharing, and to enable them to bring about change through collective action. The work can be political, because it often involves working towards equality, social inclusion and social justice with people who experience powerlessness and inequality as part of their everyday lives.

4. A Broad Perspective on Health

A social model of health is adopted, where health is perceived broadly and holistically as positive wellbeing including social, emotional, mental and societal aspects, as well as physical. It is not seen merely as the absence of disease and is not limited by medical or epidemiological views of what constitutes a health problem or issue. Health is seen to be affected by social, environmental, economic and political factors.

COMMUNITY PARTICIPATION

Participation is a word that is used widely to mean a range of activities, from those that are merely tokenistic to those which are firmly rooted in the concept of empowerment. Partnership, public participation and public decision making are all key issues in health services and local authorities. However, in reality some organisations may make decisions without having any wish to engage with the public (see Scriven 2007 for a detailed overview of collaboration and partnership working with communities).

Community Participation in Planning

The amount of community participation in planning health work organised by a statutory agency (such as an NHS or local authority) can vary along a spectrum of none to high, as shown in Table 15.1. In the health service, such participation can be called public involvement, engagement or service user involvement (see Rifkin 2014 for an interesting discussion on the value of community participation for health outcomes). See also Chapter 4, Fig. 4.1, Public Health intervention ladder, with examples.

TABLE 15.1		
Community Participation in Planning Public Health Promotion Work		
Level 1	No participation	The community is told nothing and is not involved in any way
Level 2	Very low participation	The community is informed. The agency makes a plan and announces it. The community is convened or notified in other ways to be informed; compliance is expected
Level 3	Low participation	The community is offered 'token' consultation. The agency tries to promote a plan and seeks support or at least sufficient sanction so that the plan can go ahead. It is unwilling to modify the plan unless absolutely necessary
Level 4	Moderate participation	The community advises through a consultation process. The agency presents a plan and invites questions, comments and recommendations. It is prepared to modify the plan
Level 5	High participation	The community plans jointly. Representatives of the agency and the community sit down together from the beginning to devise a plan
Level 6	Very high participation	The community has delegated decision making authority. The agency identifies and presents an issue to the community, defines the limits and asks the community to make a series of decisions that can be embodied in a plan which it will accept
Level 7	Highest participation	The community has control. The agency asks the community to identify the issue and make all the key decisions about goals and plans. It is willing to help the community at each step to accomplish its goals, even to the extent of delegating administrative control of the work
Level 8	Beyond participation	Community-owned health initiatives

Ways of Developing Community Participation

Community participation can be encouraged and supported in many ways at different levels. If you work for a public sector agency, such as a local authority or a health service, the following suggestions may be useful:

Be open about policies and plans. Publicise your policies, invite comments and recommendations on your plans, and involve representatives on planning and management groups. This is an intrinsic part of policy.

Plan for the community's expressed needs. When planning health promotion and public health services, help the community to express its own needs.

Decentralise planning. Set up planning and management of health promoting and allied services on a neighbourhood basis, encouraging and enabling the public's involvement.

Develop joint forums. Develop joint forums, such as patient participation groups in doctors' practices, where lay people and professionals can work together in partnerships. Mental health services often have joint forums to involve service users in service development.

Develop networks. Encourage individuals or groups to come together, thus increasing their collective knowledge and power to change things. Value interagency links and gain the support of workers from different organisations because competition and lack of understanding of each other's roles and cultures can hinder progress.

Use electronic/social media networking. Social media networks can provide community information and a means of communication within and between communities (email, Facebook, Twitter, Instagram, blogs and websites), which go some way towards addressing the problem of social exclusion caused by lack of information. Not only can groups and individuals find and supply information on the internet, they can discuss issues and participate in democratic processes. See Resnick et al (2010) for ideas of how to encourage community participation to virtual internet-based health interventions.

Provide support, advice and training for community groups. Provide opportunities for lay people to develop their knowledge, confidence and skills.

Provide information. Provide information about health issues, details of useful local and national organisations, leaflets, posters, books, social media and websites.

Provide help with funding and resources. Help local groups to obtain funding from statutory agencies and provide other sorts of practical help, such as a place to meet or facilities.

Provide help with evaluation. Being able to show real changes in community resources, services and health outcomes increases respect and confidence from communities, funders and agencies.

Support advocacy projects. Support projects that enable people who are otherwise excluded to have a voice, such as mental health advocacy schemes (see website under references).

Exercise 15.1 offers the opportunity for you to consider how you can encourage community participation in your work.

EXERCISE 15.1

Developing Community Participation in Your Health Promotion and Public Health Work

Consider the following list of ways in which you can encourage community participation in health improvement:

■ Be open about policies and plans
■ Plan for the community's expressed needs
■ Decentralise planning
■ Develop joint forums and networks and social media activity
■ Offer support, advice and training for community groups
■ Provide information
■ Facilitate coproduction and asset mapping
■ Provide help with funding and resources
■ Provide help with evaluation
■ Support advocacy projects.

(If you are not sure what is meant by these, look at the previous explanations and what follows.)

To what extent do you think these things are desirable?

To what extent do you do these things already?

From this list, can you identify ways in which you would like to increase community participation in your work?

Can you identify any other ways in which you would like to increase community participation in your work?

Given that there may be some obstacles to doing what you would ideally like to do, can you identify a practical way forward for acting on at least one of the things you would like to do?

Work individually, in pairs or small groups.

COMMUNITY DEVELOPMENT IN PRACTICE

However much you might seek people's participation, it may be that they feel so alienated, dissatisfied or overwhelmed with problems that they reject participation. In this situation, it is necessary to develop a climate and culture where participation can happen. You need to encourage, enable and support people, and community development is a way of doing this. Evidence suggests (although measurement is difficult) that an asset approach (see O'Leary et al 2011) encourages autonomy, strengthens social networks and other aspects of social capital and is a prerequisite for good health (Foot 2012).

Assets-Based Community Development

Community development requires community participation but also involves working with people to identify their own health concerns and to support and facilitate them in their collective action. An assets-based approach to community health improvement makes value of, enhances and develops community capacity, skills, knowledge, connections and potential (Foot & Hopkins 2010). It has been argued that an assets-based approach provides an opportunity for Local Authorities to respond to community inequalities (Evans & Winson 2014), and at the core of an assets-based approach is sustainability (see O'Leary et al 2011 for a global perspective on the various assets-based approaches).

Exercise 15.2 is designed to help you to consider what community development work and asset based approach means in practice.

Assets-based community health development approach means adhering firmly to the principles of community-based work. See Box 15.1 for some of the key principles of an assets-based approach. Health promoter or public health practitioners adopting an assets-based approach act as facilitators in a coproduction process (NHS 2011). The Scottish Coproduction network has been active in the development of this approach and set up a range of tools to enable the facilitation process (Scottish Coproduction Network 2016, NESTA 2012, NEF 2011). See Case Study 15.1 as an example of coproduction in action.

Recent developments in enabling communities to understand their own needs and to identify the community resources that can be drawn on to meet those needs have

EXERCISE 15.2

Thinking About Community Development and Asset Based Approaches

(Adapted from a questionnaire by Adams and Hawkins (undated and unpublished) and reproduced by kind permission.)

Working individually, or in pairs or small groups, work through the following questionnaire. If you are working with other people, discuss the reasons for the answers you give. You do not have to reach a consensus. When you have listened to each other's views, you can agree to disagree.

Tick whether you think each of the following statements is true or false:

Community development is about:	True	False
1. Fostering community cohesion and social capital.	☐	☐
2. Helping people to understand the root causes of their ill health.	☐	☐
3. Enabling a statutory authority to show it cares.	☐	☐
4. Getting involved in a political process to target inequalities in health.	☐	☐
5. Doing away with experts and professionals.	☐	☐
6. Confronting forms of discrimination such as racism and sexism.	☐	☐
7. Saving money on services by helping people to help themselves and to utilise available assets.	☐	☐
8. Promoting equal access to resources, such as health services.	☐	☐
9. Enabling a community worker to become a leader/spokesperson for the community.	☐	☐
10. Helping people to develop confidence and become more articulate about their needs.	☐	☐
11. Campaigning for a better environment such as improved housing, transport and play facilities.	☐	☐
12. Controlling social unrest, by providing, for example, activities for bored young people.	☐	☐
13. Helping people from lower socioeconomic groups to change their attitudes and behaviour.	☐	☐
14. Recognising and valuing the assets of skills, knowledge and expertise of individuals and groups in the community.	☐	☐
15. Beginning a process of redistributing wealth, power and resources.	☐	☐

Now add any other points you think 1) community development and 2) asset-based approaches to community health improvement is, or is not, about.

BOX 15.1

ASSET-BASED APPROACH TO COMMUNITY HEALTH DEVELOPMENT

- Begins with assets within communities
- Identifies intrinsic strengths and opportunities
- Invests in citizens and develops capacity
- Emphasises the role of community
- Focuses on the common good within communities and empowers individuals to coproduce
- Supports individuals to develop their own potential
- Sees community residents as solutions

(Adapted from Evans and Winson 2014)

---

included a number of innovations, such as asset mapping, and to enable asset mapping, WITTY and Social Mirror:

1. Asset Mapping

Asset mapping is a key process in an assets-based approach to working with communities for health

improvement. Community assets are seen as any factor or resource which enhances the ability of individuals, communities and populations to maintain and sustain health and wellbeing and to reduce health inequalities. These assets can operate at the level of the individual, family or community as health protective and promoting factors and are categorised into the social, financial, physical, environmental or human (employment opportunities, education and social networks) within a community and which enhance health and wellbeing:

Asset Categorisation (adapted from Foot and Hopkins 2010, and Evans and Winson 2014)

Assets of Individuals (e.g. knowledge, networks, time, interests, passions, self-esteem, resilience)

Associational Assets (e.g. formal and voluntary organisations and informal networks)

Organisation Assets (e.g. local services within the community and staff assets)

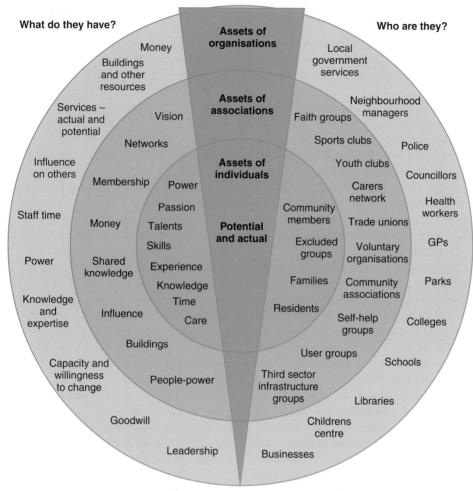

What do they have?

Who are they?

Assets of organisations

Assets of associations

Assets of individuals

Potential and actual

Money

Buildings and other resources

Services – actual and potential

Vision

Networks

Influence on others

Membership

Power

Passion

Staff time

Money

Talents

Skills

Power

Shared knowledge

Experience

Knowledge

Knowledge and expertise

Influence

Time

Care

Buildings

Capacity and willingness to change

People-power

Goodwill

Leadership

Local government services

Neighbourhood managers

Faith groups

Sports clubs

Police

Youth clubs

Councillors

Carers network

Health workers

Community members

Trade unions

Excluded groups

Voluntary organisations

GPs

Families

Community associations

Parks

Residents

Self-help groups

Colleges

User groups

Schools

Third sector infrastructure groups

Libraries

Childrens centre

Businesses

FIG. 15.1 ■ What are health assets? *Source: Asset-Mapping and more – an outline proposal for a pan-Scotland Learning Set; Slide share. http://www.slideshare.net/pashe/asset-mapping-and-more.*

Physical Assets (e.g. greenspaces, land, buildings, streets, markets, transport links)

Economic Assets (e.g. skills and talents, such as employment generation)

Environmental Assets (e.g. a community that delivers security, social justice, sense of cohesion and harmony)

Cultural Assets (e.g. music, drama, creative expression opportunities)

See Fig. 15.1 for more details on community asset categorisation.

Mapping the assets within a community will require a number of processes including data analysis, questionnaires, community mobilisation through social media and coproduction. A range of tools have been developed to assist with asset mapping. All are available online including the NICE 2014 briefing and the Brighter Futures Together Factsheet (2016). An excellent example of asset mapping is Evans and Winson 2014, the coproduction example in Case Study 15.1 and the example of using a mapping tool in Case Study 15.2.

2. WITTY (What's Important To You?)

WITTY is an app for iPad that can help community members understand the positive assets and factors which they have and can better use in their day-to-day life. WITTY was developed as an output of the

CASE STUDY 15.1

Dipping Toes into Coproduction

Case study produced by Paul Ballantyne, Development Manager, Scottish Community Development Centre – 29 May 2015

This is my 'story' of trying out asset mapping with the Health Improvement team in Inverclyde and also facilitating a session with them on coproduction. My colleague Nancy Greig, Development Manager in the People Powered Health and Wellbeing Programme at the Health and Social Care Alliance Scotland (the ALLIANCE), cofacilitated the sessions.

The team is part of the Inverclyde Community Health and Care Partnership. It has 15 members and recently reorganised so that they could work on topics and other portfolios, regardless of age and stage wherever possible across the Inverclyde area. The team had initially asked the Community Health Exchange (CHEX) in the Scottish Community Development Centre (SCDC) to facilitate these sessions, but they were unable to do so and passed the request on to me in the SCDC team.

I wanted to find out beforehand what the existing levels of knowledge and skills were within the team in relation to asset mapping and coproduction. So, I agreed to a survey monkey questionnaire with the team leader, but for various reasons this wasn't carried out before the session. This meant that knowledge and skill levels only became apparent as we went through the exercises. The feedback revealed different levels of knowledge but more importantly different 'starting points' and therefore varying expectations about what was wanted from the sessions.

During the first session, participants took part in a 'What keeps me healthy' exercise and then two asset mapping exercises: 'WITTY' (what is important to me) and Social Mirror. WITTY helps people create a visual map of assets and other things in their lives that help them stay well, connected and happy. Social Mirror helps people identify social networks – who they know and are connected to – to help offer insights into how they can work with people to improve health.

Participants produced a number of asset maps, some covering geographies and identifying various partners; others were more specific to localities and people.

We had a useful discussion about these, particularly challenging the participants to think differently about how they go about their work and to be more specific about with whom exactly they would do asset mapping and in what context.

In the coproduction session, we looked at general ideas about what coproduction is, using the New Economics Foundation (NEF) Self Reflection Framework toolkit and the Governance International (GI) Coproduction 'Star.' We then moved into small groups each reviewing a recent case study produced for the new C-production Resource in Scotland. Each group then presented their findings, saying what they liked, found useful, could learn from and so on. We then did an action plan exercise to identify how and where participants could take these ideas forward in their own work in Inverclyde.

This session worked much better than the previous one, possibly because it felt much more practical, based upon real-life case studies.

I learned a few important lessons from both sessions, some of which were from my own personal reflection but others importantly from feedback from the participants:

- If participants know each other well then do the 'what is important to me' exercise quickly and share results in pairs or small groups rather than a large group.
- Be realistic about the time it takes to do the asset mapping exercises and allow good time for participants to reflect on what they have produced and what it means before moving into 'action planning'.
- Trying out asset mapping with colleagues is not the same as doing it for real with partners and people with lived experience.

Continued on following page

CASE STUDY 15.1

Dipping Toes into Coproduction (Continued)

■ Think about how people can take their ideas forward beyond the initial sessions and how other opportunities for support and sharing learning can be created.

■ Action planning needs decent time to get beyond the 'top lines' and describe in specific and practical ways how people will involve others in asset mapping and working together in a coproductive way.

■ And finally, asset mapping and coproduction need to be seen as a way of working rather than 'projects'. They need to be embraced as part of the job, rather than an 'extra' to be done over and above existing roles.

(See http://www.coproductionscotland.org.uk/resources/further-resources-and-information/reports-and-publications/tools-and-methods/ (Accessed 29 August 2016) for the NEF Self Reflection Framework toolkit and the GI Coproduction 'star'.)

CASE STUDY 15.2

Social Mirror

Social Mirror used digital tools to link people from the community to local projects that could help their health and wellbeing. Knowle West Media Centre (Bristol, UK) worked with the Royal Society of Arts (RSA) to develop an application that would give people a social prescription which would direct them to community activities or groups instead of being prescribed drugs or other health interventions.

Launched in February 2013, the application was used in the William Budd Health Centre over a 12-month period. Patients were asked to complete a short questionnaire on tablet computers and were then given their 'social prescription'. The project came out of RSA research in the area, where more than 350 people in Knowle West were interviewed to find out about their social networks. The project aimed to improve the wellbeing of people aged 18 to 30 and over 65 by increasing their community involvement and helping them build social connections.

WHAT DID DOCTORS THINK ABOUT IT?

There is lots of evidence that social activity can have a very positive effect on physical and mental wellbeing. Some evidence suggests that loneliness and isolation can be as detrimental to health as smoking.

Bristol GP Dr Marion Sterner said about the project: 'This sort of initiative makes you enjoy your job more because it feels like it's getting to the heart of problems':

■ What participants said:

'I can't say enough about it because it has changed my life... if I hadn't done it I wouldn't have known about these walking groups. After I retired I felt like a recluse, 3 days a week I didn't go out of the flat. I've now lost a stone in weight, I can talk to people quite freely which I didn't before... I've stopped drinking alcohol – I don't need it to help me sleep as the walks tire me out'. David Bird

■ What group leaders said:

'They come and meet other people like themselves and compare notes to their heart's content, it's much less isolating for them. I reckon I keep people out of doctors' surgeries because of depression. They come here once a week and we are like a family'. Mary Hall, Lipreading Group at Knowle West Health Park

Source: Knowle West Media Centre 2016

'Social Assets in Action Project', a partnership project between the Institute for Research and Innovation in Social Services (IRISS), East Dunbartonshire Community Health Partnership and East Dunbartonshire Council, with support from the third sector (IRISS 2013).

3. Social Mirror

Social networks reach into all areas of life, yet drawing insights from network information is often complex. The Social Mirror project looked at the transformative power of social networks and tested a social prescribing tool to see the potential for its use in the context of community health and wellbeing.

Starting in January 2012, the RSA developed a tablet application prototype to measure and visualise social networks and ran a pilot study to test the impact of community prescriptions on the subjective wellbeing of individuals in the Knowle West area of Bristol (UK). By testing the app's effectiveness in different contexts, such as among GPs and other health practitioners, the RSA evaluated the impact of social prescriptions on people's mental wellbeing, their sense of attachment to and participation in the local community, and their use of public services (RSA 2016). See Case Study 15.2 outlining the use of Social Mirror.

Some Implications of the Community Engagement Approach

If you choose to adopt a community engagement approach, it is important to appreciate the implications and that areas of tension are likely to surface. These are identified in the following section as are suggestions for trying to prevent them.

1. Different Priorities and Agendas

Priorities chosen by communities may not be the same as those of local statutory agencies or the funding organisation. For example, health priorities for health promoters may be influenced by government targets with lifestyle risk factors for major illnesses and low uptake of health services dominating the agenda. Community priorities, on the other hand, may be about social conditions, such as poor housing and lack of good public transport. Conflicting agendas must be clearly understood and dealt with at the outset of any community development work.

2. Threat to Local Health Workers

If local people gain confidence, become assertive and more articulate through the process of community development, they could voice concern and criticism about local health services. Furthermore, the prospect of members of the community taking an active role in policy making and planning may be alien to many managers in statutory agencies. A thorough educational grounding in the rationale and principles of community-based work is required, although setting this up and getting people to listen may in itself be a difficult task.

3. No Instant Results

It takes time to get to know a community and to build up trust with local people, and it may be years before there is any tangible outcome. A common problem is that projects with fixed-term funding for a year or two are often expected to achieve substantial outcomes in these short timescales, which is unrealistic. Securing long-term funding, with achievable objectives, is fundamental to success.

4. A Token Gesture or an Easy Option

Well-meaning authorities who prioritise inequalities in health may consider a community health project as a way of addressing the issue. The inequalities issue is complex, involving deeply rooted causes of poor health; a community health project can make a valuable contribution, but it can also divert attention from political solutions to the problems.

5. Evaluation Conflicts

Outside agencies may expect to see results in terms of normative outcomes such as improved immunisation rates, a measurable change in community behaviour (less binge drinking, vandalism or crime, for example) or lower rates of hospital admission. However, the objectives of a community development project are rarely couched in such terms and are more likely to be concerned with far less easily measured results such as increased public participation in health planning or better communication between the community and statutory agencies. Open debate about the process, principles, aims and possible outcomes is essential (see UNESCO 2009 for an excellent guide to evaluating community-based projects).

COMMUNITY HEALTH PROJECTS

A community health project aims to improve health usually by combining a number of approaches such as self-help, community action and/or community engagement and development. They are generally expert-led rather than initiated by the community but should involve participatory approaches and can also employ asset mapping (see Chapter 5, planning and evaluating health promotion and public health).

It is important to adopt a systematic approach to planning a community health project. Fig. 15.2 summarises the planning and evaluation flowchart taken from Chapter 5, highlighting issues relevant to community health project work. This is not a comprehensive guide to setting up and running community health projects; it is intended to be complementary to the information in Chapter 5.

See Chapter 5 for more details on planning and evaluation methods.

Stage 1. Identifying Needs and Priorities

At this stage, two particular issues are: how do you get to know the community, and who do you consult?

Getting to know the community and its needs. An asset mapping process would be appropriate here. Get all the relevant information you can about the health of the community. Search out data from local health services and the local authority. Try contacting neighbourhood centres, community groups, voluntary organisations and tenants' associations. People who might be able to put you in touch with these include those working in health and social services, local churches and schools, the local Council for Voluntary Service and the local Council for Racial Equality. Talk to members of the public, perhaps at local markets and festivals, or conduct a small survey. It might be necessary to hold public meetings to elicit full participation.

Talk to local professionals, but bear in mind that professional perceptions will often stem from a problem-centred view of a locality, for example, police may talk about crime and social workers may talk about the numbers of children on the at-risk register.

Local newspapers are a useful source of information about the needs, interests and activities of a locality, and may even have a library service to select material on a particular issue for you. Another approach is to walk, not drive, around the neighbourhood. Groups of young people on street corners, smells from fast-food shops and the range and price of goods in shop windows can reveal a lot about local lifestyle and socioeconomic conditions.

Consulting before setting up. Consult with local health and social service workers at a very early stage and also elicit community participation so that they have ownership of the project. Only do this if you are confident the project is likely to secure funding, as you could raise community members' expectations falsely and diminish their trust.

Stages 2 and 3. Setting Aims and Objectives, and Deciding the Best Way of Achieving Them

Key issues here are about being flexible and realistic. It is important to have full participation from the people you have already made contact with and the management group/steering group of the project (if there is one). These people are vital to setting realistic, achievable aims and objectives, and working out the best means of achieving them.

Flexibility is vital because community health improvement work is essentially a developmental process, so you need to review and, if necessary, modify your objectives regularly. Objectives may change, and indeed should change, if new opportunities arise and/or previous objectives no longer seem achievable or compatible with changing needs.

Be realistic: this applies to identifying what you plan to achieve and when. For example, if you are planning a community development approach, ensure that you have a realistic time scale; 3 years is suggested as a reasonable minimum.

Stage 4. Identifying Resources

Funding. Funding can come from statutory organisations, such as the local authorities or the health service, sometimes in partnership (GovUK 2014). Projects may also be funded

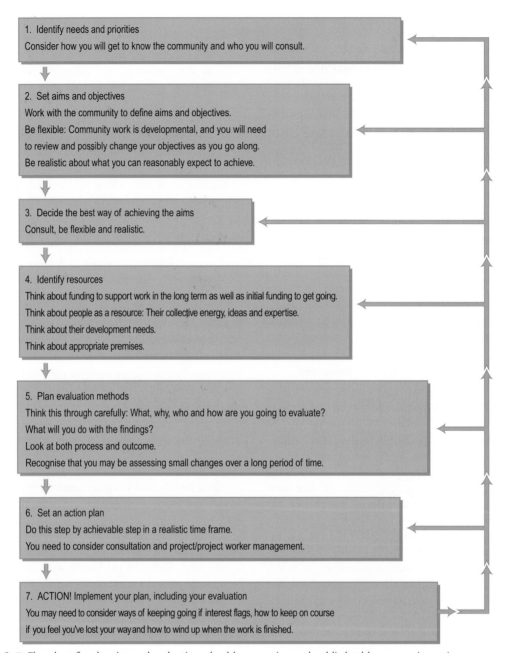

1. Identify needs and priorities
Consider how you will get to know the community and who you will consult.

2. Set aims and objectives
Work with the community to define aims and objectives.
Be flexible: Community work is developmental, and you will need
to review and possibly change your objectives as you go along.
Be realistic about what you can reasonably expect to achieve.

3. Decide the best way of achieving the aims
Consult, be flexible and realistic.

4. Identify resources
Think about funding to support work in the long term as well as initial funding to get going.
Think about people as a resource: Their collective energy, ideas and expertise.
Think about their development needs.
Think about appropriate premises.

5. Plan evaluation methods
Think this through carefully: What, why, who and how are you going to evaluate?
What will you do with the findings?
Look at both process and outcome.
Recognise that you may be assessing small changes over a long period of time.

6. Set an action plan
Do this step by achievable step in a realistic time frame.
You need to consider consultation and project/project worker management.

7. ACTION! Implement your plan, including your evaluation
You may need to consider ways of keeping going if interest flags, how to keep on course
if you feel you've lost your way and how to wind up when the work is finished.

FIG. 15.2 ■ Flowchart for planning and evaluating a health promotion and public health community project.

from the voluntary sector through funding from government grants and independent funds, such as the Big Lottery Fund (see http://www.biglotteryfund.org.uk for the full range of Reaching Communities funding and also for case studies and evaluation reports). Uncertain funding arrangements can increase difficulties in planning and evaluating work, and can divert efforts from project work to fundraising. It is important to think about long-term funding, otherwise there is a danger of work being dropped when funding runs out.

People. By bringing people with a common interest or experience together, you may find that the collective energy of the group generates ideas for future action. Your role may also begin to change from being an initiator/facilitator to being a supporter.

It is also important to think about what training and development is needed, who will do it and how it will be funded. Not only project workers but also the project management committee (if there is one), local lay people and health professionals may need help in understanding what this type of work is all about.

Premises. You need to consider what premises you need: Rooms for large and small meetings, a room for a crèche, a place to keep and use equipment such as video equipment and photocopiers, a library/place where people can look up information and use computers with access to the internet and email. Is there access for wheelchairs, pushchairs and prams? Running water and toilets? Facilities for making refreshments or meals? Good access by public transport? Well-lit premises so that people feel safe going there after dark?

You also need to consider the nature of possible premises. If you are offered space in a clinic, for example, this may mean that people perceive the project to be part of the statutory health services.

Webpage/Facebook and other social media. Many community health projects now have webpages and other social media presence, so it is important to consider who will fund and develop this resource. See, as an example, the Pilton Community Health Project Facebook page in the references section at the end of this chapter.

Stage 5. Planning Evaluation Methods

It is vital that evaluation is planned at the outset, as this will avoid misunderstandings and false expectations. All parties (funders, managers, workers, participants) need to agree on key issues. It is important to note that good health impact assessments move beyond the purely technical assessment of impacts on outcomes, to include community views (Buck & Gregory 2013):

- Why are you undertaking an evaluation? Who and what is it for?
- What will you be evaluating?
- How will you do it? What methods will you use?
- Who will do it? Will you evaluate yourselves or will you use someone who is not involved in the work as an external evaluator?
- Who will be involved in the evaluation process? Will it involve the community, the workers, the funders, the steering group?
- What will you do with your evaluation findings? Will you publish a report or disseminate via the social media? Who will the evaluation report be distributed to? Who will own it? Will findings be widely disseminated to the community?

(For an excellent guide to evaluating community projects, see Bates & Jones 2012.)

Identify evaluation conflicts and ensure that your evaluation looks at process, impact and outcome, and identifies realistic ways of assessing what may be very small changes over long periods of time. It will probably not be possible to evaluate every element of a project so it may be necessary to prioritise which elements will be assessed.

It may be helpful to think in terms of charting changes as they occur, using a framework to record these systematically.

Stage 6. Setting An Action Plan

There are many things to consider here, but the main one is to identify what you plan to do, step by step.

You may need to build the following activities into an action plan:

Reviewing aims and priorities. It is necessary to review continuously the aims and priorities originally set down for the project and compare them with those of the people who are now involved. You may need to modify the original aims and regularly check that the agenda is meeting community needs.

Consulting and being accountable to the community. The community participation established at the outset needs to continue throughout. Once the project is established, you have a continuing responsibility to involve the community. This could be through meetings, newsletters, electronic networks and open days, for example.

Arranging a management committee or steering group. A management committee or steering group should provide a secure foundation for the project, taking responsibility for its continued development, its policies and management tasks such as fundraising and recruiting. It should also provide support for the project workers. Usually these are members of the group; they should not be expected to run the management committee themselves, but sometimes this is the case. This is not desirable because it leads to confusion about who is managing whom, and puts an unreasonable burden on the workers.

A management group could consist of both local workers, such as health visitors and social workers, and local people, perhaps representing the community groups involved in the project.

It may be helpful to get the members of a management committee/steering committee together for a day to talk through the issues, clarify aims and foster a sense of teamwork.

Writing job descriptions. Paid project workers need clear job descriptions, specifying what is included. For example, does the job include fundraising, doing your own typing, servicing or even running the management committee meetings, keeping the accounts, evaluating, writing progress reports?

Ensuring support for the project workers. Recognise the value of networking as a means of informal training and support. Networking requires making time and other resources available to meet people doing similar work and to link with other community health projects in different parts of the country. This enables information and ideas to be shared and problems discussed. Access to email, social media and the internet is essential. The need to ensure that project workers are not isolated is crucial.

Networking also means that more people will know about the project and you may get more support.

Formalising your project group. It may be helpful at some stage to look at the costs and benefits of formalising a project group that started off as a loose collection of interested people. The advantages of having a formal organisation are that it can apply for financial help and for recognition as a legitimate body; the disadvantages might be that control could be exercised from outside.

Dealing with opposition. The health issues the project is concerned with will probably have a local history and be likely to have both won and lost support in the past. You need to identify opposition and plan a strategy for dealing with individuals or groups who may oppose the project.

Stage 7. Implementing Your Plan

As the project is implemented, it may run into difficulties because of a) flagging interest, b) lack of direction and c) the project coming to an end.

Keeping going. Over time, the community may lose its enthusiasm. You need to be sensitive to the many ways in which a project can lose direction and, in such circumstances, you may be able to help by:

- drawing the issue to the attention of relevant statutory agencies and conveying the response to the group
- helping the group to produce its own public health materials, such as posters, leaflets, website or video, and distributing them
- looking at other public health material on topics of interest
- encouraging members of the project to talk about their work to other people, such as groups of interested professionals and students
- sending emails to everyone to remind them of meetings
- providing practical support such as access to a computer
- introducing new members.

Working out what to do next. If you feel that you have lost direction, it can help to write down what information you have found, what contacts you have made, what needs and aims you have identified and what you have done so far. Then seek the views of your management/steering group (if there is one) or the impartial views of someone who has not been involved. Exercise 15.3 may help to provide a focus for working out what to do next.

For a range of community health case studies, see the Big Lottery Fund (2011).

EXERCISE 15.3

Planning Community Health Improvement Work

The following exercise may be useful when you are starting community health work or taking stock part way through a community health project.

Complete the following statements as fully as you can:

The key issue is …

The people I need to consult/participate with are …

The documents I need to read are …

I can get to know more about the community by …

The information that is likely to be available is …

I intend to look for this information by …

Work done on this issue elsewhere is …

The people who are likely to be supportive are …

The people I should avoid offending are …

The period of time I can spend on this issue is …

The amount of time I can give it during this period is …

The person/people I will consult/participate with in order to work out what to do next are …

Leavings and endings. There comes a point when your involvement has to stop, maybe because you change your job or the priorities of your work, or because the project work has been taken on by local people. Occasionally, you will need to recognise that you have done all you could do and that there is now no potential in the project. Ending your involvement provides the opportunity for a final evaluation of what has been achieved and what your own contribution has been and for making recommendations for future action.

DEVELOPING COMPETENCE IN COMMUNITY WORK

To be a successful community health worker, you need a range of competencies. You will also need to be committed to the principles and ideals of community-based work: the centrality of the community, your own role as a facilitator rather than an expert, the importance of addressing inequalities and a broad perspective on health (see Chapter 1, section on inequalities in health and on models of health.)

To adhere to these principles, you will need knowledge of key issues, such as the extent and cause of inequalities in health, the effects of racism, sexism and other forms of oppression on health, and awareness of the structures, policies and powers which influence the lives and health of communities. You will also need to be clear about your own particular political ideologies.

See the previous section on getting to know the community and its needs; Chapter 3, section on agents and agencies of health promotion and Exercise 4.1 in Chapter 4 on analysing your philosophical position on health promotion and public health.

Other areas of knowledge include familiarity with local health resources: who and where to go to for information, advice and materials on health issues. Knowledge of local health services and social services is vital; so is understanding how local statutory and voluntary agencies work, and how to use the system effectively. An understanding of the community itself is, of course, vital.

A range of competencies are required. It is important to have competencies in raising awareness of inequalities and discrimination, and being able to counter these by taking positive action when appropriate and working in an antidiscriminatory way.

See Chapters 5, 7, and 8 for planning and managing; Chapter 10 for communication; Chapter 11 for using communication tools and Chapter 13 for working with groups.

Other skills link to working with people: being able to communicate well, facilitate groups and run effective meetings, good team working and partnership skills. You also need skills of planning and management, using and producing social media and public health materials, and advocacy skills for working for political change.

PRACTICE POINTS

- Community-based health promotion and public health involves engaging with communities (rather than individuals) over a period of time to enable them to increase control over, and improve, their health. It may involve community development work, specific community health projects and group work.
- A key principle is that community work is bottom-up, not top-down. This means that you respond to issues that the community identifies rather than working on issues identified by people outside the community, such as health workers from statutory agencies.

- Community health workers take on the role of facilitators rather than health experts to develop the community's abilities to both identify their assets and to meet health needs.
- Work is often focused on addressing inequalities and working with people who are disadvantaged.
- Health is interpreted holistically to encompass social, emotional and societal wellbeing.
- Community participation is fundamental to health planning and health promotion activity.
- You need particular skills and processes for successful community engagement work and community health projects. You need to be aware of the potential conflicts and difficulties inherent in this kind of work.

REFERENCES

Bates G, Jones L 2012 Monitoring and evaluation: a guide for community projects. Centre for Public Health, Liverpool, JMU. http://www.cph.org.uk/wp-content/uploads/2013/02/Monitoring-and-evaluation-a-guide-for-community-projects.pdf.

Big Lottery Fund 2011 Case study brochure: Reaching Communities and Reaching Communities Northern Ireland. https://www.biglotteryfund.org.uk/-/media/Files/…/er_rc_case_studies.pdf.

Brighter Futures Together Factsheet 2016 Map assets in your community. http://www.brighterfuturestogether.co.uk/brighter-futures-together-toolkit/map-assets-in-your-community/.

Buck D, Gregory S 2013 Improving the public's health: A resource for local authorities. London, Kings Fund.

Department of Health 2010 Healthy Lives. Healthy People Our strategy for public health in England. London, HMSO.

Evans M, Winson A 2014 Asset-based approaches to public health: a conceptual framework for measuring community assets. Birmingham City Council, University of Birmingham.

Foot J, Hopkins T 2010 A glass half-full: how an asset approach can improve community health and well-being. Improvement and Development Agency, London.

Foot J 2012 What makes us healthy? The assets approach in practice: evidence, action, evaluation. Jane Foot, http://www.assetbased-consulting.co.uk/uploads/publications/WMUH.pdf.

GovUK 2014 Apply for funding for community projects. https://www.gov.uk/apply-funding-community-project.

IRISS 2013 WITTY (What's Important To You?). http://www.iriss.org.uk/resources/witty-whats-important-you.

Knowle West Media Centre 2016 Social Mirror. http://kwmc.org.uk/projects/socialmirror/.

NEF 2011 Coproduction Self-Reflection Framework: a working reflection tool for practitioners. New Economics Foundation. http://api.ning.com/files/VqSMh5MT5ZMNc9040-7x-3tlsar02l0JTvoqW7EeoW6MoLSEhi*CKaDWNipgAPhL0zyoXMHLIKSzAiH2Q2pyKnf0GbgscwEG/Coproductionaudittool.pdf.

NESTA 2012 People Powered Health Coproduction Catalogue. New Economics Foundation / NESTA / Innovation Unit, London.

NHS 2011 'Co-production for health – a new model for a radically new world' Building new approaches to delivery to achieve better health outcomes at the local level - Final report of a national colloquium. http://www.chimat.org.uk/resource/item.aspx?RID=118818.

NHS confederation 2015 What are Community Health services?. www.nhsconfed.org/communityservices. Accessed 28 August 2016.

NICE 2014 Community engagement to improve health. https://www.nice.org.uk/advice/lgb16/chapter/Introduction.

O'Leary T, Burkett I, Braithwayte K 2011 Appreciating Assets. (IACD & Carnegie UK Trust). www.carnegieuktrust.org.uk/publications/all-publications?search=appreciating%20assets&year=2011.

Resnick PJ, Janney AW, Buis LR, Richardson CR 2010 Adding an online community to an internet-mediated walking program. part 2: strategies for encouraging community participation. Journal of Medical Internet Research 12(4). Online e71. http://dx.doi.org/10.2196/jmir.1338.

Rifkin SB 2014 Examining the links between community participation and health outcomes: a review of the literature. Health Policy and Planning 29(suppl 2):ii98–ii106. http://dx.doi.org/10.1093/heapol/czu076.

RSA 2016 Social Mirror. https://www.thersa.org/action-and-research/rsa-projects/public-services-and-communities-folder/social-mirror.

Scottish Coproduction Network 2016 Tools and Methods. http://www.coproductionscotland.org.uk/resources/further-resources-and-information/reports-and-publications/tools-and-methods/.

Scriven A 2007 Developing local alliance partnerships through community collaboration and participation. In: Handsley S, Lloyd CE, Douglas J, et al. Eds., *Policy and practice in promoting public health*. London, Sage.

UNESCO 2009 ON TARGET: A Guide for Monitoring and Evaluating Community-Based Projects. http://unesdoc.unesco.org/images/0018/001862/186231e.pdf.

WEBSITES

38 Degrees website with a video on the work of the organisation. https://home.38degrees.org.uk/.

Community health services forum page. http://www.nhsconfed.org/members-and-partners/community-health-services-forum.

Community Organisers case studies and stories. http://www.corganisers.org.uk/stories.

For a list of tools for asset mapping, see North Yorkshire Partnership website. http://www.nypartnerships.org.uk/index.aspx?articleid=29644.

For a range of information on community action, see the National Association for Voluntary and Community Action NAVCA. https://www.navca.org.uk/.

For examples of community development/UK Community Foundation. http://ukcommunityfoundations.org/programmes/fourteen.

Mental Health Advocacy Scheme. http://www.advocacyscheme.co.uk/.

Scottish Coproduction Network – Coproduction case studies. http://www.coproductionscotland.org.uk/resources/resource-case-studies/.

Video case studies – IRISS what is coproduction. http://www.coproductionscotland.org.uk/resources/video-case-studies/.

YOUTUBE

NHS England Transforming Participation in Health and Care – Sir David Nicholson CEO NHS England. 2013. https://www.youtube.com/watch?v=2-7CZ4xvWCM&feature=youtu.be.

TWITTER

National Association for Voluntary and Community Action. https://twitter.com/navca.

FACEBOOK

38 Degrees, people/power/change. https://www.facebook.com/peoplepowerchange.

Pilton Community Health Project. https://www.facebook.com/PiltonCommunityHealthProject/.

16

INFLUENCING AND IMPLEMENTING PUBLIC HEALTH POLICY

CHAPTER CONTENTS

SUMMARY

The focus of this chapter is on how public health policy at local and national level is made, how it can be influenced and how health promoters and public health practitioners can challenge health-damaging policies. The characteristics of power and the politics of influence are discussed and illustrated with a case study. There are sections on developing and implementing policies, a case study on the politics of influence and an exercise on policy implementation. The chapter ends with a section on planning a policy campaign (see Chapter 7, section on linking your work into broader health promotion plans and strategies).

Health promoters and public health practitioners have an important role in influencing and implementing policies that affect health. A policy is a broad statement of the principles of how to proceed in relation to a specific issue and can be at a number of levels, from international (see NHS European Office 2016), to national, regional and organisational level. At international level, the WHO has produced a number of directives designed to influence national policy, such as

Health 2020 (WHO 2016a, see the following text; for a detailed discussion of conceptual policy frameworks and the history of public health policy, see Baggott 2015).

EUROPEAN HEALTH POLICY FRAMEWORK: HEALTH 2020

Health 2020 is the new European health policy framework adopted by the 53 member states of the European Union. It builds on the experiences gained from previous health for all policies, is evidence-based and makes the case for investment in health. It aims to support action across government and society to significantly improve the health and wellbeing of populations, reduce health inequalities, strengthen public health and ensure people-centred health systems that are universal, equitable, sustainable and of high quality. It gives policy-makers a vision, a strategic path, a set of priorities and a range of suggestions about what works to improve health, address health inequalities and ensure the health of future generations. The policy framework is based on the **values** enshrined in the WHO Constitution: the highest attainable standard of health as a human right. It acknowledges the **interconnectedness** of local, national, regional and global health actors, actions and challenges, and recommends a unity of approach. Health is seen as a resource that enables every person to realise his or her potential and to contribute to the overall development of society, and that poor health wastes potential, causes despair and drains resources across all sectors of society. The policy framework presents ways in which policy-makers can more effectively and efficiently address today's social, demographic, epidemiological and financial challenges by resetting priorities, catalyzing action in other sectors and adopting new approaches to organizing the health sector. Many partners need to come together to achieve better and more equitable health and wellbeing; the policy framework is designed to help overcome some of the principal barriers to partnership working. It provides a range of suggestions to show what works in engaging stakeholders based on research and experience in many countries. The policy framework suggests ways to identify important health gaps and focus individual and collective efforts on ways to reduce them by working across government to fulfil two linked strategic objectives:

■ Improving health for all and reducing health inequalities
■ Improving leadership and participatory governance for health (WHO, 2016a).

(See the YouTube film, *The Journey from Ottawa to Health 2020* and the Health 2020 website referenced at the end of this chapter for more detail on Health 2020.)

To influence policy, health promoters and public health practitioners need to understand international policy imperatives such as Health 2020, how power is distributed and exercised between people at various levels and be able to use that knowledge to further shape policy decisions. In other words, you need to be political. Being a policy activist involves working with statutory, voluntary and commercial organisations to influence the development of health-promoting public health policies. It also includes working for healthy public policies (Scriven 2007) and economic and regulatory changes that might require campaigning, lobbying and taking political action.

MAKING AND INFLUENCING LOCAL AND NATIONAL HEALTH POLICY

Working for policy change is an integral part of public health action with health promoters and public health practitioners well placed to press for the introduction of policies at both national and local levels and influence how they are implemented. The development of local health policies cannot be divorced from the central government's policies that shape the organisation and funding of health service, local authority and voluntary agency work at a local level. National policy is in turn influenced by consultation with and representations from a wide range of stakeholders including health services, local authorities and voluntary agencies and key public health member organisations. In the UK, these will include The Faculty of Public Health (FPH) and the Royal Society of Public Health (RSPH), who advocate on key public health issues, influencing policy change at the highest level, and working closely with policymakers. Public health research is also a key influence on policies and should form an essential step in the policy development process (Fig. 16.1).

It is vital that those working to promote health have a good understanding of national public health policy and the various drivers that shape public health policy statements and strategies. Given the scale of the challenge presented by the global growth in noncommunicable diseases and the complexity of inequalities in health, all governments need to draw on the range of available policy tactics, from strong state action including welfare and regulation to behaviour and environmental approaches.

Local and National Public Health Policy Themes

Politics is a major influence on public health and the policies that affect population health, particularly policies linked to welfare and health service reforms. The UK government's Welfare Reform Bill (2012) has come in for major criticism in terms of the health impact it is likely to have on those who rely on benefits. There are increased numbers of the disabled, families and children now living in poverty as a direct result of the reforms (see the Poverty and Social Exclusion and the Child Poverty Action Group websites in the reference section for a full analysis of the impact of the welfare reforms).

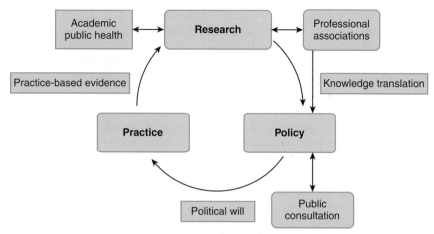

FIG. 16.1 ■ Policy continuum.

National health policies have a major impact on action at the local level. Currently there are a number of strategies permeating UK health policy agendas which guide or determine health promoting interventions. These are summed up in Fig. 16.2 and include directives that range from encouraging behavioural change to those that restrict choices through legislative and fiscal action.

Behavioural Change as a Policy Directive

Influencing people's behaviour is nothing new to governments, which often use tools such as legislation (such as a ban on smoking in public places), regulation (legislation is a directive proposed by a legislative body while a regulation is a specific requirement within legislation, such as fines for adults smoking in cars that contain children under 18) or taxation (a tax

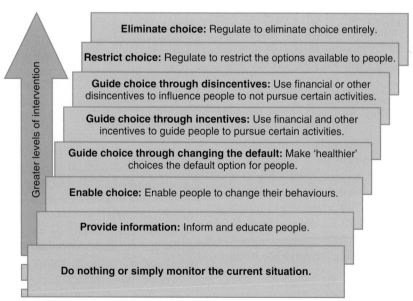

FIG. 16.2 ■ Ladder of health promoting strategies embedded in public health policy and practice. *(Source: Local Government Association (LGA; 2013) and Nuffield Council on Bioethics-Full report Public health: ethical issues (2007): http://nuffieldbioethics.org/wp-content/uploads/2014/07/Public-health-ethical-issues.pdf).*

on cigarettes) to achieve desired behavioural change policy outcomes. Behaviour change ideology even permeates discussion of the broader determinants of health: 'A high-performing health system supports individuals to make positive decisions about their own health and acts to maximise its positive impact on the broader determinants of people's health' (Gregory et al 2012). Government sponsored campaigns, such as Change4Life (see websites and Facebook pages in the references at the end of the chapter), and approaches, such as social marketing where PHE's social marketing programmes contribute to the prevention agenda by driving lifestyle change across a wide range of health related behaviours (PHE 2015) are seen as a key instrument of prevention at the heart of the NHS Five-Year Forward plan. 'The economic prosperity of Britain all now depend on a radical upgrade in prevention and public health' (NHS England 2016).

Nudging and choice architecture is another approach visible in some policy directives (DoH Ireland 2015). Choice architecture refers to the design of different ways in which choices can be presented to consumers and the impact of that presentation on consumer decision making (see Thorndike et al 2012 for an example of a choice architecture intervention). Fig. 14.3 in Chapter 14 has examples of nudging. It is important to note that behaviours do not exist at the individual level only. When replicated across a community or society, they are referred to as culture, such as the binge drinking culture or the differences in smoking culture across socioeconomic groups in the UK. Policy history suggests that wide scale cultural behavioural change is driven by a mix of both broad social argument and small policy steps. Smoking is perhaps the best example. In the UK, the behavioural equilibrium has shifted from widespread smoking to a minority activity. A combination of nudging, choice architecture and restricting choice, including health information; effective national media campaigns (and the prohibition of pro-smoking advertising); expanding bans on smoking in public places; and changing social norms have formed a mutually reinforcing thread of policy tactics to change smoking behaviour at a national level (Dolan et al 2010).

Place-Based Health

This is a dominant tactic in current health policy in England which involves planning by place for local populations in a way which is sustainable and transformatory. Sustainability and Transformation Plans (STPs) will cover (i) specialised services, (ii) primary medical care and (iii) better integration between health and local authority services including prevention and social care, reflecting local agreed health and wellbeing strategies (NHS England 2015). Selby and Kippen (2016) argue that place-based health will result in energy, money and power shifting from institutions to citizens and communities. They envisage that place-based health will become an enabler for a reform programme that starts to deliver on joining up health and social care for a population in a place with the ultimate aim to improve the public's health and wellbeing and reducing health inequalities.

IMPLEMENTING NATIONAL HEALTH POLICIES AT A LOCAL LEVEL

National strategies for health are outlined and referred to in Chapters 1 and 4.

There will be government guidance for the range of statutory policies which will need to be implemented at the local level. In England over the past 4 years these have included Joint Strategic Needs Assessments (JSNAs) and Health and Wellbeing Strategies (JHWSs; Department of Health 2012). The rationale is that leadership and delivery of public services should be made as locally as possible, involving people who use them and the wider local community. Health and Wellbeing Boards take the lead with the overall purpose of the JSNAs and JHWSs to develop local evidence-based priorities for commissioning which will improve local health and wellbeing and reduce inequalities for all ages. The outputs, in the form of evidence, the analysis of needs and agreed priorities are used to help to determine what actions local authorities, the local NHS and other partners need to take to meet health and social care needs and to address the wider determinants that impact on health and wellbeing. Local public health policies will emerge from the JSNAs and the JHWSs.

Another significant influence currently on local public health in England is the Public Health Outcomes Framework (PHOF). The vision is to improve and protect the nation's health and wellbeing, and improve the health of the poorest fastest by action on outcomes and four domains:

Outcome 1: Increased healthy life expectancy, taking into account the health quality and the length of life

(Note: This measure uses a self-reported health assessment, applied to life expectancy.)

Outcome 2: Reduced differences in life expectancy and healthy life expectancy between communities through greater improvements in more disadvantaged communities

(Note: These two measures would work as a package covering both morbidity and mortality, addressing within-area differences and between-area differences.)

DOMAIN 1: Improving the wider determinants of health

Objective: Improvements against wider factors that affect health and wellbeing, and health inequalities

DOMAIN 2: Health improvement

Objective: People are helped to live healthy lifestyles, make healthy choices and reduce health inequalities

DOMAIN 3: Health protection

Objective: The population's health is protected from major incidents and other threats, while reducing health inequalities

DOMAIN 4: Health care, public health and preventing premature mortality

Objective: Reduced numbers of people living with preventable ill health and people dying prematurely, while reducing the gap between communities. Indicators for each of these domains are across the life course (DoH 2012b). Public Health England provides PHOF data updates on a regular basis. To access these, see the Public Health website in the reference section at the end of the chapter.

It is clear from the previous English examples that public health and health promotion is a significant component of the UK government's health policy agenda. It is important to be up-to-date with your government's policy directives and the dominant themes, and from these to interpret the sort of policies that would need to be implemented at a local level to improve the health of communities and local population groups.

CHALLENGING POLICY

As a heath promoter or public health practitioner, you may find you are expected to implement policies that you perceive as health damaging or contrary to health promotion or public health principles. This can be difficult because such policies can emanate from national government, your employing organisation or even your direct manager. To challenge may create a conflict of loyalty between wanting to press for what you see as right and what is decreed to be right by government and/or your employing authority. To protest may be seen as too political. There is no easy answer to this issue, but there are some positive steps worth considering:

- Use your vote. At the next general or local election, look at the health implications in the policy manifestos. Raise questions about health policy with doorstep canvassers, at public meetings and by writing to candidates. All this can be done in your capacity as a private citizen rather than a health worker.
- Use your professional association or trade union. These groups can raise issues at a national and local level, and can be a powerful voice. You can play your part by joining and supporting their activities, and raising the issues you feel strongly about.
- Use your representative. There are many people whose job is to represent your interests. At national level, it is your Member of Parliament (MP). So if you want to raise an issue at this level, lobby your MP: send letters, telephone, attend politicians' surgeries. At local level, do the same with your local elected councillor. You could also contact your professional association or union local branch representative.
- Use your collective power. If you are concerned about a health-related policy issue at your place of work, it may help to find out if colleagues feel the same. If they do, join together so that you raise the issue collectively: this can give it more impact. Or at a national level, join with others who share your concern to improve health and challenge health-damaging policies. For example, the Royal Society of Public Health (RSPH) have more than 6000 members drawn from every area and profession across public health including environmental health, nursing, food hygiene, health promotion, health protection and dentistry, forming an international network of public health professionals committed to influencing policy and practice. 38 Degrees is a virtual collective people power organisation that

enables individuals and groups to network and to establish campaigns or to vote on policy issues of importance to public health. At the time of writing, current campaigns include action against the abolition of the human rights act, a campaign to keep European workers in the NHS and a crowdfunded investigation into secret plans by the UK government to make funding cuts to the NHS (Ilot 2016; for further information on 38 Degrees, see the 38 Degrees website reference at the end of the chapter).

However, many areas of policy development are not controversial and can be a positive and rewarding part of the day-to-day work of health promoters and public health practitioners. The main thrust is likely to be in developing, changing and implementing local policies. To do this, you need to understand the characteristics of power and influence and be competent at exerting influence when necessary.

Characteristics of Power and Influence

Power is the ability to influence others. There are four generally recognised types of power that are relevant to health promotion and public health policy work:

1. **Position power** is the power vested in someone because of their position in an organisation. For example, a Director of Public Health has position power.
2. **Resource power** is the power to allocate or limit resources including money and staff. It often goes hand-in-hand with position power. For example, a senior health service manager has both position power and the power to regulate the use of resources. You have a source of power if you have the authority to control the allocation of any resources. Every health promoter and public health practitioner will have some power because people want the skills or services on offer.
3. **Expert power** is power related to expertise. Directors of Public Health and health promotion specialists have the expert power associated with their specialty.
4. **Personal power** is the power that comes from the personal attributes of a person including strong personality, charisma and ability to inspire. It is closely related to leadership qualities

and intelligence, initiative, self-confidence and the ability to rise above a situation and see it in perspective. However, effective leaders are not always charismatic, and what makes a leader effective in one situation may cause them to be less effective in changed circumstances.

You may sometimes be in the position of wanting or needing to exert influence on people who have a stronger power base. For example, a health visitor may wish to influence a general practitioner to adopt a policy of supporting the running of antenatal clinics in the local ethnic minority group's community centre, or a community worker may want to lobby local councillors about the need for more recreational facilities for young people on a housing estate. To do this requires skills in influencing and negotiation (see Enix 2016).

Before attempting to influence someone who has position or resource power, first consider the basic questions in the planning process, such as: What are your aims? What resources do you need? Is the investment of your time in influencing others going to be worth it? Could the aim be achieved more easily another way? (See Chapter 5, planning and evaluating health promotion.)

The Politics of Influence

There are four key elements of a strategy aiming to change policy:

1. Planning
2. Making allies
3. Networking
4. Making deals and negotiating.

Planning

Three particular aspects of planning are useful to consider: undertaking a force field analysis, identifying stakeholders and considering your timing:

Undertake a force field analysis. A force field analysis identifies the helping and hindering forces and helps pinpoint how you can influence the process to make progress towards policy change or implementation. You identify how you can increase the power of the helping forces and decrease the power of the hindering forces. Use the diagram in Fig. 16.3 to set out your own force field analysis.

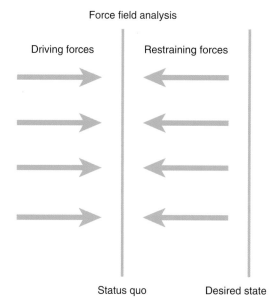

Force field analysis

Driving forces   Restraining forces

Status quo   Desired state

FIG. 16.3 ■ Illustrating a force field analysis. *(Source: The Bates Blog (2013))*

Identify the stakeholders. The stakeholders are those people with a vested interest in the issue who wish to influence what is done and how it is done. They are obviously powerful forces in the situation. It could be difficult to identify all the stakeholders, because some of them may not wish to be visible and try to work covertly through others.

Time your action. It is also important to consider when to introduce a proposal or when to delay. If people are already preoccupied with other major issues, it might not be the right time to make a new proposal. On the other hand, if a proposal will help other people to attain their own objectives, it will be a good time.

Making Allies

Identify which of the stakeholders could be allies and gain their trust and confidence to establish and maintain an alliance. It helps to pay attention to their concerns, values, beliefs and behaviour patterns, and to see what you need to do to form an effective working alliance.

For example, if you are concerned about the way in which people with disabilities are treated in an organisation, you might identify the person in charge of human resources as a key stakeholder. So find out if they are concerned about it and if they think it is important for the organisation. What kind of way do they work, are they likely to respond best to a lively discussion on the subject or to a well-argued paper on the need for policy, backed up with facts and figures? Do they like time to make decisions? Will they be happy to leave you to take the lead, or will they want ownership of the initiative?

Networking

Many people working in organisations belong to one or more interest groups who meet to discuss, debate and exchange information on issues that concern the members. By playing an active role in these networks, people can extend their influence. Networks provide access to information that can help with making a case, to people with experience of successful influencing and to other resources. There are different types of networks:

Professional networks. Members are from the same profession. Professional networks may attempt to influence government, employers and organisations to reconsider their policies or to develop new policies for the future. Professional networks institute criteria for professional practice and are active in the professional development of their members. The Faculty of Public Health is a professional network.

Elitist networks. Membership is normally by invitation only. Members of such networks may have considerable power and influence, often through their position in organisations. An example of such a network might be the UK Public Health Network, which is a collaboration of umbrella organisations representing public health across the four nations that make up the United Kingdom. The four Chief Executives of the Faculty of Public Health, Royal Society of Public Health, Association of Directors of Public Health and UK Health Forum act as a coordinating group to oversee the Network, which prioritises mapping the policy priorities and work priorities for the organisations in the Network and developing a collective view of key UK-wide priorities for public health (see website references at the end of the chapter for details).

- Pressure groups. Members wish to pursue certain objectives, which may be environmental, social or political. There are a number of public health pressure groups, such as Action on Sugar, which have been influential in the introduction of a UK government childhood obesity strategy, which unfortunately the pressure group feels does not go far enough in tackling some of the major issues (Wollaston 2016). See the website and Twitter pages for the Action on Sugar pressure group in the references at the end of this page.

Influencing Policy by Making Deals and Negotiating

Making deals is common practice in most organisations. Individuals or groups agree to support a policy proposal in return for agreement on something that benefits them. In order to make deals successfully, it pays to know the person with whom you are dealing, paying careful attention to their values and intentions and what you could realistically expect from them.

Negotiation is the art of creating agreement on a specific issue between two or more parties with different views. Successful negotiation takes place when there is a desire to solve problems and the parties genuinely commit to going through a number of steps.

There are many guides on how to improve your negotiation skills. While these are mainly written for the business community, the skills are also relevant to health promotion and public health. See, for example, Enix (2016).

On Being Political

A final point is about political behaviour, which refers to finding out about who holds power and working to use this information to change a situation. When is it acceptable and when is it unethical?

Being political can be considered devious and manipulative. Some people may view it with suspicion and will therefore not be easily influenced by such behaviour. To manipulate covertly or coerce, lie or deliberately withhold information that affects others is unethical and unprofessional. But to ignore the politics within organisations is unwise, because it results in failure to make a realistic appraisal of situations and failure to make the best of the opportunities for promoting health. Furthermore, it is possible to be political without losing professional integrity, for example, by ensuring deals are made as the outcome of open negotiations and those relationships should be based on genuineness, trust, goodwill and mutual respect. Case Study 16.1 offers an example of the politics of influence in practice.

CASE STUDY 16.1

The Politics of Influence – Health and Safety at Work

Bob is an environmental health officer working for Midshire City Council. His aim is to improve the implementation of the health and safety at work policy of the council. He makes a list of the *helping* forces and the *hindering* forces:

Helping:
- The existing safety officers
- Existing codes of practice, for example, sight checks for VDU operators
- A councillor who is a health lecturer at the university
- A human resources officer interested in improving the working environment for staff
- An existing commitment to appoint an occupational health nurse.

Hindering:
- The cost of any improvements (the council has severe financial constraints)
- Staff time to attend health and safety training
- Problems with recruiting an occupational health nurse
- Deficiencies in the structure of council buildings (poor ventilation, open-plan offices, lack of showers for those staff wishing to take physical exercise during the day)
- Lack of councillors' commitment to improve health and safety conditions for staff
- Lack of access to council buildings for disabled people.

The Politics of Influence – Health and Safety at Work (Continued)

He identifies the stakeholders as:
■ the staff themselves
■ the trade unions
■ departmental managers, senior and chief officers
■ the councillors
■ the public health specialist and the health promotion specialist from the Local Authority (LA).

He further identifies key stakeholders as:
■ officers in the department of engineering because they enforce building regulations
■ council members on the health committee

■ the director of personnel.

He then identifies ways of increasing the helping forces and decreasing the hindering forces. Through making an ally of the interested human resources officer, he is able to increase the commitment of the director of human resources, who is also a chief officer. One short-term outcome is that an occupational health nurse is recruited. Another outcome is a plan agreed by the human resources department and the trade unions for training staff in health and safety.

By joining a local network of people interested in health promotion, he is able to find out what is going on elsewhere, and this gives him some useful ideas including sources of help in stress management training which he incorporates into the training plan.

He makes a deal with the engineering department by agreeing to assist with monitoring construction sites of new buildings to prevent accidents on the site. In return, they agree to assist with a plan for improving soundproofing and modifications to open-plan offices. Their commitment grows after a report shows that accidents on construction sites are reduced. He discusses with them the issue of raising with council members the plan for modifying council buildings.

Finally, he makes an ally of the councillor at the university by offering to provide an input to some of the courses. This councillor is on the health committee and provides him with useful advice on how to approach the committee and how to prepare documents for its consideration.

Developing and Implementing Policies

Many public health policies are about health issues that relate to workplaces or other settings such as schools, communities and hospitals. Other policies focus on health issues in a range of contexts, such as the UK Childhood Obesity Strategy (HM Government 2016) where action has to be taken across settings and involve a number of different types of interventions

including voluntary agreements with the food industry. For some health issues, such as alcohol in the workplace, it is common practice to have a policy (see TUC 2010).

Policies on Promoting Health in Workplaces

The benefits of promoting health at work are well established, and reviews of the literature identify the major benefits as a decrease in absenteeism and staff turnover, and an increase in productivity and morale (Kirsten & Karch 2011; O'Donell 2014). The European Network for Workplace Health Promotion (ENWHP 2013) has a range of publications that will support policy development that encourages employers and trade unions to take on a wider concept of health at work including giving priority to issues such as smoking, alcohol and stress. The World Health Organization (WHO) also has a number of guidelines on supporting workplace policy development (for example, WHO 2010).

In the UK, there are a number of agencies that support the promotion of health and wellbeing in the workplace. The Health and Safety Executive is also a source of information on all statutory policies governing health and safety in the workplace (see the HSE free guides under the web references). Many other organisations have an interest in workplace health, for example, the British Heart Foundation Blog on health at work in the references at the end of this chapter.

Policies on Promoting Health in Hospitals

Health Promoting Hospitals (HPH) is a WHO initiative designed to improve health and environmental conditions for both staff and patients by reviewing and implementing a range of health promoting policies. HPH consists of more than 28 National/Regional Networks and individual hospitals and health services members. The International HPH Network totals more than 700 hospital and health service members all over the world (see website reference at the end of the chapter). It can be difficult in practice to inform and involve everyone in an institution as large and complex as a hospital, and with this in mind the The New Haven Recommendations on partnering with patients, families and citizens to enhance performance and quality in health promoting hospitals and health services (INHPH 2016) are designed to inform policy development linked to health-promoting hospitals.

Promoting Health in Urban Settings: Healthy Cities

The WHO's Healthy Cities initiative promotes comprehensive and systematic policy and planning with a special emphasis on health inequalities and urban poverty, the needs of vulnerable groups, participatory governance and the social, economic and environmental determinants of health. It also strives to include health considerations in economic, regeneration and urban development efforts. It aims to work from the bottom-up, not from the top-down, and to involve collaborative work between local government, health authorities, local businesses, community organisations and, of course, individual citizens. The UK Healthy Cities Network (UKHCN) is part of the global movement for urban health that is led and supported by the WHO. Its vision is to develop a creative, supportive and motivating network for UK cities and towns that are tackling health inequalities and striving to put health improvement and health equity at the core of all local policies (see website in reference section; see also Chapter 15 for principles of working with communities).

Policies on Promoting Health in Schools and Universities

The European Network of Health Promoting Schools (ENHPS), now known as Schools for Health in Europe, sets out to show that schools can be powerful agents for change through the adoption of whole-school approaches. This means that the school promotes health not only by curriculum policies which include sufficient time for social, personal, economic and health education for the pupils, but also by wider school policies that ensure that the school promotes a sense of positive self-esteem and the health and wellbeing of teachers and other staff, parents and the wider community who have contact with the school. An evaluation has found there was evidence that the WHO HPS framework is effective at improving some aspects of student health (Langford et al 2015).

The UK National Healthy Universities Network was established in 2006 and aims to offer a facilitative environment for the development of a whole university approach to health and wellbeing. The Okanagan Charter for Health Promoting Universities and Colleges was launched in 2015 at the International Conference on Health Promoting Universities and Colleges. The Charter sets out a radical and far-reaching vision designed to influence organisational policies within the University sector (see full details on the Schools for Health and Health Universities websites in the references at the end of the chapter).

Policies on Promoting Health in Prisons

The WHO coordinates the Health in Prisons Programme to promote health in prisons (WHO 2016). See NHS Commissioning Board 2012, PHE 2014a, 2014b and the Welsh Government 2015 for examples of policies and guidance on public health in prisons and secure settings in the UK.

For a useful overview of the theoretical basis for health promotion and public health using a settings approach, see Dooris et al (2014).

Guidelines on Developing and Implementing a Policy

Many health promoters and public health practitioners have a role in developing and implementing polices in specific settings such as those previously discussed. An example of such a policy is the workplace healthy eating draft policy outlined in Exercise 16.1.

EXERCISE 16.1
A Draft of a Workplace Healthy Eating Policy

A healthy eating at work policy for:	Workplace A
Effective from:	00/00/00
Next review date:	00/00/00

Notes

This section of the policy could include information on some of the following topics:

- How and why a good diet affects productivity and performance at work
- How the organisation can create an environment that supports and encourages healthy eating
- How the support of health at work initiatives can demonstrate that the workforce is valued and the work-life balance is respected.

The need for a healthy eating at work policy

Healthy eating is essential for good health and contributes to positive wellbeing. Many of the leading causes of disease and disability in our society, such as obesity, coronary heart disease, diabetes, and certain forms of cancer, mental ill health and osteoporosis, are associated with poor nutritional choices. A healthy, balanced diet contains a variety of different types of food, including: lots of fruit, vegetables; plenty of starchy foods such as wholemeal bread and wholegrain cereals; some protein-rich foods such as meat, fish, eggs and lentils; and some dairy foods. We should also be drinking about six to eight glasses (1.2 litres) of water, or other fluids, every day to stop us getting dehydrated. The workplace is an important setting in which people can increase their intake of healthy foods to benefit their health and protect against illness. A healthy, balanced diet also helps people to recover more quickly from the illnesses they may get. What we eat and drink, not only has a physical impact on our body, but can also contribute to our mental health, resulting in improved levels of concentration, mental alertness and ability to cope with everyday stresses and strains and therefore perform better in work.

Example aims are given on the right. These can also link to policies on mental wellbeing, smoking and physical activity, as well as national public health policies and initiatives.

Aim of the policy:

- To support and encourage employees to make healthy eating choices
- To increase the opportunities for employees to learn more about nutrition
- To create a workplace culture that encourages employees to incorporate healthy eating into their daily routine, thus creating a lifestyle behaviour
- To set out a coordinated approach to increase the availability of healthier eating options
- To achieve recognition for a healthy workplace through the Workplace Wellbeing Charter, Healthier Catering Award or Public Health Responsibility Deal.

The objectives should be SMART (Specific, Measurable, Achievable, Realistic and Time-specific). See the examples opposite. Each objective should be followed by what the organisation will do – 'policy actions' – to meet the objectives

Objectives

To implement a healthy eating policy that raises awareness of the benefits of healthy eating.

Policy actions:

- Develop healthy eating pages on intranet and provide educational leaflets and resources on healthy eating
- Appoint a healthy eating champion, to be responsible for workplace healthy eating programmes
- Ensure healthy eating is included in any health and wellbeing groups with senior management attendance
- Provide courses and seminars on the benefits of healthy eating and the risks of poor nutrition
- Hold healthy eating promotional events such as Fruity Friday.

Continued on following page

EXERCISE 16.1

A Draft of a Workplace Healthy Eating Policy *(Continued)*

To implement a healthy eating policy that supports employees to make healthier eating choices in a variety of ways.

Policy actions:

- Encourage employees to make healthy eating choices through the use of promotional and motivational resources, e.g. encouraging employees to make healthy choices from the canteen menu
- Provide food storage and preparation areas in all departments
- Provide information on local or onsite weight management groups
- Organise fruit and vegetable box delivery schemes
- Investigate the demand for and feasibility of extending canteen opening times to include breakfast
- Designate 1 week each year as Healthy Eating Week, with a range of organised activities
- Provide access to water in all meeting and training rooms.

To remove barriers and enable employees to make healthy eating choices.

Policy actions:

- Review current provision of services in vending and catering facilities
- Engage senior management in the development of the policy
- Provide cool storage areas for lunchboxes and snacks
- Work with on-site caterers to trial more healthy choices, reducing salt and trans fats. Develop a traffic light system in canteens as easy reference for employees to see the foods which are healthier
- Increase access to healthy foods for shift workers by introducing healthy options in vending machines
- Develop links with local food providers who will deliver healthy food options to the workplace
- Endorse the eating of meals away from desks
- Provide fruit bowls in each department
- Offer fruit instead of biscuits during meetings
- Provide access to cool drinking water for all employees.

Explain how this policy will be communicated throughout the organisation.

Communication

All employees will be made aware of the healthy eating policy and the facilities available. The healthy eating policy will be included in the employee handbook and employee information or induction packs. A specific focus group will be established to take forward the actions from this policy to compliment other health at work policies. Regular updates will be provided to all employees via their line management.

Regular review and monitoring are vital to assess the effectiveness of a healthy eating policy. How will you track progress?

Review and monitoring

Employees participating in any of the healthy eating activities will be regularly asked for feedback. Healthy eating will be integrated into a 'health at work audit', which will be undertaken annually. The policy, status updates and evaluation reports will be circulated to management and be available on request through the workplace health champion. The policy will be reviewed six months from implementation and then annually after that to ensure that it remains relevant.

Date:

Signature:

Source: Rochdale Borough Council 2016

Having read the sample policy consider these questions:

- What steps are involved in the development of the policy?
- What else might have been done?
- What are the significant points to note about the development of a public health policy from this example?

1. Preparation Of The Policy

The formulation of a policy by any organisation is a corporate matter, so the usual starting point is to convene a working group. This group:

- clarifies its terms of reference and elects a Chair.
- identifies the need for a policy
- identifies the committee, department or senior person who has overall responsibility for taking the policy forward
- identifies key personnel to consult with and convince of the need for a policy
- establishes a timescale for policy development
- prepares a draft policy and consults widely
- prepares the final draft policy for approval.

In the case of a workplace policy, it is important to involve trade unions. This can be achieved either by including trade union representatives on the working group or by setting up an effective framework for consultation and negotiation. This may be crucial in persuading the workforce to look positively on the new policy.

It is also important that an identified senior member of staff or manager, with political influence, acts as a champion for the policy. This person will be crucial in getting the commitment of other managers to the policy.

2. Implementation of The Policy

This starts with planning, which will include:

- setting aims and objectives
- setting up a system for monitoring and evaluation
- identifying resources and defining key implementation tasks
- defining the role of key personnel
- developing an action plan.

Key personnel should be encouraged to participate actively in identifying their roles and in discussing

boundaries and overlap in roles so that the potential for conflict and confusion is reduced. For example, managers have the primary responsibility for ensuring that their staff are fully conversant with workplace policies and understand what is expected of them. Nevertheless, the trade unions also have a role in informing the workforce of the policy. These sources of information hopefully will be complementary and spell out the same, not contradictory, messages. The open discussion of these issues will help to increase commitment to making the policy work.

Any policy that is not the subject of regular review risks becoming obsolete. So the working group must reconvene at intervals to consider issues such as the following:

- Does the workforce know about and understand the policy?
- Have attitudes changed to the health issue covered by the policy? If so, how? How do staff feel about the policy?
- Has the behaviour of individual staff changed? Does this include changes in working practices and/or individual lifestyles?
- Are staff getting the help they need?
- Are managers and trade unions supporting the policy?
- Are indicators showing that the policy is making progress towards the attainment of its aims and objectives? For example, in the case of a workplace policy, has sickness reduced? Has work performance improved? Is morale better?
- How can we improve the effectiveness of the policy?

3. Education and Training

This is a continuous process, not a one-off event. Wherever possible, it should be integrated into existing provision for professional and managerial staff development. The purposes of education and training include the following:

- Securing the commitment of management (such as elected members, chief officers and senior management in the case of a local authority).
- Obtaining the commitment of the whole workforce or group at which the policy is aimed

(such as the prison population or the staff of a business).

■ Providing those responsible for implementing the policy with the necessary skills.

■ Overcoming prejudices, discrimination and stereotyping where relevant (for example, in policies on alcohol and HIV/AIDS).

■ Encouraging and assisting the workforce, or the particular groups of people the policy is concerned with, to make choices and individual lifestyle changes.

4. Evaluation

This should include evaluation of both process and outcomes. It will require the collection of information, both baseline and ongoing.

See Chapter 5, section on planning evaluation methods for further suggestions.

CAMPAIGNING

You, or clients with whom you work, may feel strongly about changing policy or practice about a public health issue and decide that the way forward is to mount a campaign.

Policy campaigns can range from short-lived local campaigns with the objective of making a single change to long-term national campaigns. Examples of a national pressure group campaigning for policy change is Action on Smoking and Health (ASH), which is a campaigning public health charity that works to eliminate the harm caused by tobacco. ASH has a list of policy issues on their website (http://www.ash.org.uk), which includes inequalities in health.

Some pressure groups (such as Shelter) may provide direct services as well as acting as a pressure group.

Principles of Campaigning for Policy Change

Some important principles to keep in mind if you are setting up a policy campaign are the following:

■ **Be persistent:** Success requires persistent effort, so you must be committed and prepared to put in a lot of time and energy over a long period.

■ **Be professional:** Give care and attention to details (such as well-written campaign materials

with the name of the campaign clearly evident), and ensure that activities such as keeping records are undertaken properly.

■ **Keep a sense of perspective:** Your campaign may be vitally important to you, but being perceived as fanatical will do your cause no good.

■ **Reflect your ideals:** It is no good, for example, campaigning for changes to equal opportunities policy if your own organisation does not have good access for people with disabilities.

■ **Be positive:** Use positive, rather than negative language and arguments.

■ **Join with others:** Rival pressure groups campaigning on similar (or even identical) issues waste a lot of time, effort and other resources. If someone is already campaigning on your issue, join them rather than setting up a rival organisation. Or if there is more than one organisation working on similar issues, form a coalition.

■ **Involve as many people as possible:** This not only harnesses support but also informs people about what is wrong and what needs to change.

Planning a Policy Campaign

When you plan a public health policy campaign, it helps to go through the same planning process as you would with any other kind of health promotion activity.

See also Chapter 5 for help with planning that applies to planning a campaign:

■ Identify your aims clearly
■ Decide the best way of achieving them (public meetings? press coverage? lobbying MPs and local councillors? a petition? use of social media?)
■ Identify your resources (do you need to fundraise?)
■ Clarify how you will know if your aim is achieved (set milestones and specific outcomes?)
■ Set an action plan of who is going to do what and when.

As a concluding point to this chapter on policy, and to the book as a whole, I would like to share the views of Popejoy (2016). He argues that population health outcomes are the result of a complex interplay of variables, not all of which have been studied adequately to help us arrive at a set of policy solutions.

Health promoters and public health practitioners have much to do in developing and/or influencing the evidence base to underpin public health policy.

PRACTICE POINTS

- Recognise that you and all health promoters and public health practitioners have a role in influencing policy at national, local and the organisational level.
- Influencing policy requires careful planning and timing. You need to know how national and local health promotion and public health policy is created, developed and changed, and how you can have a voice by commenting on proposals and plans.
- Know the rights and standards you can expect from NHS and LA services, and comment on those which you and your clients receive.
- Challenge health-damaging policy by working with others, using your vote and by collective action.
- Identify how you could be more effective in influencing policy through reviewing your skills in planning, networking, negotiating and joint working.
- Start policy change by identifying key stakeholders and looking at issues from each of their viewpoints; use techniques such as force field analysis to establish how to move forward.
- When campaigning on health issues, pay attention to careful planning and be persistent, professional and positive; involve as many other people as possible.
- Keep the ethical aspects of activities in mind when campaigning, lobbying and working towards changing health policy and practice; work with other people to build up trust and mutual respect.

REFERENCES

Baggott R 2015 Understanding health policy, 2nd edn. Cambridge, Polity Press.

Department of Health 2012a Statutory guidance on joint strategic needs assessments and joint health and wellbeing strategies. https://www.gov.uk/government/uploads/system/uploads/attachment_data/file/223842/Statutory-Guidance-on-Joint-Strategic-Needs-Assessments-and-Joint-Health-and-Wellbeing-Strategies-March-2013.pdf.

Department of Health 2012b The Public Health Outcomes Framework for England, 2013–2016. https://www.gov.uk/government/uploads/system/uploads/attachment_data/file/216159/dh_132362.pdf (Accessed June 2016).

Department of Health Ireland 2015 Nudging in public health – an ethical framework. A report by the National Advisory Committee on Bioethics. http://health.gov.ie/wp-content/uploads/2016/04/Nudging-in-Public-Health-Ethical-Framework-Dec-2015.pdf. (Accessed 23 March 2017).

Dolan P, Hallsworth M, Halpern D, King D, Vlaev I 2010 MINDSPACE: Influencing behaviour through public policy. London: Cabinet Office, Institute for Government.

Dooris M, Wills J, Newton J 2014 Theorizing healthy settings: a critical discussion with reference to Healthy Universities. Scandinavian Journal of Public Health 42(15 Suppl):7–16.

Enix A 2016 Negotiation: 8 essential negotiation skills to increase your influence and persuasion. CreateSpace Independent Publishing Platform.

ENWHP 2013 European network for workplace health promotion. Image Brochure http://www.enwhp.org/fileadmin/user_upload/pdf/ENWHP-image_brochure-final.pdf.

Gregory S, Dixon A, Ham C 2012 Health Policy under the coalition: A midterm assessment. London, Kings Fund.

HM Government 2016 Childhood obesity strategy: a plan of action. https://www.gov.uk/government/uploads/system/uploads/attachment_data/file/546588/Childhood_obesity_2016__2__acc.pdf.

ILot L 2016 NHS secret plans. Press Release. https://home.38degrees.org.uk/2016/08/26/nhs-secret-plans-press-release/.

INHPH 2016 The New Haven Recommendations on partnering with patients, families and citizens to enhance performance and quality in health promoting hospitals and health services. http://www.hph-hc.cc/fileadmin/user_upload/HPH_Declarations/New-Haven-Recommendations.pdf.

Kirsten W, Karch RC 2011 Global perspectives in workplace health promotion. Massachusetts, Jones and Bartlett Publishers.

Langford R, Bowell C, Jones H et al 2015 The World Health Organization's Health Promoting Schools framework: a Cochrane systematic review and meta-analysis. BMC Public Health 15:130.

LGA 2013 Changing behaviours in public health: To nudge or to shove? London, Local Government Association.

NHS England 2015 Delivering the forward view: NHS planning guidance 2016/17–2020/21. London, NHS England. https://www.england.nhs.uk/wp-content/uploads/2015/12/planning-guid-16-17-20-21.pdf.

NHS England 2016 The NHS Five-Year Forward View – executive summary. https://www.england.nhs.uk/ourwork/futurenhs/nhs-five-year-forward-view-web-version/5yfv-exec-sum/.

NHS European Office 2016 The EU and Health Policy. http://www.nhsconfed.org/regions-and-eu/nhs-european-office/about-the-eu/the-eu-and-health-policy.

Nuffield Council on Bioethics 2007 Public Health: Ethical Issues. http://nuffieldbioethics.org/project/public-health/.

O'Donell MP 2014 Health promotion in the workplace, 4th edn. Amazon: CreateSpace Independent Publishing Platform.

Popejoy WM 2016 book review of Health Inequalities: Critical perspectives. Perspectives in Public Health 136(5):307.

Public Health England 2014a Public health in prisons and secure settings. https://www.gov.uk/government/collections/public-health-in-prisons.

Public Health England 2014b Health & Justice report 2014. https://www.gov.uk/government/uploads/system/uploads/attachment_data/file/434951/HJ_report_11_6.pdf.

Public Health England 2015 Social Marketing Strategy 2014-2017: One year on. https://www.gov.uk/government/uploads/system/uploads/attachment_data/file/445524/Marketing_report_web.pdf.

Rochdale Borough Council 2016 Health Eating at Work Policy: Sample Policy. http://www.rochdale.gov.uk/pdf/2732_WelfareAtWork_EatingAtWork_HR.pdf.

Schubert C 2016 A note on the ethics of nudges. http://voxeu.org/article/note-ethics-nudges.

Scriven A 2007 Healthy public policies: rhetoric or reality. In Scriven A Garman G (eds) Public health: social context and action. Open University Press, Maidenhead.

Selby D Kippen H 2016 The journey to place based health. PHE Blog https://publichealthmatters.blog.gov.uk/2016/03/17/the-journey-to-place-based-health/.

The Bates Blog 2013 Leading Transformational Change: Using the Force Field Analysis. http://www.bates-communications.com/bates-blog/bid/94065/Leading-Transformational-Change-Using-the-Force-Field-Analysis.

Thorndike AN, Sonnenberg L, Riis J, Barraclough S, Levy DE 2012 A 2-Phase Labeling and Choice Architecture Intervention to Improve Healthy Food and Beverage Choices. American Journal of Public Health 102(3):527–533.

TUC 2010 Drugs and Alcohol in the workplace: Guidance for workplace representatives. London, TUC.

Welfare Reform Act 2012 http://www.legislation.gov.uk/ukpga/2012/5/contents/enacted/data.htm (Accessed: 23 March 2017).

Welsh Government 2015 Policy implementation guidance mental health services for prisoners. HMSO, London.

Wollaston S 2016 Public health is in crisis – and Theresa May is failing to act. Health Policy, The Guardian Newspaper 1 September 2016.

World Health Organization 2010 Healthy workplaces: a model for action: For employers, workers, policy-makers and practitioners. Geneva, WHO.

WHO 2016a Health 2020: the European policy for health and well-being. http://www.euro.who.int/en/health-topics/health-policy/health-2020-the-european-policy-for-health-and-well-being.

WHO 2016b Prisons and health: Partnership for Health in the Criminal Justice System. http://www.euro.who.int/en/health-topics/health-determinants/prisons-and-health.

WEBSITES

38 Degrees new campaign page. https://you.38degrees.org.uk/petition/new?source=google-start-a-petition38&gclid=Cj0KEQjwr7S-BRD96_uw9JK8uNABEiQAujbffMIYBHvBZT7aoaSbpSqh2Pf-srsd3Kk0yz-gg73RmBR4aAtuE8P8HAQ.

Action on Sugar pressure group http://www.actiononsugar.org/.

Child Poverty Action Group discussion on the Welfare Reform Bill. http://www.cpag.org.uk/welfare-reform.

Collaborate, a policy and practice hub supporting cross sector collaboration in services to the public http://collaboratei.com/2016/03/new-report-place-based-collaboration-that-can-transform-health-and-care/.

Details of the Public Health Network. http://www.ukpublichealth-network.org.uk/about-ukphn/.

HSE free guides on health and safety at work and other employment policy issues. https://www.citation.co.uk/free-guides.

NHS Change4 Life website http://www.nhs.uk/change4life/Pages/change-for-life.aspx.

Poverty and Social Exclusion (PSE) discussion on the Welfare Reform Bill. http://www.poverty.ac.uk/news-stories-benefits-welfare-system-government-policy-disability-child-poverty-housing-government.

The European Network for workplace health promotion. http://www.enwhp.org/the-enwhp.html.

The Health Foundation's work on health policy and economic analysis - http://www.health.org.uk/collection/informing-public-policy#sthash.ngUHfJIM.dpufhttp://www.health.org.uk/collection/informing-public-policy.

The NHS Confederation Network Pages, meeting specific needs of different specialist groups through its networks. http://www.nhsconfed.org/networks.

TUC pages on Drugs and Alcohol in the workplace. https://www.tuc.org.uk/workplace-issues/health-and-safety/drugs-and-alcohol.

WHO 2020 website. http://www.euro.who.int/en/health-topics/health-policy/health-2020-the-european-policy-for-health-and-well-being/about-health-2020.

BLOGS

British Heart Foundation health at work blog. https://www.bhf.org.uk/health-at-work/blog.

Health Promoting Universities Network website. http://www.healthyuniversities.ac.uk/.

https://publichealthmatters.blog.gov.uk/2016/03/17/the-journey-to-place-based-health/.

NHS Voices is where leaders from all parts of the healthcare sector come together, raise and improve understanding of the issue, share ideas and opinions, and debate solutions. http://www.nhsconfed.org/blog.

Public Health England Blog, Public Health Matters. Duncan Selbie and Henry Kippin, 17 March 2016. The journey to place based health.

The European Schools for Health Network. http://www.schools-for-health.eu/she-network.

The International Network of Health Promoting Hospitals and Health Services website. http://www.hphnet.org/.

UK Healthy Cities Network page. http://www.healthycities.org.uk/.

YOUTUBE

Over the past 25 years, the Ottawa Charter has had a profound effect on public health, described as a tipping point for global health development. This meeting of free thinkers in Ottawa reframed the way people look at health and wellbeing and provided a legacy for crafting a new common European Health Policy - Health 2020. The video takes us through the 25 year journey and the conferences that addressed each: WHO Regional Office for Europe: The journey from Ottawa to Health 2020. https://www.youtube.com/watch?v=gJ1H2ojwb2Q.

WEBINARS

The Health Foundation webinars on a range of health policy issues. http://www.health.org.uk/node/126.

TWITTER

Action of Sugar pressure group. https://twitter.com/actiononsugar?ref_src=twsrc%5Etfw.

FACEBOOK

Change4Life Wales. https://www.facebook.com/C4LWales.

INDEX

Note: Page numbers followed by *f* indicate figures, *t* indicate tables and *b* indicate boxes.